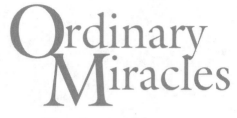

Ordinary Miracles

True Stories About
Overcoming Obstacles &
Surviving Catastrophes

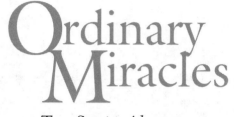

Ordinary Miracles

*True Stories About
Overcoming Obstacles &
Surviving Catastrophes*

Edited by

Deborah R. Labovitz, PhD, OTR/L, FAOTA
The Steinhardt School of Education
New York University
New York, New York

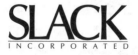

An innovative information, education and management company
6900 Grove Road • Thorofare, NJ 08086

The work SLACK publishes is peer reviewed. Prior to publication, recognized leaders in the field, educators, and clinicians provide important feedback on the concepts and content that we publish. We welcome feedback on this work.

Library of Congress Cataloging-in-Publication Data

Ordinary miracles : true stories about overcoming obstacles & surviving catastrophes / edited by Deborah Labovitz.
    p. ; cm.
Includes bibliographical references.
  ISBN 1-55642-571-6 (alk. paper)
  1. Occupational therapy--Case studies.
  [DNLM: 1. Disabled Persons--rehabilitation--Personal Narratives. 2. Occupational Therapy--Personal Narratives. WB 320 O65 2002] I. Labovitz, Deborah.
  RM735.45 O735 2002
  615.8'515--dc21

                                  2002009147

Printed in the United States of America.

Published by: SLACK Incorporated
                     6900 Grove Road
                     Thorofare, NJ 08086 USA
                     Telephone: 856-848-1000
                     Fax: 856-853-5991
                     www.slackbooks.com

Contact SLACK Incorporated for more information about other books in this field or about the availability of our books from distributors outside the United States.

Last digit is print number: 10 9 8 7 6 5 4 3 2 1

CONTENTS

Contents

Section Four Adults: Navigating the Perils of Illness and Injury 121

Contents

Part Two: Life's Unpredictable Events

Contents

Contents

PREFACE

This is a book about optimism and hope. The stories in it are about people who have courageously overcome adversity and whose lives have been improved through resourcefulness and creativity. In many ways, this reflects my own personality and the philosophy of my profession of occupational therapy. I believe that every problem has a solution, and we just have not discovered the best one yet for those problems still unsolved; that not only is the glass half full, but refills are on the way. When people tell me that "those who can keep their heads when all about them are losing theirs just don't understand the gravity of the situation," my response is that only those who can keep their heads—and find a ray of hope—can ultimately fix the grave situation. I believe that even if we cannot control the circumstances we are in, we can control our reaction to those circumstances and can turn tragedy into triumph with our own strength and with the help of others.

My optimism was sorely tested on September 11, 2001. As a New Yorker whose office faced the World Trade Center, less than a mile away, I watched in horrified shock and disbelief as the Twin Towers burned and then collapsed. I saw and smelled the smoke. My horror was deeply personal as well as generalized. On my way to work that fateful morning, I had witnessed the attack from the street corner as I exited the subway at 9:05 a.m. and saw both Towers already in flames. The two-block walk to my office from that corner became a nightmare of fear: my son's office was on the 30th floor of Tower Two, and I did not know if he was already there and, if so, whether he would be able to escape from the burning building.

Thankfully, he was one of the lucky people. He had not yet arrived at his office and was thus spared a terrifying escape from the burning buildings, or an even worse fate. I learned later that he had been two blocks away when Tower Two collapsed, and that he had managed to take refuge in a small storefront restaurant to escape the choking clouds of ash and dust and the panicking crowds. At the time, however, I had an unforgettably anxious 2 hours, not knowing where he was, before he was able to find a working pay phone and call. He spent the next 4 hours walking the six miles to his home.

This book was in the last stages of completion on September 11, 2001. I must admit that the tragedy affected me deeply. Perhaps it was because of my family's close escape; perhaps because I work daily in New York and saw the devastation first hand; perhaps because, like all Americans, I lived with the nonstop television coverage of the event for days afterward; perhaps because, like most human beings, I simply could not comprehend the magnitude of the crime or the extent of the loss.

Preface

It was difficult for me to resume life and work as usual, and particularly challenging to continue to compile and edit these stories—stories about individual people who overcame adversity, unconnected to the tragedy. The people and the stories seemed not to reflect the immediacy and immense scope of the disaster.

As an occupational therapist, I believe in the power of "doing." To cope with the tragedy and to contribute to the recovery, I needed to act. So I volunteered my time, donated funds, read articles about the heroes and the victims, and examined the photographs. I attended tributes to heroes and visited street corner and police station and firehouse memorials, and I began collecting more stories, two of which appear in this book. These activities were and continue to be very satisfying and helpful to me.

Ultimately, however, it was resuming work on this book with its message of hope that was the most powerful and important activity that helped me begin to heal and to recapture my optimism. I came to realize that these stories, about the large and small miracles of life, about the courage and creativity of individuals, about the ability to recover from disaster, were exactly what I needed to begin my healing process. These stories represent the wonder, joy, and hope that makes life worth living. They are the embodiment of life and the future. They make it possible to go on, to hope, and to continue to face the future with optimism. In gratitude for the ability to be comforted by these stories and what they represent, and to continue my efforts to help others recover from individual and community tragedies, I will be donating a portion of the profits from this book to organizations that help people cope with adversity.

In this time of national need for healing, I hope that reading these stories and learning about the resourcefulness and optimism of the people in this book will help others heal as well. I offer them to you with my optimistic wish that they help you as they helped me.

Deborah R. Labovitz, PhD, OTR/L, FAOTA
New York, March 2002

INTRODUCTION

These are the stories of ordinary people whose lives have been saved in seemingly miraculous ways. Some very special people helped them not only to survive, but to cope with life-threatening catastrophes and terrible circumstances and make it through tough times. This book is about hope and about how people can work with what happens to them to take charge of their future.

Catastrophes occur with unexpected swiftness, and in an instant can change our lives forever. Other difficult or even dreadful circumstances may develop slowly, but relentlessly, and over time can change our lives forever.

But do miracles that save us ever happen in ordinary life? Ask Brett Duffey. On that breezy spring evening in 1989 in Myrtle Beach, South Carolina, 20-year-old Brett, a Marine air traffic controller on leave, was enjoying vacationing with his dad in a posh high-rise hotel overlooking the beach. When he stepped out onto the balcony of his 12th-story room to view the sunset, he noticed some attractive young ladies on the balcony two floors above him and leaned out to exchange friendly greetings. As he was talking, his foot slipped and the 6' 3", 250-pound Marine lost his balance and plummeted through space, 12 stories down to the ground below.

Obviously, Brett knew in that split second as he plunged from the balcony that his life was over. So casually, so quickly, so incredibly impossible! He had only intended to watch the sunset and flirt with some cute girls, and now he was going to die. And yet, miraculously, Brett did not die. He landed—with 16 broken bones and a closed head injury that left him in a coma for 6 weeks—but alive. Brett literally hit bottom.

And then what happened? Ten years ago he was given a 5% chance of survival. Today he is a college graduate and a father with an exciting new career. Brett credits his miraculous recovery to the incredible hard work, motivation, creativity, and resourcefulness of his rehabilitation team, especially the occupational therapists. How was Brett able to rise again to live, love, and learn? When you read Brett's story, you will find out how his occupational therapists helped save the day.

The true stories in this book are about miracles that happen to ordinary people. Some of these miracles are large and highly dramatic events: surviving a plane crash, a bus bombing, or a landmine explosion. Others involve courageous recoveries from sudden tragedies: diving accidents, drive-by shootings, automobile accidents, or Brett's fall from a 12-story balcony. Sometimes the miracles are important achievements:

moving about in a powered wheelchair, driving an adapted car, riding a horse, or returning to work. And still other miracles are small and quiet events: regaining the ability to play with toys, speaking and communicating with others, or even tying shoes after an accident, an illness, or a developmental problem has made those things virtually impossible.

The people whose experiences these were believe in miracles.

Consider what Katherine and Frank Mayer know about miracles.

In August 1996, the Mayer family was anticipating a fun-filled vacation, but as they loaded the family car outside their suburban New Jersey home, their excitement turned to horror. Jason, one of their 4-year-old twins, lost control of his Big Wheel on their sloping driveway and rolled into the street in front of an oncoming truck. It happened so quickly that Justin, Jason's terrified twin brother, and the rest of the family could only watch helplessly as Jason and the Big Wheel were dragged 55 feet underneath the truck. Finally, Jason's dad, Frank, managed to jump the fence, run down the street, catch up with the truck, and get the driver to stop.

Jason's mom, Katherine, was sure that Jason was dead, snatched away from the family in that split second between enjoying the sunshine as he played in front of the house and his plunge into the street. Miraculously, Jason did not die. His battered body with its extensive injuries was airlifted to a specialized children's hospital where the expert medical team saved his life several times over the next 3 weeks.

Months of therapy helped Jason regain the skills he lost in the accident. How did this happen? Jason's remarkable recovery was engineered by his occupational therapist. She creatively used Justin, Jason's twin, as her most effective therapeutic tool to motivate Jason to participate in the painful but necessary rehabilitation activities. How she did this, and why the Mayer family considers it a special miracle, is one of the inspirational stories you are about to read.

Miracles can happen to everyone, people from all walks of life. Sometimes they occur under extraordinary and at other times routine circumstances. All of the miracles in this book share one thing in common—success. All of these stories are tributes to the ability of people to triumph over adversity and to succeed when life is hardest.

While all the stories deal with successful solutions to problems, success means different things to different people. For some, the success was the first step on the road to recovery. For others, it was achieving their highest lifetime goals despite having some disability. For some, the success was living a productive, happy, or meaningful life in their last years, months, or even days. For others just starting out, success involved the accomplishment of tasks that unlocked barriers and made possible the beginning of a productive, happy, or meaningful life.

Introduction

In this book you will meet 96 remarkable people—people born with disabling conditions, people who got sick, people who became injured, people who grew old. They all required help to learn or relearn the skills needed for the "job of living," and they all received that help from an occupational therapist. In turn, they improved at doing their own jobs of living.

How did this happen? Could it happen to you or me? What does any of this have to do with miracles?

The lives of the people in these stories have been changed by the chance to learn—or relearn—the skills they needed for their own jobs of living, no matter what, no matter where, no matter how. You will be amazed at their courage, energized by their achievements, and awed at the miracles they have managed to accomplish with a little bit of help from occupational therapy.

Their examples will inspire you and reassure you that successfully surmounting seemingly insurmountable obstacles is possible for all of us when faced with adversity.

Who are these remarkable people, and who are the occupational therapists who entered their lives and had such a profound impact?

These powerful vignettes, written by the people who had the experiences, their families, or their occupational therapists, illustrate the ways in which ordinary and famous individuals surmount the seemingly insurmountable, defy the odds, and redesign their lives to achieve meaningful fulfillment following what could have been a life-shattering event. These episodes recount the large and small miracles of healing and adapting made possible when courage is combined with resourcefulness, creativity, and an indomitable will to succeed.

Some will bring a tear to your eye; some will bring a smile to your lips. All will inspire you with the knowledge that, as the people in the stories discovered, ordinary miracles do happen. You will read about people whose stories are the stuff of high drama:

- Rambo, an El Salvadorian national soccer star whose feet were amputated after a wartime landmine explosion
- Cruz, a young man paralyzed from the neck down by a random drive-by gang shooting
- Karen, a doctoral candidate who was plunged into confusion and unbearable head pain when a truck plowed into her car

There are others in the book whose rehabilitation started with small but nonetheless important things:

Introduction

- 83-year-old Mrs. S, a new resident of a nursing home, who could not find a satisfying place for herself in it after having taken care of her family all her life
- Aaron, a 61-year-old businessman recovering from a stroke, whose dream was to walk his daughter down the aisle at her wedding
- Bob, who needed a way to continue to live with his aging dog Barney, despite Barney's problems with managing his daily backyard activities

You will see how babies and children get a good start in life:

- 6-month-old Fayda, whose weakened body kept her from using her hands to manipulate her toys and play with her older siblings
- 15-month-old Sam, who needed to be kept perfectly still for several days until his spinal surgery began to heal
- 2-year-old Jack, whose tiny hands had stiffened into tight fists from an unknown cause
- 3-year-old Cecilia, whose body was "frozen" in strange positions and who was also completely unable to speak
- 2½-year-old Erin, who had a stroke while still in the uterus, who followed the therapeutic paws of Max, the therapy cat who lives and works in a children's occupational therapy clinic

If you do not know what the profession of occupational therapy is, or what an occupational therapist does, read on. You will find out about the many ways that people learned the skills for their job of living from occupational therapists who entered their lives after an illness, injury, birth condition, emotional problem, or the normal aging process made it necessary for them to have help with their daily tasks of life.

Some of the occupational therapy encounters were quite short—just enough time to help the people learn to do something that was really important to them. Other occupational therapy lasted weeks, months, or even years, as people's changing abilities and needs required redefinition of the goals of their continuing occupational therapy treatments.

In the array of stories of the many different people and their varying needs and solutions can be found the essence of occupational therapy: treating whole people within the context of their family and their environment to help them build the skills they need for the job of living their lives.

The people who have experienced this remarkable treatment and its results believe in miracles.

So, are other miracles really possible? And if so, under what circumstances? These stories confirm that the answer is a resounding yes when a spirit that refuses to capitulate to hardship combines with the informed ingenuity of the caring professional occupational therapist.

Adversity can happen to any of us. These stories reflect the positive side of life and can provide hope to those who are now facing their own physical and emotional challenges, give insight to those who have family or friends in similar situations, and inspire confidence in all of us.

There is no right or wrong way to read this book. Some of you may choose to read it straight through from beginning to end. Others may be searching for particular stories that speak to some event in their life or the life of someone they know. In order to decide how to proceed, it may be helpful to know how the stories in the book are arranged.

The book is divided into three parts. In *Part One, The Journey Through Life*, you will be introduced to people at various stages in their lives—infants and children and their parents, teenagers, adults, and senior citizens who have successfully met some of the challenges and overcome some of the obstacles that are not uncommon to particular phases of life.

Accidents, traumas, and catastrophes, however, are indiscriminate and rarely respect age and stages of life. In *Part Two, Life's Unpredictable Events*, you will meet people whose common link is the way in which they coped with such life-altering events outside their control.

Finally, in *Part Three, Retrospectives*, you will get to know people who have learned to live productive lives and can look back at years of accomplishment despite lifelong health conditions and challenges.

Whichever approach you choose, read on to enjoy the company of these remarkable people.

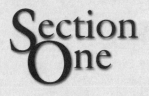

Section One

Infants & Toddlers

Getting Off to a Good Start

Getting Off
to a Good Start

Meet twelve infants and toddlers with a variety of birth conditions, illnesses, developmental problems, and other obstacles that jeopardize their abilities to grow and thrive, and see how the situation was turned around by the action of parents and therapists working together to help children flourish.

Chapter One

Fayda Sits in the Corner

Patricia Petersen, MA, OTR

It was an ordinary day in our household. Fayda sat in her high-chair dabbing at Cheerios with her palm. After several dabs, she would bring her hands to her mouth and lick the Cheerios off her wet palm. At 6 months old, Fayda was enjoying her new-found ability to feed herself. Fayda was in many ways an ordinary child. She enjoyed exploring her environment with her hands, feet, arms, and legs, but mostly with her mouth. She would spend many happy minutes sitting in her highchair playing with her food.

Every so often, however, Fayda would let out a loud and piti-ful cry. I would turn to investigate and try to ascertain what was the source of her distress. Sometimes a toy had fallen over the side of the tray attached to the highchair. A quick retrieval would set things right, and Fayda would resume her play. But there were other times that she would cry differently. Not so much a cry as a plaintive wail. She didn't sound frustrated or mad, but hurt. Several times when this happened, I was not immediately sure what had caused her sorrow. Her toys would all be on the tray. Her food would be within easy reach. Nothing seemed amiss. I would search the floor again to see if I could find anything that she had dropped. Nothing was on the floor. Everything was on the tray. Then I noticed her arms were at her sides.

Chapter One

Of course, having her arms at her sides does not seem to be an obvious cause for distress, but Fayda with her arms at her sides was Fayda left without the ability to touch. Fayda had been born without the usual formation of muscles in her shoulders and upper arms. As a result, she did not have the ability to lift her arms from her side, and place them on the tray of her highchair. When properly seated, with her arms placed in front of her on the tray, she would happily play with whatever was provided for her enjoyment. However, once her arms left the tray and returned to her sides, she could no longer grasp or play with any of the enticements lying before her eyes, just out of reach.

Realizing the difficulty that Fayda was having keeping her arms on the tray, I tried to devise some sort of propping system to allow her arms to remain at the level of the tray. The combination of pillows and blankets worked well enough until her torso began to slip down and tilt to the side. Once the delicate balance was lost, all the pillows and blankets were just so much stuffing around her limp body. Somehow, I thought, we needed to find a way to keep her upright so that this tilting-slipping process would not end again with her arms, useless, at her sides.

At our next visit with Fayda's occupational therapist, I mentioned the trouble that we were having with the highchair and Fayda's frustration with not being able to keep her arms on the tray. Terri had worked with Fayda on those muscle problems since she was 2 months old and was familiar with both her persistence and her lack of tolerance for frustration. Terri immediately agreed that we needed to find a solution to the problem of the tray.

Terri asked about the highchair: Did it have straps for the waist? The crotch? Did the tray wrap around the arms? Was it adjustable? Did the chair tilt? I described the highchair in as much detail as I could, and Terri listened attentively. When I was finished, Terri asked me to describe what I had done to try to help Fayda with keeping her arms on the tray. I explained about the pillows and blankets and mentioned that they seemed effective until Fayda began to tilt and eventually slip down in the seat.

Terri's response was almost immediate. She asked if I had ever heard of a corner chair. I had not, but was interested in anything that might help the problem. Terri asked me to wait for a few minutes while she looked through the storage closet in which she kept that type of chair.

When Terri returned, she had in her arms a curious-looking chair and a low table. The chair was constructed of two perpendicular pieces of wood, attached to a third piece that formed the base. The three pieces together formed what amounted to a corner, thus the name—corner chair. Inserted into this corner arrangement were two cushions which formed the seat and back of the chair. Terri placed the chair on the ground and set the table directly in front of the chair. Terri then asked me to put Fayda into the chair.

I set Fayda down into the chair, and Terri assisted me with fastening a large Velcro strap around Fayda's torso. The strap held her snugly against the seat back. Terri explained how the strap gave excellent support to Fayda's body, which might prevent the slipping and sliding I had described. It would also help her conserve her strength, which she had been previously using merely to hold her body erect.

Terri then placed some toys on the table in front of the chair. Fayda almost immediately raised her arms and began to play with the toys on the table. I was astounded. Never before had she been able to raise her arms up to near shoulder level without full assistance. This time she just raised her arms and reached for the toys. The body support she was getting from the Velcro strap and the sides of the chair did the trick! It truly seemed like a miracle. Terri suggested that we borrow the chair and table and try it at home.

When we brought the chair home and set it up, Fayda's older brother and sister were immediately interested in this new piece of equipment in the house. We put Fayda into the chair and placed some of her toys on the table. She began playing with the toys just as she had at the therapy clinic. Even more amazing than that, however, was the fact that Fayda's brother and sister came and sat down on the floor near her and began playing with her. This was the first time in her life that Fayda had been able to play with her siblings without being held by an adult for support.

They played together for almost an hour, never seeming to tire of handing toys to Fayda, which she would touch, mouth, and throw off the table, only to have them retrieved by her brother or sister and placed again on the table. Each day this scene was repeated, and as Fayda played with her toys on the table, we began to notice that her arms were growing stronger. The support from the Velcro strap around her torso allowed her to conserve the strength that before she had needed to use to remain upright. Now, instead, she could use that strength for moving her arms. From that point on, we began referring to the chair and table that Terri had loaned us as the "miracle chair," for the change it had made in our family was really something of a miracle.

Fayda's chair became the focal point of daily activities in our family, with Fayda sitting grandly in the middle of the living room where everyone would stop and play. As Fayda continued to grow and develop, she eventually outgrew her need for the miracle chair. We came to see that the real miracle was Fayda herself and the amazing progress that she has made with the help of her occupational therapist and others. Fayda is now an active 4-year-old girl who attends a neighborhood preschool and sits in any chair she chooses.

Chapter Two

Sam Gets a Halo

Cindy Wright, MA, OTR

Ask just about anyone what a halo is, and you can be sure he or she will start talking to you about angels with big white wings and a golden ring above their heads. But when I think about a halo, I think about the one my 15-month-old son, Sam, started to wear after having lengthy micro- and laser surgery on his spine. Of course I think that Sam is an angel—or at least my special angel—but he is also a real flesh-and-blood little boy, and his halo was an occupational therapy device designed to help a wiggling child keep his head and neck from moving so his spine could heal.

I had been an occupational therapist for nearly 20 years, both as a clinician and as a faculty member teaching others to be occupational therapists. I have a particular interest in helping children and an expertise in mental health. It never occurred to me, however, that I might need to call on those skills for myself and members of my own family, until Sam was born and developed serious medical problems. As a family, my husband, Sam's big brother, and I were faced with the biggest treatment challenge I had ever had to deal with.

After an uneventful pregnancy and delivery, Sam arrived on July 15, 1992. He was healthy, beautiful, and very welcomed by Mommy, Daddy, and Big Brother. Over the next year, however,

Sam developed numerous medical problems, such as poor weight gain, low muscle tone, delayed motor development, and emerging curvature of his spine. We spent countless hours and hundreds of dollars seeing various specialists who ordered tests, but found nothing. It was a frightening, frustrating, and incredibly stressful experience.

Finally, when Sam was a year old, he was seen by a neurologist for a follow-up visit. When she discovered several positive signs of neurological dysfunction that were not present previously, she immediately ordered a special full-body x-ray called magnetic resonance imaging, or MRI. The MRI revealed a 2½-inch lipoma (fatty tumor) surrounding his spinal cord from his neck to the middle of his shoulders. Although not a life-threatening condition, it was certainly a very serious life-altering situation; continued squeezing of Sam's spinal cord by the tumor could lead to permanent nerve damage or even paralysis. We were referred to a neurosurgeon who felt that surgery might be an option, but because Sam's condition was unusual, he wanted to consult with a few leading pediatric neurosurgeons before making a final decision. Another grueling 3 months went by before we finally received word that surgery was the only hope we had for improving Sam's condition.

When I received the initial diagnosis, I was shocked, but also relieved that we finally had something concrete to deal with. My professional self kicked into high gear, and I immediately began researching information on spinal cord injury. I began to anticipate the resources that we might need, and I made lists of professional contacts that I might need to call on. Not only was this information useful, gathering it was my own occupational therapy. This purposeful activity made me feel that I was doing something useful and helped me to cope with a future full of unknowns. I believed that my occupational therapy knowledge and experience were coming together now for the sole purpose of allowing me to help my child. It became my destiny and my source of strength.

My husband and I met with the medical team for a pre-surgery conference in October 1993. At this time, the procedure and what we could expect as possible outcomes were discussed in detail. The neurosurgeon was cautious in his optimism and told us that his goal was to remove as much of the tumor as possible in order to prevent further cord constriction. Nonetheless, he fully expected Sam to be left with some degree of permanent nerve damage that would then require treatment.

My husband was distraught over this news, and I suddenly understood that he had never allowed himself to consider anything for Sam except a full recovery. I realized that I needed to share some of the information that I had collected with him, and we talked about other family members who were living with disabilities. My commitment to our son and my convictions regarding the benefits of the therapy seemed to rub off on my husband, and he was calmed by the knowledge that we were part of a team all working for Sam's best interests. Here again, almost without realizing it, I was using the mental health skills I had learned as an occupational therapist to help my own family.

On November 10, 1993, Sam underwent 10 hours of micro- and laser surgery to remove some of the tumor. Approximately 60% of the tumor was removed. The remaining 40% was so deeply entwined with the spinal cord tissue that it could not be removed without risking significant nerve damage. Sam was moved to the spinal unit after surgery and was placed on full bedrest for his 8-day hospital stay. Sam was 15 months old. Full bedrest for a 15 month old? They had to be kidding.

But no, they meant every word. We were cautioned not to let him move about at all until the site of the surgery had begun to heal. Any movement might mean additional damage and dislodging the stitches from the surgery, which could lead to paralysis. Forty-eight hours after surgery, the last effects of anesthesia and medication wore off. Sam awoke bright-eyed, happy, and ready to move. He began lifting his legs to the side of the crib and attempting to roll over, all things that had been impossible for him to do prior to surgery. Of course, everyone was thrilled that the outcome of surgery appeared to be so positive. But, now we were faced with a major dilemma. How do you keep an energetic 15-month-old child perfectly still and on his back in a crib for a week?

We certainly tried. I brought mobiles and hanging crib toys from home. My family searched for new push-button books, musical toys, and anything with lights and sound. We brought in lots of family visitors to take around-the-clock shifts to watch him and play with him. Our older son, who was 4 at the time, also became part of the team and entertained Sam with songs and chatter. We read stories, played with puppets, and watched Barney. But Sam was restless and raring to go! He didn't like being fed lying down, and it was very messy. He desperately wanted to be picked up, and we were all missing that important cuddle time.

The orthopedic surgeon told us that a custom-designed body brace that would allow his spine to be totally immobilized for proper healing would be constructed for Sam prior to discharge. Sam would have to wear this brace for 24 hours a day for 3 months, but while wearing it, his movement of the rest of his body would not be restricted. When he was in the brace, we would be allowed to hold him and he could get out of bed. However, it was going to take at least 3 days for the orthotist to construct and fit this brace. What would happen in the meantime?

I spoke with the orthopedist and requested an occupational therapy consultation for the purpose of constructing a temporary splint. Most people think that a splint is something to support a broken arm or leg or to wear on your wrist. But splints can come in all sizes and shapes to fit all body parts.

Sam's doctor was new to our medical team and was unaware of my occupational therapy background. However, he was very respectful of my knowledge and seemed quite impressed that I had formerly been on the occupational therapy faculty at the medical center. I told him that several of my former students were on staff at the hospital, and I felt certain that together we could design a custom-fitted splint that would satisfy the orthopedic concerns. He wrote the order for it immediately.

Within an hour, one of my former students and her colleague arrived to evaluate the situation. The two therapists worked most of the day constructing a combination cervical collar and halo headpiece that kept Sam's head and neck from moving. He was not too happy to be in the splint initially, but as soon as I lifted him from the crib and held him on my lab, he was all smiles, just like an angel in a painting. There wasn't a dry eye in the room when my husband and I hugged our baby for the first time in 4 days. At that moment, I truly realized what a tremendous impact occupational therapy can have on a life.

Sam began a 3-year rehabilitation program 6 months after surgery, and there were many wonderful therapeutic moments. But, in my mind, nothing compares to that first moment of independence and nurturing 3 days after surgery that was the beginning of our journey. I will always be grateful to the occupational therapists who made that moment happen.

Sam is now within the normal range for his age in all developmental areas. He has a progressing spinal curvature, which will require additional surgery, and he has bowel and bladder control problems due to the nerve damage, and for all of these problems he continues to be seen by a team of specialists. We are thankful for the excellent progress that he has made, and there is no doubt that occupational therapy has continued to positively affect our family through the long process. It is particularly gratifying that I was viewed as both mother and collaborator in Sam's therapy program. I appreciate the compassion and respect I have received. It has been enlightening to be on the receiving end of therapy, and I am incredibly proud of my profession.

Chapter
Three

Jack's Hands

Beth Cooper, OTR

Pop! Pop! As my husband helped me hold our 2-year-old son, Jack, I slowly and gently pried open the tightly clenched fingers of his right hand and moved each finger carefully to extend it. The noises were the sounds of the ligaments in the knuckles and the other two joints of each finger gently letting go and releasing to allow the fingers to move smoothly. I didn't yet know why his fingers had been clenching together tighter and tighter every morning over the past several days, but the one thing I did know from my occupational therapy training was that if I didn't force them to open they might stay clenched and eventually might never open again. When they were painful and tight, moist heat helped to loosen them up so I could get them to extend. Once they were extended, his hand remained open and busy, and his fingers looked fine and worked normally for the rest of the day. No occupational therapist could have had a better-tempered client; even at 2, Jack seemed to sense that I was worried about his hand, so he would try to cheer me up by telling me, "It's okay, Mommy, this other hand still works."

Jack has amazed us since the day he was born at 10 pounds 10 ounces, and my husband has been busy planning his future football career ever since. He had always been very healthy except for a high fever that lasted for 3 days a few weeks before our saga began, so I didn't think too much about it the morning when Jack woke up with his right hand closed in a tight fist. Soon his fingers were opened and busy. The next morning, however, his fingers were stiff and tightly flexed again. During breakfast, his fingers remained closed as he tried to stick the handle of his spoon into his little hand. My husband and I wondered if perhaps he'd hurt his hand somehow. From an occupational therapist's perspective, his hand was intact. There appeared to be no edema or swelling, no color changes, no abnormal temperature, no pain, no problem.

I took Jack to the pediatrician who examined him and ordered an x-ray of his hand, which was negative. Then he sent us to an orthopedic surgeon. He found nothing wrong, but confirmed that Jack would make a good football player some day. Another round of x-rays was ordered on Jack's hand a few days later. I was able to get the secretary to make me copies of his x-rays for his grandparents and his baby book, something perhaps only an occupational therapist could really get excited about. This turned out to be a good idea.

Jack's right hand became increasingly stiff and then more painful to open as the days and weeks went by. I found my knowledge as an occupational therapist priceless in my desperate quest to keep Jack's hand from contracting and losing function, as none of the doctors had given us any advice about treatment. Each day my husband and I held him down in the morning to range his fingers very carefully, just to keep them from staying flexed all day. The feeling of opening them was like trigger-fingers popping open in all of his joints. We applied moist heat each day. I relied on all my psychological training to keep him motivated to use his right hand, especially to feed himself, and to let me range it every day.

One morning, about a month after the hand saga started, we had already ranged Jack's right hand and I was getting ready to leave for work. Suddenly, I noticed Jack fumbling to eat, this time with the fingers of his left hand tightly fisted as well. I frantically called my husband and the doctor. What had started out seeming to be a sprain of one hand now looked like it could be an overall rheumatological or neurological problem. I made resting hand splints to keep my precious toddler's fingers extended while we waited for another doctor's appointment. The pediatrician requested a blood test to check his sedimentation rate, but it was only slightly elevated. Another blood test seemed to rule out a virus. Jack was put on big doses of ibuprofen, a pain killer, and muscle relaxant.

Appointments were made quickly with the pediatric rheumatologist and the pediatric neurologist at the large teaching hospital nearby. The pediatrician informed me that we were lucky to get to see these specialists so fast and that they were quite interested in what they might find. The pediatric rheumatologist even called me before the appointment and talked for 15 minutes about Jack's hands. I had worked at the hospital as a new graduate after finishing occupational therapy school, and at that time I had enjoyed the exposure to unusual diagnoses and interesting cases. However, to be the mother of the case in point and capable of understanding their medical jargon was a living nightmare for me.

On the day my husband and I took Jack to the hospital to meet the pediatric rheumatologist, I did not range his fingers open. I felt that the physicians needed to see and feel for themselves this "trigger-finger popping feeling." I still believed that the problem was in the fingers themselves. However, the doctors did not seem to agree. They did not stop to feel Jack's fingers and had no comment about the splints or the ranging we were doing. The rheumatologist concluded that the problem had to be neurological, my worst fear. We spent that entire afternoon with the pediatric neurologist. He ordered blood for tests and wanted a full head and neck MRI, a special high resolution x-ray procedure requiring the patient to hold totally still for 45 minutes, which, for a 2 year old, would need to be performed with sedation. With great trepidation we scheduled it for the day of Jack's third birthday, 2 months off. Before we left the parking lot for the drive home that day, I stopped to help Jack open his fisted little hands. Not one of the doctors or assistants had felt them.

All our family and friends had been praying for Jack. With heavenly guidance I think, it occurred to me the next day to call a well-known homeopathic doctor in the area. He examined Jack, looked at the x-rays I had brought along, and paid special attention to his fisted hands. He concluded that the problem might be due to a simple virus from Jack's illness weeks before when he had had the high fever. He thought that the virus had settled into the ligaments around the joints in Jack's fingers, and he prescribed a remedy for him that looked like a little jar of sugar pills.

In 3 days we started noticing less stiffness, and in a week Jack could range his own fingers open independently. In about 6 weeks the stiffness was completely gone. When the neurologist called to tell me all his blood tests had come back negative, I took delight in telling him that Jack was well and he could cancel the MRI. We later found out that the homeopathic remedy was Rhus tox (poison ivy—no joke!). It had been a miracle for Jack.

Another month went by. Jack walked up to me one morning, held out his hands, and said, "Mommy, look at these little hands." With my heart in my throat, I asked him what was wrong with them. Jack's reply was simply, "They're just growin' and growin'," and off he went to play.

Postscript: Writing this story has reminded me in a vivid way what a difficult and trying time we overcame with God's help and the support of a lot of family and friends. I believe that my knowledge as an occupational therapist kept Jack from experiencing the trauma of clenched, contracted fingers in both hands. The compassion and empathy I feel now for others in the midst of a similar medical journey has taken me to a higher level as a therapist.

Chapter Four

Cecilia Gets Unglued

Lisa E. Cyzner, PhD, OTR/L

Usually when people are described as "getting unglued" it means they have lost control of themselves and are having a tantrum, a rather negative event. However, in Cecilia's situation, getting unglued was actually a very positive result of our work together. Losing control and having tantrums certainly happened frequently to Cecilia, as I found out later. But my first impression of her, on an early September afternoon in 1996, was that it would be impossible for me to treat her unless I could get her unglued from her mother. On that day, this beautiful 3-year-old girl entered my office with her head buried deeply in her mother's side, her arms securely locked around her mother's waist. "This is Cecilia," her mother said, as she gently began to disentangle herself from her daughter's grip.

Earlier that summer, Cecilia had been diagnosed with a regulatory disorder, which caused her to have little or no control over her behavior. People with this condition lack the ability to use information that comes in through their senses, which directly affects their ability to function. Cecilia was impulsive, hyperactive, had no awareness of safety, and engaged in unprovoked hitting. In addition, she craved sensory input. Her clinical psychologist determined that her behaviors were indicative of a type III regulatory disorder: motorically disorganized and impulsive. That gave a label to her muscular incoordination and her sudden angry, seemingly uncontrollable flinging herself about. But it didn't tell her parents what to do about this vexing and troublesome behavior.

At our initial meeting, once I was able to pry her loose from her mother, Cecilia was virtually nonverbal, releasing an occasional stifled growl as her only means of voluntary communication. Her body language and visible behaviors told me a lot about her. The child who crouched before me literal-ly seemed frozen in time as she stood with her left leg and right arm rigidly bent and drawn tightly against her body. These and other strange kinds of behaviors had led her parents to seek a medical diagnosis and then to look for treatment for Cecilia's condition.

Cecilia sought out every opportunity for what is called proprioceptive input, the deep-pressure sensation that lets us know where our bodies are in space, by squeezing her body under tables or wedging herself into tight crevices. Without warning, she instantly would be consumed with rage. In her mother's own emotional account of Cecilia's medical and psychological history, and her own desperate search for answers, she wrote of her child, "This disorder is affecting her temperament and personality development in a negative way. We were told that she would 'grow out' of this. We are wait-ing patiently and losing hope at this point in time. It is very hard to watch your child suffer without being able to offer her some comfort."

I believed that I had only one choice in choosing a course of therapy for Cecilia. I had to become her link to the sensory experiences that she craved. More importantly, I had to become the family's source for guidance on how they could interact successfully with their daughter. Much of her family's interaction with Cecilia to this point consisted of their being the objects toward which Cecilia directed her aggression. I had to help them provide Cecilia with the necessary sensory input to organize herself and to help her regulate her own responses to sensory stimulation from the environment, so that Cecilia would begin to function more like a typical 3 year old.

Typical activities for most children, such as putting on a coat and prepar-ing to go outside, were very difficult for Cecilia. In fact, her parents had grown accustomed to allocating 2 hours to help Cecilia prepare for an outing, first calming her down, then dressing her, and often having to carry her from place to place because she would become too agitated to walk by herself. This was life as they knew it.

After we began our occupational therapy sessions, life soon began to change, for both Cecilia and her parents. After a few weeks, Cecilia slowly began to speak to me, expressing many of her thoughts. "There's something in my belly button that makes me growl... something in my body that makes me not move, like when my leg goes up [referring to her posturing]," Cecilia told me.

At that point, I realized that somehow she held the answers to her own treatment. Only she could help me to help her. Even if she did not or could not tell me her needs verbally, she expressed them through other behaviors. For example, if she entered my office crashing her rigid body against the walls, I filled the treatment room with activities that would provide her with the same type of deep-pressure input. If she went into a rage and couldn't calm herself down, I became her external regulator, again providing the deep pressure she needed to soothe herself, by enveloping her entire body in a firm embrace, and I taught her mother to do the same. "Hold me, hold me!" Cecilia would scream, and we did, again and again.

By January, I felt that it was time to move ahead in her therapy. Because so much of Cecilia's early life, and also the first few months of occupational therapy, had focused on her responses to sensory stimulation, she was missing out on many experiences of a normal childhood. "Lunch with Lisa" (often with her mother, too) became not only Cecilia's special time with me on Friday afternoons but mine with her as well. Treating Cecilia in a natural environment had been one of my personal therapy goals for her. During our meals together, I began to see her evolve into her own person. She would ask me what I was having for lunch, and I would show her, offering her tastes of foods she may have been reluctant to try before due to their sensory qualities. In return, through my modeling and my reducing my spoken prompts over time, she would independently offer me tastes of her food.

Our lunchtime experiences also provided opportunities for us to work on initiating conversation and social interaction. Before we began therapy, Cecilia was accustomed to employing behaviors that were mostly nonverbal but still suggestive of her needs or desires. She grabbed food impulsively without asking. Often, she invaded others' personal space without realizing it because of her difficulties knowing where her body was in space in relation to other people or objects.

Cecilia also jumped and bounced around the room, both as a means for seeking sensory input and for signaling that she was finished eating, rather than simply saying that she was done. Together, her mother and I modeled alternatives for Cecilia so that she began to learn other ways of making her needs and desires known to those around her. Soon, she began to use these alternatives more independently.

Eleven months after her treatment began, Cecilia had blossomed into a "big girl," as she liked to refer to herself. Of course, I cannot claim that occupational therapy was the sole reason for these changes in her, but I can say with confidence that our therapy activities have allowed Cecilia to more fully explore the environment, which she once perceived as hostile. Her movements have become much less inhibited by her posturing, and her rages are subsiding (although she is still working on this area). She is quite verbal now and asks questions out of curiosity, much like any other 4-year-old child. She is just beginning to interact with other children, learning how to take turns and to share with others. And she has stopped holding on to her mother's waist, preferring instead to explore her environment freely on her own.

While continuing to address her sensory processing needs, I am also working to improve other performance areas that affect her daily routine, including fine motor, visual motor, and gross motor coordination skills. During each session, in her unique way, she provides me with the insight I need to learn more about her behavior. In return, I try to help Cecilia learn more about how to help herself.

Cecilia is entering a new phase in her development—preschool—and new challenges await her. But now Cecilia no longer needs to hold on tightly to her mother's waist and bury her head in her mother's side when starting a new experience. Going to school should be a lot more fun for her.

I'm delighted to report that Cecilia and her mom remain as strongly bonded emotionally as before. However, Cecilia no longer needs to rely on the vice-like grip that kept them bonded physically as well. Cecilia now enjoys the freedom of being "unglued" from her mother.

Chapter Five

I Can Do It

Toby Black, MA, OTR/L

"I can do it." These are four short words. But every time I hear them spoken by Peyton, I hear so much more—I hear the pluck, determination, and courage of a very special little boy. I have never actually heard Peyton's mother, Sandra, use these words, but they say just as much about her.

I first met Peyton and his family at an orthopedic clinic. He was only 2½ months old, but his blue eyes and impish smile, which were all I could see at first while he was swaddled in a blanket, attracted my attention. As his mother removed the blanket, none of my occupational therapy training quite prepared me for the shock at the sight of his hands. Flexed, with tiny, perfectly formed fingers that almost touched his forearm, these hands seemed totally out of place on this pink faced, adorable baby boy. I learned that Peyton also had some urogenital abnormalities, which are associated with this genetic syndrome.

I later found out that Peyton was not the first member of his family with these kinds of problems. His 3-year-old brother could not turn his forearm so that the palm of his hand faced up, and he also had the same urogenital difficulties. His maternal grandmother had had lifelong problems with her hands that were finally relieved only after surgery. Peyton had many of the same problems, though his were far more severe. Peyton's parents, and particularly his mother, Sandra, were having great difficulty coping with the genetic implications and a sense of guilt that she had perhaps unwittingly been the source of her children's disabling condition.

During the next year, a hand specialist evaluated Peyton and later performed corrective surgery on the boy's clubbed hands. Then, as a 14-month-old toddler, Peyton was referred to me for occupational therapy for his hand function. Remembering my initial shock at the sight of his hands, I was pleased to see the positive results of the surgery. Peyton still had to wear hand braces around the clock and was not able to move his fingers independently of one another. But as he quickly made me notice, he did not allow this to limit his hand use, and all of his other developmental milestones for growth were right on target.

However, things were not going as well for Peyton's mother, Sandra. She and Peyton's father joined a support group of parents whose children had the same genetic condition. I was told about the informational newsletters that the group published and the telephone conversations that Sandra had with the other parents. But she continued to worry about and deal with Peyton's recurring respiratory pneumonia and ear infections, which are typical for children with Peyton's condition at his age. Sandra knew that Peyton would outgrow those bouts of illness, but that did not relieve her from being housebound when he was sick or diminish her sense of isolation from her friends and neighbors for weeks at a time. I could see the light dim in her eyes, and I knew Sandra was hurting emotionally.

And so, in addition to treating Peyton, I began meeting with Sandra one-on-one, without her children present. This gave her the opportunity to vent her frustrations and speak about the guilt she felt about carrying the defective gene that had caused her boys' condition. She needed time to cry and express her feelings. Nonetheless, Sandra was a very special mother. Despite her own understandable depression, she continued to put on a happy face around the boys. From that point forward, I was on parallel tracks, treating Peyton and continuing my individual meetings with Sandra.

At age 3, Peyton still had blue eyes and an impish smile, which he flashed at me more and more as he was becoming quite a tease. He continued to wear his hand braces without complaint and allowed me to do stretching and passive exercises, where I gently guided his hands through various positions, with good humor and a smile. His legs were now bowed, and at the recommendation of a specialist whom Sandra located, Peyton wore leg braces for a year to help correct his bone alignment. Peyton still lacked the protective response of reaching out with his hands to break his fall, which most of us take for granted. When he felt himself falling, he continued to hold his hands close to his body, which meant that he could never prevent falls. Once he fell, there was always a danger of injuries to his arms and shoulders. But none of this stopped him from trying to get me to chase after him during our occupational therapy sessions.

Peyton's urological symptoms required more surgery, and because of the surgeries and respiratory illnesses, many formal occupational therapy sessions had to be canceled. So we shifted to more informal play therapy. Peyton and I focused on finger activities such as finger painting, color forms,s and theraputty/clay activities. Peyton was particularly proud of his squeeze scissors, which he shared with his friends. Peyton also now did not want to be babied by having someone dress him. So we adapted his clothing, using loops on his pants, so that he could pull them up all by himself. He was an independent little guy who would work at an activity until he could master it.

In the meantime, Sandra began to focus more on what she wanted for herself. She confided in me that she wanted to complete her college degree so that she could go back to paid employment outside her home when Peyton entered first grade. To do so, however, she would have to enroll Peyton in the local public school's preschool program, and she was very conflicted about it. Peyton was a bright child, but he continued to develop many colds and ear infections. He no longer wore leg braces, but still could not protect himself with his hands when he fell. I was pleased that Sandra was focusing on something she wanted for herself after 4 years of putting her own desires on hold for the sake of her family. I encouraged her to visit the school and have a frank talk about Peyton's abilities and needs with the teachers, which helped ease her concerns. Finally, with the help of a backup babysitter for emergencies, Sandra was able to go back to school. Her parents and her husband were all very supportive, filling in when needed to allow her time to study.

Peyton continued to develop well. The time had come for Peyton to learn to use a pencil. He was a lefty and managed to develop a grip that seemed to work for him even though his limited finger movements affected the positioning of his hand. Peyton loved to draw, but he disliked writing. As a compromise, we focused on tracing stencils as a way of helping him to learn to increase his hand pressure on the pencil. As he pushed my guiding hand away, it was then that I first heard him say, "I can do it!"

More time passed, and Peyton was now ready for his first computer. I introduced him to one with a touch screen, which his parents were delighted to purchase for him, and together we looked for ways to adapt the keyboard to accommodate his limited finger movements. We should have known better. With his typical grit and stubbornness, Peyton refused to use any adaptations and was determined to learn to use the keyboard his own way. As usual, Peyton seemed to know better than the rest of us the best way he could complete activities like working on a computer. When he figured it out, he triumphantly shouted the by-now-familiar "I can do it!" chant.

Chapter Five

It was a special day when Peyton started kindergarten. He was small compared to his classmates, but was always in the middle of all the action. He now expressed clothes preferences, including jeans with a zipper and snap and a baseball cap. However, the snap proved to be an insurmountable challenge; Peyton just did not have the hand strength to push it closed. So we settled on Velcro instead, and Peyton ended up dressed just the way he wanted to be.

By the summer after kindergarten, Sandra had "done it!" She had completed her degree and was working as the office manager for an attorney. She continued to bring Peyton to his therapy appointments and at times shared with me her concerns about whether Peyton would be able to handle the challenges of first grade. Peyton's hands both had begun to develop a severe ulnar drift, so that on the little finger sides they were pointing noticeably outward, and this could no longer be controlled by his elaborate hand braces. The only solution was additional extensive surgery.

But Peyton was not one to worry about himself. His concern was that his mother would miss him when he went back to school. He already had his dinosaur lunch box and backpack. Together, we had settled on an adapted brightly colored pencil grip to help him hold the various writing instruments he would need to use in the classroom. Far from being embarrassed by it, Peyton was so proud of it that he offered to share it with an admiring friend.

I knew that the year of first grade was going to be a challenge for all of us. Peyton was going to temporarily lose his writing ability due to the upcoming surgery. His occupational therapy rehabilitation would become more intense than anything he had experienced so far. With some trepidation, therefore, I asked him if he was ready to work on some other hand skills. I should not have worried. Peyton gave me his special look of determination and exclaimed, "I can do it! You help me, but I am the one who does it. He then picked up his pencil and carefully wrote his first name: PEYTON, followed by the words: CAN DO IT.

Today, Peyton uses a speech-activated program for his computer, has excellent academic skills, and plays the French horn in the school band. Peyton's grit and determination sure have showed me how positive thinking and a good old-fashioned "can-do" attitude can make all the difference in the world when it comes to overcoming physical challenges.

Chapter Six

When He Smiles, the Room Lights Up

Judi Hoggatt, MA, OTR

Like many other occupational therapy professionals that work with developmentally challenged infants, I sometimes have moments of doubt. I have listened to, cried with, and agreed with devastated parents of special needs children who state that "This just isn't fair." However, in the very back of my mind, there is always a shred of hope for another story like the Ford's.

When Cynthia and Larry Ford found out they were expecting, they were delighted. Cynthia watched her diet and did all the right things. Cynthia's diabetes, which up till then had been controlled with diet and medication, now required that she take insulin injections. She learned how to do this and was able to stay in good control of her blood sugar until 37 weeks into her pregnancy, at which time her sugar increased to a very dangerous level. Also she was concerned because she had been trying to elicit movement from the baby but was getting little response. She saw her obstetrician and voiced her concern over the noticeably decreased fetal movement. Because of her high blood sugar and the baby's slowdown, Cynthia was hurried to their suburban hospital for an emergency cesarean section. Everyone there rushed into action, especially when on the fetal monitor, the baby's heart rate decreased just before surgery began.

Chapter Six

This was certainly not the beginning that the Fords had planned. Larry and the grandparents were in the waiting room, agonizing. Meanwhile, in the delivery room, a severely sluggish and lethargic Kody was born. His Apgar scores that measure various aspects of a newborn's functioning, were very low—only 1 at 1 minute, 1 at 5 minutes, and 2 at 10 minutes out of a normal infant score of 10. A full neonatal code signifying a life-threatening emergency was undertaken. Kody received five doses of epinephrine, and chest compressions to keep his heart beating and mechanical ventilation to help his breathing was begun. The prognosis looked grim. However, normal heart rate was obtained at 15 minutes and gasping respirations were noted at 30 minutes. The delivery room was full of doctors and hospital personnel. But there seemed to be some type of disagreement between the doctors. Finally, the Fords' obstetrician convinced the rest of the team that there was a chance to save him. Kody was air lifted to Texas Children's Hospital, a major city children's hospital, where the most severely ill children are treated.

Once at TCH, several major problems were identified during the immediate period. Kody was on paralyzing medications for a week and remained on a ventilator to breathe for him during this time. His medical chart grew heavier and heavier, as did his parents' hearts. His list of diagnoses continued to increase—severe birth depression, pulmonary hypertension, pneumothorax, low blood pressure, significant hypoglycemia, cardiorespiratory arrest, neonatal seizures, left parietal intercranial hemorrhage, gastroesophageal reflux, failure to thrive, and hepatomegaly.

To his parents, this sounded like a foreign language. They met a variety of doctors, each with another diagnosis and a poorer prognosis. Cynthia and Larry, in desperation, finally insisted on a family conference, asking that each doctor treating Kody be present and report their findings. This took some real coordinating, but it was finally arranged. In hindsight, the Fords wonder how they ever found their way home after the meeting, so dire were the predictions. They talked and prayed and prayed and talked. They had been told that Kody would probably be blind, probably have very limited movement and maybe not even be able to turn himself over. Due to major reflux, his stomach contents regurgitated up into his esophagus. The doctors predicted that Kody would be unable to take a bottle, so there was an urgent need to surgically implant a gastrostomy tube so that Kody could safely receive nutrition. They were told that there was significant brain abnormality that could interfere with his intelligence, and he would have noticeable developmental delays. He had a heart defect and would need to be followed by a cardiologist. He would be seen as an outpatient, but he could probably receive some therapy at home through an early childhood intervention (ECI) program. The Fords made the decision to bring Kody home and to do whatever they needed to do to help Kody develop to his fullest potential, whatever that was.

They learned what they had to do—tube feeding, applying his hand splints, what to do if... Then, the Ford family finally got to come home. A nurse came to the house twice a week at first, but after they became proficient with handling Kody's feeding and medical needs, the Fords were on their own. Crying in frustration sometimes, the parents were overwhelmed, but in the back of their minds and hearts, they still had hope.

They called their local ECI program, Keep Pace, in Klein, Texas, and after the assessment process, started having weekly visits from Karen Glosson, OTR. Meanwhile, Cynthia kept doing all the things she had been told to do but she began to notice little differences in Kody. After occupational therapy sessions, Kody's thumbs no longer had to be pried out from under his curled fingers. And even when Cynthia made no noise at all, Kody would turn his head to follow her when she moved, something that seemed very odd for a child with supposedly severe visual problems.

Kody also began to suck and seemed to be acting as if he wanted to be taking a bottle. How could this be, they wondered. Karen, his occupational therapist, began working on oral motor skills because Cynthia had stated that what she wanted most was to be able to feed Kody normally. However, the problem was that Kody was a mouth breather, so to fill his mouth with a nipple was to cover his airway. Karen taught Cynthia and Larry some strategies to encourage Kody to breathe through his nose. Cynthia worked with Kody diligently to practice these techniques, and soon, to their delight, Kody learned to breathe through his nose. Seeing this, his doctor gave the okay for them to work slowly toward normal feeding by mouth.

Cynthia and Larry were beginning to notice more positive changes, but the medical community seemed to have their minds made up about Kody. He continued in the programs to which he was originally assigned. One day when Cynthia took Kody to his routine eye exam, she tried to get the resident to really look at Kody because she thought he was seeing. The resident tried to placate her by quickly scanning Kody. Then, as they do in the movies, the resident seemed to do a "double take." He quickly left to get the chief ophthalmologist, who also could find nothing wrong with Kody's eyes. They checked and rechecked, but it appeared that Kody's visual problems were gone!

Cynthia had long since discarded Kody's hand splints, as his thumbs and fingers were opening and closing, holding rattles, and picking up little pieces of string and lint. He still did not seem too crazy about toys, but then, he had mom and dad to entertain him.

Within 2 months of working with Karen, Kody returned to the medical team. Cynthia asked that the G-tube be removed. The team, ever cautious, held out for one more month, but then agreed to remove it. Cynthia's dream was coming true.

Chapter Six

Karen's schedule changed, and I became Kody's therapist when he had to switch therapists. Now that Kody was able to use a bottle, Cynthia and Larry had a new goal. They wanted Kody to walk. This was almost more than they had ever dared to dream, but they said it out loud, and so Judi wrote it as their top priority. Of course, there were other goals, but that was the main one.

Today Kody is 11 months old. He is able to pull up independently (never mind that he was not supposed to even roll over), he cruises between furniture, and with a big rolling push toy, he is able to walk 10 to 15 feet by himself. He has two words: "Dada" (which always gets a smile from daddy Larry) and "bye-bye" along with lots of babbling, bubble blowing, and raspberries. He can see and hurry over to the smallest piece of something on the floor that he should not have. He uses a modified pincer grasp with his thumb and forefinger to pick up very small things. He eats a variety of baby food and is beginning to eat small pieces of table food. He can follow and locate items under several layers (if he is interested in the item). When he smiles, the room lights up, between his smile and his parent's smiles. Even the doctors and therapists are smiling these days. No trace of heart problems, visual problems, or feeding problems are seen today. Is Kody a miracle? Was it maturity? Did he just heal well? We don't know, but we sure are glad that he proved everybody wrong.

So, when things look the very blackest, I am fortunate to have the Kody Ford story to show that miracles sometimes do happen, and you never can tell to whom they might happen.

Chapter Seven

Just Say No

Jane C. Chamberlain Olsasky, OTR/L

We've all heard the anti-drug slogan, "Just Say No." But for a child like Samantha, first exposed to drugs while in utero long before she was born, there was no chance to say "No." Samantha is a soft-spoken 3 year old with blue eyes and blonde hair who loves stickers, dolls, and stuffed animals. She prefers to wear dresses and shorts rather than turtleneck sweaters and slacks with elastic waistbands, even in cool weather. She dislikes loud noises and is so sensitive to them that she will sometimes wake up during the night if she hears even the sound of the furnace turning on. She loves to be pushed on the swing, but is cautious when walking up and down the stairs. Samantha exhibits these behaviors because she was exposed while still in the womb to methamphetamines, drugs that are known as "crank." Things used to be much worse for Samantha and her parents. The good news is that Samantha has shown marked improvement in her social and emotional skills as a result of occupational therapy intervention to treat her inability to tolerate loud noises, postural imbalance, and even a light touch on her skin without becoming tense and screaming loudly.

I saw Samantha for the first time in 1994 when she was 6 months old and have followed her yearly since that time. She was placed in foster care when she was 3 days old. At 16 months, she was adopted by this same loving foster care couple who, in addition to taking foster children, also had six children of their own. Samantha's gross motor skills have been weak. At 2 years of age, Samantha, unlike most active 2 year olds, refused to stand on one foot even with assistance and could not jump in place. She displayed extreme shyness, clung to her mother, would not talk, and did not play with toys for the first half-hour of the 2-hour occupational therapy evaluation.

After talking to her parents, watching her at play, and asking her mom a few questions, I suspected that Samantha had moderate sensory defensiveness. I explained that moderate sensory defensiveness doesn't affect the child's total body functions, but may only disrupt a few key areas of a child's life, such as dressing, bathing, and eating. Children with this condition may also have difficulty socially, coming across as overly aggressive or as totally isolated to others.

Samantha's mother could relate to that! She told me that Samantha preferred to wear diapers or loose T-shirts to bed, would not tolerate having blankets on top of her, resisted having her hair washed, avoided getting her hands messy, and disliked wearing tight fitting clothing such as turtleneck sweaters and slacks with elastic waistbands. Needless to say, all of this made daily life with Samantha a real hassle. She was at a loss to explain why Samantha behaved that way, but she didn't think that Samantha was doing it deliberately.

Samantha's mother was also concerned with her daughter's aggressive behavior, which she noticed appeared to occur periodically as a response to her extreme sensitivity to light touch and her fear about changes of position or any movement. I told her parents that the area in the brain that carries the sensation for pain and light touch, such as a tickle, also carries the sensations for temperature. Those who are sensitive to light touch may become overheated easily and uncomfortable. Apparently that's what happened to Samantha.

Samantha had other behaviors that puzzled her parents. She would not get on or off elevators unless she was held, and she screamed during the process; she feared stepping off a curb, so she would get down on her hands and knees to cross it; and she hated being placed in a playground swing. These fears of having her feet leave the ground or having her head tipped backward, known as gravitational insecurity, affected her play skills as well as her social and emotional skills. These behaviors certainly made it hard to take her anywhere. In short, daily life with Samantha was a constant battle.

Samantha and her parents needed help. I recognized all of her behaviors as her attempts to make sense of her world and to respond to the confusing messages she was getting through her senses. So, for 2 months in the fall of 1996, I treated Samantha once a week for 1 hour using a sensory integrative approach. I was trying to help Samantha be able to play with other children by not being as aggressive, to help Samantha feel more comfortable with her body's position in space so that she could play on at least one piece of playground equipment without fear, and to help Samantha become less jumpy when touched so that she could tolerate her hair being washed without distress.

In my first treatment session, I tried building rapport with Samantha and giving her parents information about Samantha's sensory defensiveness. Samantha sat on her mother's lap, hugging her teddy bear, watching me intently but not talking.

I explained to her mother that children with gravitational insecurity, that is, being uncertain about where their bodies are in space, need to feel comfortable first with movement in straight planes and with being low to the ground. Samantha was encouraged to lie on her stomach over a 4-inch cylinder while throwing a ball in a bucket. However, Samantha was not motivated to play this game that day. Fortunately, Samantha gradually became more attentive and interactive during the next couple of treatment sessions as I tempted her by using puppets. I also let Samantha watch her mother and me playing with moving equipment including a 20-inch diameter ball.

In addition to activities to develop her vestibular system, which controls her sense of movement and changes in head position, I gave her activities to develop her proprioceptive system, the system that gives her information about where her body is in space from her muscles, joints, and skin. Samantha was given opportunities in "heavy work" play activities such as pushing, lifting, and throwing and mouth activities such as blowing a pinwheel. I instructed her parents about how to handle changes in routines, and their new ways of interacting with her helped Samantha feel more calm, alert, and organized; her sensory defensiveness decreased. After 3 weeks of treatment, Samantha was walking into the elevator herself without screaming or crying, although she insisted on holding onto the railing.

To deal with her defensiveness to touch, especially for hair-washing time, I suggested activities such as massaging her head first before applying shampoo. This helps because the head, neck, shoulders, palms of the hands, and soles of the feet are the most sensitive to touch, so firm, deep pressure is less threatening than light, quick touch. Using this technique, Samantha's parents were able to successfully wash her hair.

After 5 weeks of treatment, Samantha's mother stated that Samantha seemed less fearful in new surroundings and appeared less aggressive. After 2 months of therapy, Samantha's social skills also improved with Samantha starting conversations with me during treatment.

Toward the end of Samantha's 2 months of therapy, Samantha's mother asked for specific advice about handling a troubling aspect of Samantha's auditory defensiveness. Samantha would not stay in her bed at night, yelling "I'm scared." When I found out that Samantha's bed was near the window, where she could see the outdoor street lights and hear the traffic going by, I suggested that they move the bed away from the window and even put the mattress on the floor. It worked. After that, Samantha began waking up only two times during the night, and everyone was getting more sleep! I was particularly pleased that her parents were able to recognize situations that were hard for Samantha to handle and that they were now beginning to figure out some solutions based on the things we did in occupational therapy.

When I saw Samantha 1 year later for her 3-year-old re-evaluation, Samantha's mother could not come so Samantha's father was present. He was very proud to report her progress. Samantha now enjoyed playing with a large therapy ball, she was jumping off the bottom step, she liked swinging on a swing, and she tolerated having her hair cut; however, she still continued to prefer to wear lightweight clothing.

Her father also reported happily that Samantha now wakes up only once during the night, usually when she hears the sound of the furnace going on. And now, when her sleepy parents tell her it's time to get back into bed and go back to sleep, they are always delighted to hear Samantha say, "Yes."

Jeff Wipes His "Ticky" Hands

Jean M. Kassnel
Submitted by Lesley Larsen Kountz, COTA

At his preschool occupational therapy program graduation, my 2½-year-old, Jeff, walked up calmly to accept his "diploma," then returned to his seat to eat a party snack. When his hands got sticky, he came over to me. "Mommy, my hand ticky; please wipe." I smiled, the kind of happy smile that comes from a moment of tender joy. Happiness over a child asking to have his hand wiped? In Jeff's case, absolutely. Seven months ago, before Jeff's therapy—occupational, physical, and speech—the same scene would have ended much differently. Jeff might have screamed at the top of his lungs because of the mess on his hands or run in panic from the room.

Jeff had been a difficult child almost from birth. No mother likes to say that, but now with the progress he has made, it doesn't hurt so much to acknowledge it. From the moment he came home from the hospital, he was extremely different from his sister. He cried every time you changed his diaper; he screamed all through his bath; he only liked being held very, very close; and he never seemed to sleep. As an infant, he was either really upset or very happy; there just was no middle ground. My husband and I got used to the fact that Jeff was different, but we always attributed it to his personality, or to the fact that he was a boy, or that he was a second child.

Chapter Eight

It wasn't until after Jeff's second birthday that I really noticed how different he was from the other children his age. I knew he was behind in his speech (he only said nine words at the time), but once again I was comparing him to his sister. And didn't everyone know that boys and second children were just slower than girls and first borns? But I couldn't ignore that there were other differences as well. Jeff had difficulty paying attention, he overreacted to any change in his environment or routines, he did not like doing activities with his hands, and he became extremely upset when his hands got the least bit dirty. His hyperactivity and roughness with his sister really started worrying me. It is hard to use the words, but I was concerned not only for his safety, but worried about his physical abuse of our daughter.

At Jeff's 2-year check-up, I got up the courage to ask about his speech and other problems, rather than just treat them as boy things or second child behavior. That was the first time that someone brought up the possibility to me that Jeff had sensory defensiveness, a condition in which the receptors for touch, skin sensation, or pain are so overly alert that the tiniest touch feels like a major assault. People with sensory deficiencies cannot tolerate even the softest touch and often cannot stand dirt or mess on their hands or skin. After more discussion, listening, and reading, there was no doubt in my mind that Jeff had some serious sensory problems.

By Christmas of that year, when Jeff was scheduled to start therapy, there was hardly peace and joy in our family world. Frankly, I was at my wits' end. First, Jeff was sick for most of the month of December. His daytime waking hours were spent in almost constant crying. Just about anything he touched seemed to aggravate him and bring on another lengthy crying spell. It got so bad, I couldn't even hold my own child to calm him down. He could not tolerate anything sticky on his hands. Putting up the Christmas tree was a double challenge, making sure he did not touch it, particularly the prickly needles, while in his wilder moments, keeping him from running headlong into the tree and knocking it over.

I remember the nights most. Jeff refused to go to sleep and would come out of his room crying every 15 minutes. My husband and I would have to hold him just so and rock him, but that was not easy because the one area in which he was quite normal for his age was his growth. By the time he would finally fall asleep, my husband and I were so tired and emotionally drained that we found it hard to get into the spirit of wrapping presents. Even if we tried, it wouldn't be long before we would be interrupted by Jeff again. He would wake up four or five times during the night. We were all totally exhausted.

It was nearly impossible for me to do any shopping. Any trip with Jeff was an immediate disaster. If I put him in the shopping cart, he would start to whine and cry after only a few minutes. If I tried to distract him with something to eat, he would scream because his hands were dirty. If I let him out of the cart, he would start running around the store like one of Maurice Sendak's Wild Things. I just could not control him. I knew what the problem was, but that did not ease my embarrassment at the looks I got or comments I overheard from my fellow shoppers. Life was like the nightmare before Christmas.

Jeff started occupational therapy just before Christmas. It was not an auspicious start. On the second day, there was a Christmas party at the therapy center. I tried to bow out by explaining to Jeff's case worker that I did not think he would be able to control himself, but I was persuaded to bring him. Sure enough, he refused to see Santa Claus and clung to me. When I tried to get him to participate, he started running and screaming. Finally, he got a toy car, lay on the ground to play with it, and just shut out the rest of the world. This is what I had learned to expect from my son, but now we were at the therapy center, and I really began to despair. If the trained therapists couldn't control his behavior here, what else was there? But slowly over the next several months, I began to see a change.

I've already told you how this story ends, but now let me tell you how that wonderful graduation came about. Jeff received speech therapy twice a week and occupational and physical therapy each once a week. After only a short time, the first change I noticed was with the sticky, dirty hand problem. After tactile activities and skin brushing in occupational therapy (a technique in which the deep nerve endings are stimulated using a surgical scrub brush in various patterned movements on his back, shoulders, and arms in order to help calm and organize his sensations), instead of screaming when his hands got dirty or sticky, Jeff would hold them out and say "ticky'" to get me to wipe them clean. He still does not like his hands to be dirty for very long, but he does not have a tantrum, he simply asks for a towel.

Other occupational therapy activities included swinging on a flat swing to help him develop postural righting reflexes so he could better manage where his body was in space, being exposed to a variety of textures and materials on his hands so that his skin could get used to the feel of various kinds of stimulation, and sleeping under a weighted blanket to provide constant pressure to calm the deep nerve endings in his body and help him feel where he is relative to the floor.

Miracle of miracles, Jeff has learned to go to sleep on his own every night. He is brushed, then sleeps in sweat suits or long underwear and T-shirts under his weighted blanket. This helps him feel secure and able to tell where his body is in space. He may need a lullaby to play for an hour or so or want to read his picture books in bed, but he rarely cries or comes back out of his bedroom. Even when he awakens once or twice during the night, it is because he is lonely, like any 2 1/2 year old, or his blanket has fallen off the bed. My husband or I go in and tuck him back in, and he falls back asleep.

Jeff's speech has also blossomed. He seems to have so much to say, and his sentences have gotten much longer and more complex. Being able to express himself so much better, he is less likely to get frustrated when he wants something.

Shopping has also become much more pleasant. If Jeff eats something and gets his hands dirty or sticky while we're out, I simply wipe him up. He does not run as much as he did. He seems able to pay attention to my instructions better and notices his surroundings with interest and curiosity. We have even made a successful outing to a museum with Jeff in a stroller.

Perhaps best of all, life at home has improved dramatically. Jeff and his sister are able to play together and have fun with each other. There are moments when he gets hyperactive and acts out with her, but when he does, playing a physical game or giving him something to eat is usually enough to calm him down and defuse the situation.

I could, I guess, have followed so many people's advice and just waited until Jeff was older, hoping against hope when people told me he would "grow out" of his behaviors. But I know that children with Jeff's condition do not just grow out of their behaviors. They need help from occupational therapists to organize their brains and their bodies to get constant messages about their world. If I had waited, Jeff and our entire family would not have benefitted from the skilled and caring attention of his teachers and therapists, and I would not have had the joy of that special graduation when my little boy came up to me, held out his hands, and said "ticky."

Postscript: Jeff finished his last year in a preschool early childhood program, and he started kindergarten in an integrated classroom with extended special education services in the afternoon. He has since come a long way. His gross motor skills have reached age level. He continues to work on fine motor activities, although his tactile defensiveness seems to be almost gone. His speech is fairly normal. He continues to receive occupational therapy at school. With the help of his occupational therapists, Jeff was able to attend a regular classroom in first grade and learned coping techniques to deal with life and his education in the future. Jeff was discharged from occupational therapy at the end of first grade.

Chapter Nine

Close to My Heart

Denise E. Williams, OTR/L, CHTP

Meigui, a Mandarin Chinese woman living in America, had strong ties to her Chinese background and traditions, especially when it came to raising her daughter. When something seemed wrong with her child's development, she asked questions and sought help, but even then it was hard for her to be convinced to change her traditional ways. So occupational therapy with her daughter, Zhesheng, involved not only activities to help the 18 month old, but special efforts to gain the confidence and trust of Meigui. Thus, convincing Meigui that we occupational therapists had something to offer, and enlisting her cooperation, became our first occupational therapy goal with Zhesheng.

Zhesheng was an 18-month-old girl with cerebral palsy. She was a twin, but the other sibling had died in utero. Zhesheng herself had spent several weeks in a neonatal intensive care unit after birth. Although she had some head control, her muscles were rigid and spastic and she didn't seem to have any language skills. Unlike other babies her age or even younger, she never tried to move or roll over, regardless of whether she was on her back or her belly. Meigui realized that her daughter was slow to develop and sought help. Zhesheng was admitted to the early intervention program at a local public school and was immediately referred to occupational therapy.

At our first meeting, Meigui held Zhesheng tightly against her chest, their faces almost touching. Zhesheng seemed content until I tried to hold her. She began to scream, and the rigidity in her extensor muscles became more pronounced when I held her. She stopped screaming immediately and her muscles relaxed as soon as I returned her to Meigui's chest. Meigui confided that as soon as she brought Zhesheng home from the neonatal unit, she had held her in this traditional chest-to-chest position whenever she was awake. Zhesheng was now so used to this pattern that she would cry incessantly if held in any other position, such as facing away, even by her mother.

For several months this behavior pattern was repeated with me and with all other staff members. Zhesheng was content when being held by Meigui, screamed loudly when anyone else tried to hold her, and became calm again only when given back to her mother.

An important issue that we had to face was that during all this time Meigui seemed reluctant to follow our therapeutic suggestions. She thought that our American practices were very different from the traditional Far East Mandarin Chinese medical and child-rearing methods she had known. We therefore spent a lot of time talking with Meigui about what we wanted to do and why, and encouraging her to understand how these things would help Zhesheng. Meigui slowly developed trust and respect for the team. More importantly, she knew that Zhesheng was not getting better without our help. At last, she gave us permission to try our American methods.

Now, with Meigui's permission and cooperation, we were able to begin to unravel the mystery of Zhesheng's disorder and determine what would help her. We had tried many different strategies to encourage her participation in activities that other children her age enjoyed: playing musical instruments, toys, games, songs. Nothing seemed to capture her attention long enough to halt her unrelenting crying. Often, other frustrated school staff members would accuse me of making Zhesheng cry or would give us their suggestions for working with her. Unfortunately, their suggestions were generally based on what worked for a typical child, not one with cerebral palsy, and certainly not one who was so bonded to her mother.

With the help of Zhesheng's teacher and Meigui, I now began to devise a treatment plan that would stimulate her senses, improve her motor skills, capture her attention, and make her feel comfortable. It was a slow process, filled with trial and error.

Our first attempt was in a quiet, dimly lit room. Zhesheng, Meigui, and the teacher sat on the floor while I chose soothing music, such as New Age, Baroque, or classical tunes. While I hummed or sang quietly to Zhesheng, I massaged the soles of her feet, delivering deep pressure, a method that can be very relaxing. It was very disappointing to all of us when Zhesheng did not seem to respond well.

We felt that an important key to Zhesheng's improvement would be helping her get used to new situations without being held by her mother. Meigui tried holding Zhesheng facing outward so that Zhesheng could strengthen and control her eye muscles, develop more tolerance for new positions, and become more independent from her mother. But Zhesheng still resisted vigorously.

We realized that we had to be just as vigorous in our therapy attempts. Every week, we came up with new suggestions and theories. I consulted with other occupational therapy colleagues in the hopes of finding a successful treatment. One occupational therapist suggested that perhaps Zhesheng felt "connected" to Meigui on a general sensory level, and that she felt threatened and fearful when she wasn't allowed to make that close-to-the-heart chest-to-chest contact. With this in mind, I decided to continue the techniques we had been using, but to slow our pace so that changes were very gradual. At the same time, we began to alter Zhesheng's environment with approaches that were multisensory.

One day, I noticed that when Meigui tried to calm Zhesheng, she spoke so fast that she instead caused Zhesheng to cry even more and to become even more rigid in muscle tone. Acting on a hunch, I asked Meigui to speak slowly and to use the same phrases over and over. With Meigui following our advice, slowly, Zhesheng's crying lessened and she began to listen to her mother. After a while, she seemed less agitated when she was turned to face outward, away from Meigui.

Once we had decreased Zhesheng's fears of being separated from Meigui and had calmed her, Zhesheng gradually began to achieve other developmental milestones. She began to roll, reach for things, make prolonged eye contact, and vocalize. She could soon crawl a little, sit up with assistance, and push herself up to her elbows when lying on her belly. Even the sound of her crying had begun to change, from a striated pitch to a more resonant tone, a sign that she was calming down and also involving her rib cage muscles.

As the end of the school year approached, Zhesheng could get into a crawling position by herself and even crawl to her mother with just a little assistance. With Meigui's encouragement, Zhesheng would lift her head and look at her mother, a feat that had seemed impossible 9 months earlier. Meigui was elated.

In the rehabilitation of a child with severe disabilities, little breakthroughs and improvements are incredibly important. Though they may seem insignificant when viewed separately, they are all small steps that lead to grand leaps when pieced together. So this small step, being able to lift her head and look another person in the eye, coupled with the little steps of increased vocalizations and the ability to sit on Meigui's lap facing outward, meant that Zhesheng was now ready for interactive sessions with a speech-language pathologist.

Chapter Nine

Imagine, Zhesheng talking! Wouldn't that be something?

Our last session of the school year arrived, and I decided to use it for Meigui's parent education. She needed to learn a special home program with graphics, and I wanted to demonstrate various techniques to her and encourage her to continue the home program during the summer.

When our session ended, we stood at our classroom door saying goodbye to Zhesheng and Meigui. Suddenly, Zhesheng looked up at us, smiled, and said in perfect Mandarin, "Zai-Jien"—Mandarin for "Goodbye." We were overjoyed, elated, and completely awestruck. We had not expected this—Zhesheng making eye contact *and* bidding us farewell! We were so proud of this child, once so close only to her mother's heart, who had managed to take the first small step to let us into her heart as well.

Please note: Names were changed to protect the family's privacy.

Chapter Ten

A Healing Transformation

Elizabeth A. Haluska Ankney,
OTR/L, PC

My son, Jesse, is now a typical, functional, thriving 8 year old. This in itself is a miracle to me and to anyone who knew him "before"—that is, before occupational therapy. I am a second-year occupational therapy student and the mother of three. My youngest was a special care child and had been since birth. Our story is a perfect example of how occupational therapy can completely, dramatically improve a life. Occupational therapy literally turned our lives around, freeing my son to live the life of a normal child and giving me a genuine passion for a new career.

Soon after his birth, it was clear that Jesse had severe feeding problems. During his first feed, and all the others that followed, his swallows came out through his nostrils. He was never able to adequately suck a nipple. This was compounded by massive gastroesophageal reflux, a condition in which the contents of the stomach return back up into the esophagus.

Jesse spent the first several years of his life in and out of hospitals and children's rehabilitation centers. He has had a number of surgical procedures, which have improved his overall condition. First was a Nissen fundoplication, which is a surgical procedure to discourage reflux of stomach acid into the esophagus; next was a gastrostomy tube placement, which is a feeding tube inserted in the stomach, also called a G-tube; and several more, all of which were necessary to help him swallow and keep the food in his stomach where it belongs. Jesse's case has been the frustration of many feeding teams. Despite the obvious need for all of these surgical procedures, there still were more than a few of these swallowing teams who told me that Jesse was simply stubborn, and this was the reason for his refusal to eat.

Jesse went through many barium swallows, a process during which he swallowed contrast dye that shows up on x-rays and other radiology tests. As the dye moved through his digestive system, its progress was charted to identify where and when reflux and pharyngeal insufficiency occurred. The barium swallows helped form a diagnosis: oral motor dysfunction, abnormalities in the swallow, and chronic aspiration syndrome—he was inhaling liquids into his lungs.

Jesse underwent oral stimulation therapy in the past with a physical therapist before several of the surgeries, but he still did not improve enough to take in foods by mouth. I was left with the impression that the pharyngeal flap surgery had been our last hope to improve his feeding skills. Jesse was still dependent on G-tube feedings for one-half of his total nutritional intake. It looked as though we had run out of treatment options. There was nothing more we could try.

Then came Jesse's salvation. He started speech therapy to focus on improving his speech with a new speech-language pathologist, a man who was also an occupational therapist with special expertise in feeding problems. The new "two-in-one" therapist quickly discovered that Jesse had very sensitive oral reflexes. He had probably developed these as a defense against the great amount of reflux and aspiration he had experienced. He was not knowingly refusing to eat, nor was he merely stubborn!

I have to admit, I was skeptical at first. After all, I'd been here before. But as a parent, I was willing to do anything to make my child the best he is capable of being.

Jesse's treatment was converted to occupational therapy and he began "intra-oral stimulation" to desensitize his very sensitive gag reflexes. This involved slowly introducing a special device into Jesse's mouth so that he would gradually become accustomed to the sensation of something in that area. Jesse also performed neck rolls to increase his swallowing strength. He began to learn compensatory swallowing techniques to help eliminate further aspiration. Each week, Jesse was able to tolerate the stimulation a little further into his mouth. And each week, he ate a wider variety of new food textures and consumed larger amounts.

I couldn't believe what I was seeing: Jesse actually began to enjoy eating! After just 12 weeks of occupational therapy (which became the focus of his treatment), we discontinued his manual pump feeds. Within the year, Jesse metamorphasized into a child I barely recognized, and I am very thankful for that.

I have seen, firsthand, how occupational therapy can literally transform a life, or, in our case, two lives. There are other children in this world with problems similar to Jesse's, and because of our experience with occupational therapy, I know that there is so much occupational therapy can do for them. There is no doubt in my mind that I have to be part of this progress, making occupational therapy not a job, not a career, but a lifestyle and a mindset. I want to learn all I can, try to improve and create, and never stop learning. There are so many lives out there waiting to be turned around by occupational therapy. I'm going to be a part of it!

Postscript: Jesse is now 13 years old and a normal, healthy teenager. I am now an occupational therapist with special training and concentration in dysphasia and feeding problems. I have a new granddaughter who was born with very similar problems and is now under the care of the same team of specialists who helped Jesse. They are using his medical records to guide their treatment and I am confident that another "healing transformation" is possible for our family.

Chapter Eleven

Therapeutic Paws: A Tail of Success

Rhona Feldt-Stein,
BSc OT, OT Reg (Ont)

One day, quite unexpectedly, the stray cat living in the store next to our clinic wandered in. Before long, it had adopted us. Our practice, York Pediatric Therapy Services, Inc, has been known to use all sorts of inducements to keep their young clients motivated during therapy. Because play is a child's way of learning, fun and games are a part of all occupational therapy practices that treat children; stuffed animals routinely reside at clinics, but sometimes a live animal is even more effective at catching a child's attention. So, we seized the opportunity for her to become our "clinic cat." The appearance of a soft four-legged creature was an immediate hit with the children who attended the clinic for occupational therapy. Suddenly, "therapy" was a fun place to come. But nights and weekends were lonely for our new feline therapist without any children around, and soon it was apparent that she needed a companion to fill the hours. Enter Max.

Max had good timing. That little brown tabby and white ball of fluff just seemed to know he was needed. As I made my way out of the barn where I had come to choose a kitten, his meowing trailed after me, begging me to stop, as if to say, "Hey, wait up for me." When I finally did, he trundled over and dutifully lay at my feet as an offering. I guess you can say, he chose me.

So Max eagerly joined our two- and four-legged staff at the clinic. As a 6-week-old kitten, Max accepted his role as entertainer and toy with complete resolution. The children would pick him up and carry him upside down, and he tolerated this with nary a cry or complaint.

But then an amazing transformation occurred. Max seemed to realize that our occupational therapy clinic wasn't only for fun, we had business to accomplish. So he began to train himself to be a therapist like the rest of us! Max could easily motivate a stubborn child to use both hands to pull apart two ropes to send a float zooming from one end to the other by jumping up to get the float as it passed by. He tirelessly trotted after a piece of string attached to a tricycle to entice the child to peddle it.

As he grew, Max would jump up on the table where we do hand skill activities. At times, he would just lie close by, purring away, adding just enough distraction for a child with an attention deficit to allow us two-legged therapists to complete our evaluation and to test the child's level of concentration. Finish the task and you get to play with Max! One time in particular, I was trying to get a little boy who had cerebral palsy to use his spastic arm to reach up and put a toy in the upper room of a toy house. After much fretting and my getting nowhere with him, Max jumped up onto the table and stuck his paw through the window of the room in the house. In no time flat, the little boy's arm was extended to reach out and touch his new friend.

Max's willingness to be part of the crowd is always apparent. He loves to greet people as they walk into the office and rolls his now 17-pound body onto his back, eagerly anticipating a belly rub. One thing that really bothers Max, however, is the sound of a crying child. That is how he came to meet Erin.

Erin is a 2½-year-old girl who is a petite bundle of charm and personality. Her adult-like speech and long brown curls make you laugh and want to cuddle her at the same time. Erin has been coming to our clinic since the age of 1 year for mild right-sided weakness as the result of a prebirth stroke.

At the beginning of therapy, Erin tended to hold her right arm close to her body. She could not put out her arms and hands to protect herself. She could go from sitting to a crawl position, then crawled using alternative arm and leg movements equally. Erin could begin the process of bringing herself up to tall-kneeling; however, she was not yet pulling herself up to stand or to crawl up or down stairs. Her balance was also very unstable; she, therefore, refused to get up and move. If she was placed in a standing position, Erin would hold onto another person for support, but she was not yet standing on her own to "cruise" and move around furniture.

Erin, despite her cunning ways, was very stubborn and had a temper to rival anyone. She often cried to avoid doing new or challenging activities. If she did engage in these, it was for very short periods of time. Therapy goals, therefore, were very hard to achieve.

Chapter Eleven

Enter Max. During some of the trying times, Max would often wander into the therapy gym and distract Erin during therapy. This allowed the therapist to work with Erin for extended periods of time. Max seemed to sense when and where he was needed quite naturally. When we were trying to get Erin to crawl up the stairs, Max would independently place himself on the top step, meow, and wait for Erin to get to him. Once she patted him, he would then go down and wait for her near the bottom step. This would be repeated several times without Erin's becoming disagreeable. Within a number of sessions, Erin would wait for Max to go to the top stair, crawl up and then crawl down to pat him, with very little assistance.

Max also therapeutically assisted Erin in getting her to walk. Upon request he would climb onto the seat of a wheeled secretary's chair and allow Erin to push him through the clinic. When we were trying to teach Erin more independent walking, Max would position himself about 6 to 10 feet in front of her. Every time she would get closer, he would instinctively move a little farther away and lie down. Every now and then he would allow her to catch him, pet him, and give him a belly rub. Then it was back to therapy business as he moved enticingly out of her reach to encourage her to walk toward him once more.

Max also assisted in encouraging Erin to use her right hand. Once again, he would come and position himself on the therapy mat near Erin, but on her right, so she would need to use her right hand or both hands to pet him. At other times, he would play with a toy, again on her right, thus engaging her interest. This would allow me to get Erin to use her right hand to get the toy.

Erin is now walking and using the stairs independently. She uses both her hands for many activities, although she still needs encouragement at times to use her right hand. Erin can still be quite stubborn, but this has dissipated considerably.

Despite the progressive changing of therapy goals, Max is still an "active assistant" in Erin's therapy. Whenever Erin arrives for therapy, she now comes in asking for the "Meow," and Max is always there to greet her, waiting for his next "therapy assignment."

Max, along with our other cat, and my dog Penny, who is a regular visitor to the clinic, are supplemental to our two-legged occupational therapy staff at the clinic, but they remain the most sought-after "therapists." Their needs are few—food, water, a cozy place to sleep, and lots of love and attention from us and the children—but their contributions are enormous. And best of all, their salaries are low and I pay no taxes on their wages.

Chapter Twelve

A Doll for Wendy

Fred Sammons, PhD (Hon), OTR

What do airplane parts, the space program, an aeronautical engineer, and a large doll have to do with a 4-year-old girl born without arms? Just about everything. They helped her eat applesauce all by herself for the very first time, and, with her newfound independence, to expand her skills and knowledge as she grew up, and become an occupational therapist.

Today, people without arms or legs have a full range of technological options to provide them with what they need to function fully. Wendy's story begins in 1960, before any of us had seen TV commercials showing athletes on artificial legs playing championship basketball or setting speed records running. No one had yet heard of the "Bionic Man" TV series or dreamed about voice-activated robotic arms that could pick up tiny marbles. Back then, before modern-day prostheses, a 4 year old born without arms had to rely on developing dexterity in her feet and toes in order to do things the rest of us do with our arms and hands.

In 1960, after 5 years as an occupational therapist and director of the OT Department at the Rehabilitation Institute of Chicago, I moved to Northwestern University's Prosthetic Research Center as a research associate. There I was assigned to develop workable arms for that little girl, Wendy. We had been taught in occupational therapy school about adaptive devices, but in 1960, putting a combination of the right people and things together for Wendy was as adaptive as I had ever had to get.

My role as the occupational therapist on the team was to be the "human factors person"—the one who makes the practical connections linking what the person wants to do and the device that will help her do it. In this situation, I had to connect the artificial arm, a mechanical device, and Wendy, the little girl who needed to be able to use the device in her daily activities.

The Bowden cable had been invented for aircraft controls. We soon found another, more down-to-earth use for it. We realized that it could be adapted to allow the force from the shoulder area of the good arm of someone missing one arm to be transferred across the back and down the artificial arm to the terminal or end device. This "hand at the end of the artificial arm" was generally a hook-shaped clamping device that was opened by the cable and closed by a rubber band. Our one improvement to the Bowden cable system was that we were able to line the housing with Teflon material so it was smoother and easier for the user. However, people with both arms missing presented an even more unusual challenge as we struggled to provide them with mechanical help for daily personal hygiene, leisure activities, and job requirements. They didn't have a "good arm" for transfer of force to power an artificial arm.

At Northwestern University we were affiliated with the Michigan Child Amputee Program at Mary Free Bed Hospital in Grand Rapids, Michigan. Based on the needs of their young patients, they challenged us to develop a "feeding arm" for children ages 3 to 5 who had no arms. This simplified approach allowed us to concentrate on a prosthesis that had as its primary purpose a single function, namely, getting a spoonful of food from the plate to the mouth and the spoon back to the plate for another bite.

We tried our best to work with the kinds of equipment available in 1960, and sometimes we found ourselves using the strangest, seemingly most unlikely stuff in the most unusual ways. For example, nickel cadmium rechargeable batteries were new at the time. Small low voltage but powerful electric motors were being made for the space program. Micro switches were available to fit in small places to provide control. The technique of making the socket or body shell with stockinette and polyester resin was standard procedure. Velcro brand hook and loop closure was new on the scene and not yet commercially available. All this came in handy for our newest project.

The director of the research center was Colin McLaurin, an aeronautical engineer from Canada who had invented the Canadian Hip Prosthesis, an innovative artificial device for the hip joint. From his experience with this device, we knew he was very successful at taking a creative look at problems and then coming up with simple but effective solutions.

For us, Colin devised a special kind of parallelogram linkage in the fore-arm that turned the spoon toward the mouth as it came up from the plate. The shoulder joint was set to provide adjustment for table height. The child's shoulder blade muscle—the scapula—would activate the micro switch for up and down movement.

Enter little, blonde, 4-year-old Wendy, who lived in Iowa but who traveled all the way to Michigan with her devoted parents to be part of the Michigan program. People like Wendy, born without arms, can learn to use their toes and feet with great precision, unlike people who lose their arms later in life who generally never develop such accurate foot function or get enough hip range of motion to be useful. Wendy was no exception to the rule—she was already quite adept at using her feet and toes as hands and fingers. We knew that our arm and hand prosthesis could never be as proficient as Wendy's current level of foot usage, so we encouraged her parents to continue helping her improve her foot function. Still, we knew that as she grew up, having arm and hand function that resembled that of other people would be increasingly important to her, so we were delighted when her parents agreed that she would be a per-fect candidate for the very first feeding arm we were developing for children like her with both arms missing.

Artificial arm-maker Fred Hampton, our talented research prosthetist, took a plaster cast of Wendy's upper body and made a mold for the two shoul-der sockets. Space was provided for the switches on the inside, and the sock-ets were laminated with polyester resin. We used the new product, Velcro brand closure, so the comfort and control functions could be adjusted easily.

Our machinist, Gus Weiskopf, made the parts to hold the motor and link-age inside the hollow upper and lower right arm shells. A child's hook termi-nal device held the spoon at the best angle. But the question of what to use for an arm to hold the batteries for Wendy's other side stymied our greatest minds for several days. Finally we had an idea. We went to a toy store and bought the biggest doll we could find!

The rechargeable batteries were fitted into the doll's left arm, which was then removed from the doll and attached to the left socket of the prosthesis. It was my job to connect the wiring and control systems and to be sure that the fit and function of the device were suitable for Wendy. When finished it a made a strange-looking apparatus that almost overshadowed little Wendy. But it was time to try it out.

Wendy and her folks came back for several days as we fitted the shoulder sockets and made sure they were comfortable and functional. We used apple-sauce as the first food and Wendy began eating with much success. From applesauce she went on to other foods; from eating she progressed to other activities. Then she and her parents went back home with the new prosthe-sis and the one-armed doll in tow. For me, it was always hard to say goodbye to my patients. It was like having a loved one leave on a long voyage and whom you might never see again. This time it was particularly tough, especially when Wendy turned and waved goodbye.

Many years later, I found out that Wendy had become an occupational therapist and that she was practicing in the South. My career led me to develop self-help aids—products for occupational therapists and their patients to use all over the country. One day I stopped to visit the occupational therapists using my products at a nursing home in Florida. By chance, Wendy was there! We hugged each other. She promised to tell her folks about our meeting. Before we said goodbye again, we talked about applesauce, which Wendy said always remained a favorite food, and about a large one-armed doll that Wendy still keeps to remind her of how she got her first arms.

Section Two

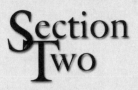

Children

Keeping on the Right Track

Keeping on
the Right Track

Read about 10 children with school-related difficulties, illnesses, or other problems that were resolved in a satisfying way by families, teachers, therapists, and the children themselves so that the children could continue to grow and develop.

Chapter Thirteen

Meet Gabriella: An OT Success Story

Barbara E. Joe

Now a thriving 10 year old living in Minneapolis, this former Romanian orphan is beating the odds. "I do not like swearing because it hurts my feelings. Words like that make my heart break. People who swear could choose other words that wouldn't hurt so much." This statement by 10-year-old Gabriella was chosen for a young writers' forum on the subject of swearing published in the *Minneapolis Star Tribune*. Any parent would be proud to have a child's words appear in print, but Gabriella's adoptive parents saw something more in their daughter's declaration: evidence of just how far she had come.

As an infant, Gabriella was placed in an orphanage in Iasi, Romania. She was 3 years old when Gale Haradon, PhD, OTR, first discovered her in Orphanage Section II, rocking back and forth in her crib, unable to walk or talk, and avoiding touch and eye contact. Her overall developmental level was less than 1 year. Gabriella was no bigger than an 8-month-old baby and weighed only 19 pounds. She could not feed herself or eat from a spoon. She was able to crawl and pull herself up but could not stand independently. When she was picked up, her legs would flex under her. "But at times," Haradon now recalls, "she flashed a certain bright-eyed, curious look that indicated her innate potential."

Haradon, in her capacity as director of professional education for an American foundation, took Gabriella and 45 other failure-to-thrive toddlers out of their cribs; introduced them to play, music, and toys; and educated their caregivers. Haradon cannot forget the day of Gabriella's breakthrough. The children's cribs were all clustered together to save space, but when Gabriella saw Haradon enter the nursery, she climbed eagerly from crib to crib, tumbling over other children, and into Haradon's waiting arms. From then on, she blossomed, learning new skills every day. A photo of her with Haradon appeared in *OT Week* (the weekly news magazine for the profession of occupational therapy, published by The American Occupational Therapy Association, Inc. "Hard Lessons from Romania," Feb. 18, 1993) in connection with a story about Romanian children's institutions.

OT Week reader Mary Kay Walsh, COTA, happened to show the article to a Minneapolis couple with an adopted son from Romania. The couple fell in love with the little girl's picture, but struggled 2 long years before her new mother finally traveled to Romania and brought 7-year-old Gabriella home.

One of the first things her mother noticed was that Gabriella not only closely examined every facet of her new surroundings, but stroked and even smelled inanimate objects. Without any experience of family life, she immediately took to eating her meals at the table with spoon and fork and sharing a bedroom with her brother. Before long, she graduated to sleeping alone in her own room.

Right after her arrival, she would cling inappropriately to any adult, but has since become more secure and independent. In those early days, she admonished a Romanian family friend—in English—"Don't speak Romanian, it's not nice." Symbolically, she took scissors to a photo her mother had snapped at the orphanage, carefully cutting herself out and chopping the rest into a hundred tiny pieces.

In a baseline occupational therapy assessment performed in April 1995, Gabriella's scores hardly registered, partly because of language barriers. The child was assessed again after starting first grade in 1995 and was found to have developmental delays. Participating in those assessments was Kay Dole, MS, OTR, NDT, director of neurodevelopment for the University of Minnesota's international adoption clinic. Since Gabriella's initial screening, Dole has advised her parents about her development, steered her toward the right school setting, consulted with her teachers, and continued to follow her progress. "It's important for adoptive parents to have access to appropriate resources, including OT," says Dole, who sees occupational therapy playing a vital role "in helping the child and family adjust to their lives, and in educating medical staff and teachers on the issue of post-institutionalized children."

Meet Gabriella: An OT Success Story

Gabriella attends third grade in a public school, 1 year behind her age level. She is the tallest child in her class. Except for participating in an English-as-a-second-language program, she receives no special services. She recently scored above average in reading, comprehension, and vocabulary, but has some difficulty with math, as well as with attending to task.

In a recent reevaluation, Dole found Gabriella falling within normal limits on the VMI (a test of motor abilities). Her fine motor skills, coordination, and handwriting showed no deficiencies. "She has made tremendous progress," Dole observes. Gabriella is certainly an OT success story. Says her mother, "Gabriella gets so much pleasure out of life, out of every facet, every little thing. We feel blessed."

Postscript: Gabriella is now 14 years old and plays the clarinet in church performances. She is an active Minnesota teenager in her adopted country.

Reprinted from Joe BE. Meet Gabriella: an OT success story. *OT Week*. 1998; 12(25): 11. ©1998 by the American Occupational Therapy Association, Inc. Reprinted with permission.

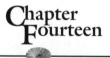

Jacob's Declaration of Independence

Donna Langmead, COTA

Four years too late is a long time, but "better late than never" is what Jacob's adoptive parents decided when they brought him home with them to Maryland from his native Russia. Jacob had been born with two very short arms so that he almost resembled a person with both arms amputated, and he needed a brace on one leg and a partial artificial limb for the other leg. No real medical care or rehabilitation services had been given to him in Russia for the first 4 years of his life. However, his ready smile, his verbal abilities (in Russian), and his obvious spirit of independence made it easy to overlook his physical challenges. His new parents had faith that the rehabilitation services available to Jacob in his new land would make quite a difference, but they were not prepared for just how much independence he would be able to achieve in the next 4 years of his life in America!

When Jacob began school, the initial sight of him automatically concerned the entire school staff. The first response from his classroom teacher was "he'll need a full-time, one-on-one assistant in the classroom with him at all times. He won't be able to do anything." Such assistants were available under the Federal law guaranteeing all children with disabilities the right to be educated in public schools with their peers, and many such students were glad to be given this opportunity to manage in the classroom. But not Jacob.

Jacob's Declaration of Independence

I am the public school system's certified occupational therapy assistant (COTA) who works at Jacob's school. When I met Jacob, I saw a very different child than the one who had made the rest of the school staff aprehensive; I saw a boy with great potential who did not see himself as different from any of his peers, a child with a wonderful spirit. He demonstrated that spirit in many ways. For example, on field day, Jacob would sign up for the 100-yard dash, not the 50-yard dash that would have been easier for him to complete. From the first day of school he was determined to be like any other child; to help him reach his goal, therefore, I started my 4-year-long project to adapt the school environment so that he could achieve the independence he wanted.

With Mom's help we adapted his clothing, starting with his pants. We worked on putting them on and taking them off, and with a lot of practice he did it. The school's bathroom needed adaptations, so I created a plastic wall urinal that he could lean into. Jacob's goal from the start was to be able to do everything by himself; he wanted to be just like all the other kids. As I continued adapting, he continued to master the challenges, one by one, the teachers put before us.

The teachers were still insistent that he needed a full-time, one-on-one assistant to be with him in the classroom. Jacob wanted none of that. I spent hours trying to educate the entire staff and trying to convince them that a one-on-one assistant would only create dependence, and that independence would be the key to Jacob's future.

With a slant board and a universal cuff to help him hold things for pencil-and-paper tasks and an adapted chair for proper positioning, we found Jacob to be quite the student. He began to learn letters, too, and soon he was writing words, then sentences in English. Adapted scissors took care of the cutting problems, the universal cuff worked for feeding, and Jacob just went on and on from there.

Meanwhile, after Jacob showed that he could participate in all of the regular school activities, I still had my work cut out for me in the special classes like music, art, media, and gym. With adaptations in these areas, Jacob continued to amaze the staff. I adapted the music room and showed the music teacher how he could play an instrument. I convinced the art teacher he could carry his own tray of paint and could create many masterpieces. I worked out a system in the library for retrieving and returning books. Even in physical education I could adapt equipment or modify the activity. Jacob was thrilled.

By first grade, Jacob, who had been riding to school in the special education transit bus, decided that he wanted to ride the regular school bus with his brothers; this became our next hurdle. The transportation company would not allow him to ride the bus without having his seatbelt buckled, especially because his short arms would not allow him to reach forward and stop himself from hitting his head on the seat in front of him if the bus stopped abruptly. No problem—I was confident that Jacob could learn to buckle and unbuckle a seatbelt. The seatbelt they insisted that he use, however, was more like a harness than a laptop belt. I was convinced that they had picked the hardest seat restraint to operate because they were sure that he would be unable to put that kind on independently, but that didn't stop us. After several weeks of practice, and a few adaptations, Jacob could put it on in 1½ minutes and take it off even more quickly, all by himself. He became a regular school bus rider. So far so good.

When Jacob was in first grade, I entered him in an international contest called "Yes I Can," sponsored by The Foundation for Exceptional Children. I told them how his spirit, his determination, and his drive to be independent and just be like any other child made working with Jacob both challenging and rewarding. Needless to say, he won! Jacob's mom received the letter saying that Jacob had won an award in the category of independent living skills. When she explained to him what that meant, she said, "You have leaned to do all sorts of things that are difficult for you but easier for other children, like going to the bathroom by yourself at school." Jacob was incredulous; he looked at his mom and said, "I didn't know they gave awards for going to the bathroom."

The local Lions Club and the American Legion sponsored his trip to Indianapolis to accept his award. Jacob, his mom, and I all flew to Indianapolis for the trip of a lifetime. Jacob won everyone's heart and demonstrated his total independence. Everyone from the Foundation marveled at his accomplishments. How exciting it was to see Jacob receive his award from the Kansas City Chiefs' defensive end, Neil Smith.

During first grade, the school staff still provided "access" to an assistant, but didn't require that the assistant be in class with Jacob full-time. This finally was a step closer to independence. I was feeling pretty good about all the areas I adapted and the education I was providing the teachers about occupational therapy and independence. But I found out that I still had some challenges ahead of me.

One day I walked into the classroom when the teacher asked the children to come to the front of the class and sit on the floor. The children took off and Jacob sat in his chair yelling, "Hey, wait for me, somebody get me out of this chair." I knew at that moment he was trapped at his desk. He was dependent on another student to push his chair out so he could get out from behind the desk, and he needed someone to push him in when he went back to sit down at the desk again. Obviously, his previously adapted chair needed some more modifications to provide Jacob with total independence. So this became our next project.

As I looked around the school environment, I realized that the heights of the desk and the table sizes varied. So the adapted chair I envisioned for

Jacob would not only need to move forward and backward (like a power wheelchair) but also up and down. A power chair was out of the question because Jacob was an independent walker and I was afraid of the stigma that a wheelchair would create for him. I started looking in catalogs and calling equipment companies. To my dismay, there was absolutely nothing commonly available on the market. Next, I contacted The Volunteers for Medical Engineering, a wonderful and creative group of Westinghouse volunteers, some who were current employees and some who were retired employees. A terrific engineer, Phil Atkinson, was able to put together my visions and his engineering skills and voila—the ideal chair was designed.

The Maryland Division of Rehabilitation Services has a program for adults with disabilities to learn a trade. It was there that I met George Stram, whose student had done a lot of the machine shop work for Jacob's original chair. Turning the engineering design into a finished chair was a true effort on the part of Phil, myself, George, Jacob, and the American Legion, who donated the money.

The chair was finally completed just before the Christmas holiday when Jacob was in second grade. The day the chair was delivered by Phil and George, I involved Jacob's classmates, teacher, and mom. It was a huge special event. The county newspaper came for pictures and did a story about our exciting project. The school system videotaped the event. This tape was later edited and narrated by Phil and me and shown on public access television.

The success of Jacob's chair was instrumental in establishing a partnership with The Volunteers for Medical Engineering and the school system. Now many other children can benefit from one-of-a-kind adaptive equipment that is not sold in stores and not available even through specialty adaptive equipment catalogs.

Then came third grade. The assistant who was once "full-time," then merely "accessible when needed," was now needed only to move Jacob's chair from one classroom to another. By fourth grade, I had convinced the staff that Jacob no longer needed an assistant at all. The teacher now moves the chair and Jacob knows he can come to me if he finds anything else with which he needs help.

From this experience I've gained many hugs and heart-warming smiles from Jacob and his family when I was able to adapt things so that Jacob was able to be like the other children. Jacob's mom, who always knew he could do anything he wanted to do, has told me many times how she appreciated my determination in educating the school staff to promote Jacob's being able to get along on his own. Fortunately, I also work in the middle school and the high school that Jacob will attend. This will allow me to continue to advocate for his independence and continue to make the adaptations needed to promote his success. I'm having great fun, and Jacob continues to thrive and to improve all the time.

Chapter Fourteen

Jacob has been truly responsible for opening the eyes of many people who have met him along the way. He showed them that a disability does not mean "I can't," but "I can" with the help of occupational therapy adaptations. The first half of his life, in Russia, and the second half of his life, here in America, have been very different. Jacob's journey from Russia to America has certainly showed all of us here what a "declaration of independence" from a determined little boy can mean.

Chapter Fifteen

Four Steps to Freedom

Leslie Rubman, MPH, OTR

This story is about a 7-year-old girl named Baila and her family. It is also about a three-story walk-up building in Brooklyn in which this large Hasidic family lives, and it is about arthrogryposis, a muscular condition that robbed Baila of her ability to walk.

I was Baila's third occupational therapist and started with her at a time when she was already gaining more mobility and autonomy. A soft-spoken child, fluent in both English and Yiddish, Baila was smart in her quiet and very determined way. Baila was always a bit shy, but was very accepting of these therapist strangers into her home and her life. Baila was one of six children at the time. Within the family, her disability was never an issue and was never discussed. Baila was always helped unconditionally when in need and was loved equally by her devoted parents and her siblings.

Going into a Hasidic home was a unique experience for me. Although I am Jewish, I lived a very different kind of Jewish life. I did not dress the same, eat the same, celebrate holidays in the same way Baila's family did. I was always fully accepted into this household, though, twice a week for 3 years, and then, when my therapist role ended, as a friend right up to the present.

Baila got around on her bottom, using her arms in extension to push and pull herself from place to place. After more therapy, she was able to come to an upright, standing position and eventually graduated to a walker, and then starting walking independently. During that time, she had a surgical procedure on her legs, a tendon transfer, followed by casts on both legs, which, in the end, helped her with mobility. The house had narrow hallways that turned out to be an asset because they gave Baila easy support when needed. Baila moved faster and faster and seemed to be enjoying her new ability to get around on her own.

Going outside, however, remained a problem. Baila needed to be carried up and down the stairs by someone. Her older sister was often her helper since her mother had younger children and groceries to get up the stairs. Oh, those steps! We all knew they were the only thing between Baila and the outdoors she loved so much. Baila adored being outside, and since walking took so much effort, she had learned to use a Big Wheel to cruise around the neighborhood. For her, this was indeed freedom.

For Baila to achieve a greater sense of independence and to ease the burden on her sister, Baila needed to conquer those three flights of stairs and make her way down without needing assistance. And what a formidable barrier they were—four sets, each with eight steps, covered in old linoleum, uneven in spots, and with wide spaces between each step. All of this terrified Baila.

I don't remember quite how, but one day I came up with the idea of building intermediary steps to place on each step to bridge the gaps. I enlisted my husband and together we built a series of those in the basement of his father's shop. We made four portable ones that could be moved from step to step, and I carted them off to Brooklyn the next week. I was very excited about trying to help Baila take her next step, literally! Baila was never comfortable showing how excited she felt, and clearly that day I appeared far more excited than she did about those steps.

We worked first on going up and eventually got to coming down. We tried all different positions, sitting, kneeling, and pivoting, going forward and backward and sideways. I could sense that Baila's fear was diminishing with each attempt, and her sense of challenge and determination was increasing. After a couple of months of diligent practice, Baila got the hang of the steps going up and down. We continued to practice together, and she practiced with her family when I wasn't there. It was working, and before another few months passed, the homemade steps were no longer needed. Baila was able to deal with the steps just as they were, independently, needing someone with her only as a safety precaution.

Those few little steps made a big difference in a young child's life and in the life of her family as well. I don't know what happened to those four wooden steps; I do know that I never had occasion to use them again. I also remember how amazed her parents were that such an idea could be thought of. Those of us in the field of occupational therapy know that a little bit of adaptation goes a long way. That wonderful family in Brooklyn now knew that to be true.

Baila is a teenager now. I know that she goes down those steps every day to the school bus by herself and has done so for the past few years. She probably continues to need help opening the two front doors, but then again, knowing Baila, she may have mastered that skill as well. She has gone to sleepaway camp and continues to be the smartest child in her classes.

The summer is over now and the children are back in school. The Jewish New Year will arrive in early October; and once again Baila and her family, and my family and I will celebrate in our different ways. My happy New Year call to Baila's mother will take place as it does every year, and we will catch up on the news and continue our friendship. We will reminisce about those steps, about how I climbed them so long ago to meet the family, and about how far Baila has been able to go since she learned to make it on her own down the steps and out the door.

Chapter Sixteen

John Goes on a Diet

Margaret D. Rerek,
MS, OTR/L (Retired)

John was 5½ when we met. He was entering kindergarten, and I was beginning my sixth year as a school-based occupational therapist and my third year in Queens, New York. John was and still is quite tall for his age and very thin. His physique was traceable not only to parental genes, but also to his marked hyperactivity. This hyperactivity was deemed disruptive enough to result in his placement into a class with other "learning disabled" kindergartners—children whose developmental lags in language, physical achievement, and behavior are serious enough to anticipate "handicapping" problems in regular kindergarten participation.

While in utero, John surely must have studied a diagnostic manual of psychological disorders, as he is a perfect textbook example of a child with attention deficit disorder with hyperactivity (ADHD), a condition that is characterized by the inability to focus attention and to keep still long enough to concentrate on tasks. He also apparently studied the chapter in occupational therapy pediatrics texts on sensory defensiveness, the behavioral responses some people make to certain seemingly harmless sensations as if the sensations were dangerous or painful. The most innocent environmental events—sounds, touches, smells, sights—completely distracted and disorganized John. He was constantly restless, sitting sideways in his chair, jumping up and running around, falling out of his chair, and totally melting down when sitting on the floor to watch and listen as the teacher sat in a chair reading stories. This told me that instead of clear and constant "messages" to and from his brain to tell him where his various body parts are (the proprioceptive system) and how to maintain his upright posture with respect to what he is looking at (the vestibular system), John's messages were confusing and inconsistent.

Once the sensory events that put a child on overload or shutdown have been identified, occupational therapy calls on a variety of activities to be scheduled to provide both calming and alerting experiences to all the senses to help the child feel safe and organized throughout the whole day. This activity program is called a "sensory diet." Initially, this approach should be intensive, involving the significant participation of family members and classroom personnel, so that it is consistent and constant in all of the child's interactions with his or her environment.

One of the elements of the diet that has been especially effective with many people with John's symptoms is "brushing," an intense massage done to the back and extremities with a surgical scrub brush. The brushing provides stimulation to deep nerves and muscles that is calming and organizing in its effects, and it is done in conjunction with other therapeutic activities and before regular task activities are begun. John needed to go on such a diet.

When I met with John's mother to discuss with her my recommendations for John's sensory diet, I learned how different the real world can be from occupational therapy theory. Her major concern about John's behavior and symptoms was that John, unlike her baby girl, resisted being touched by any-one, even his mother. He screamed and pulled away whenever she tried to give him a kiss or a hug, or even to take his hand. This disturbing behavior and the feelings it created within her was the most difficult for this loving mother to handle. However, I realized from her gaunt appearance, highly anxious manner, and new baby that it would be both useless and cruel to even suggest her intensive involvement at home in John's therapy. Without asking her, I silently decided that this would have to be one of those com-promises school-based occupational therapists must constantly make when neither home nor classroom can be part of the treatment environment.

Obviously, it is crucial to let parents know exactly what the therapeutic plan will involve. So, in addition to explaining some of the other OT activ-ities I would be doing with John, and because the brushing activity can be misleading, I simply showed her the brush and explained how and where I would and would not brush John, just to help her understand if John came home from school one day saying, "Ms. Peggy put her hand up my shirt."

John and I had a great year with one another. I brushed; he bounced, slid around the floor on a scooter board, did puzzles (at which he is great), and together we tried various activities to establish useful pencil-and-scissors skills (at which he was not so good). Through it all, John and I enjoyed each other and our time together. There were no complaints from home. However, neither his teachers nor I noted any significant reduction in those almost constant signs of his sensory defensiveness. We felt discouraged.

That's when John's mother, whom I had earlier pretty much thought I had to write off, showed herself to be more observant and perceptive than all of us professionals. Or maybe she knew best what was really important.

It was kindergarten graduation day, and of course I attended the ceremony and reception afterward. Suddenly, John's mom came running up to me, shouting, "What did you do to my son?" My heart sank, and then began to pound from wherever it landed near the floor. This is the moment that school personnel dread—a parent who has perhaps misunderstood something that went on at school and then accuses you of the worst! I felt faint, and tried to recall the name and telephone number of my malpractice insurance agent. I was sure it was the brushing that had her so upset.

I was so concerned that I had to shake my head hard to make sure I heard correctly what she said next, with the biggest smile on her face I had ever seen: "It's a miracle! It's so wonderful! John lets me touch him now."

Chapter Seventeen

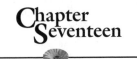

Snazzy Gets Her Driver's License
Janet Christhilf O'Flynn, OTR/L, BCP

Sister Joanna, from a Canadian convent, was the first certified occupational therapist I met. I was a greenhorn American volunteer in the Missionaries of Charity Orphanage in Lima, Peru, teaching a small preschool class every morning to the children who were able to walk and run down to the classroom. A handful of children, however, never left their beds because their cerebral palsy made them unable to sit up in a chair. That is until one Monday when I came in to find a short row of wooden chairs with seatbelts and trays and that handful of bed-bound children sitting in them. For the first time they were involved in the greetings, jokes, antics, and mischief of the preschool gang. Adults who entered the dayroom said, with surprise, "Look at all the new kids! Hello'." Or actually, "Hola! Que tal?!" Sister Joanna had measured each child and had a local carpenter build the chairs. It was a dramatic change for the children, and all the good that came for them (socializing, communicating, and strengthening) seemed an ongoing, quiet miracle.

Thanks to Sister Joanna, I entered occupational therapy school upon my return to the United States, and I have had many years of pediatric experiences and great stories since then. But one story in particular deserves to be told because it reminds me of that remarkable day in Peru. It's the story of Snazzy.

Chapter Seventeen

Snazzy was born with brittle-bone syndrome (osteogenesis imperfecta) of the most severe type. She had multiple fractures from the delivery process. When her foster parents took her home from the hospital, they were told she would not live beyond 3 months. She was placed on a water bed mattress and given excellent care, and little by little began to call on her inner strength and prove the doctors wrong. She did not grow, however, or only infinitesimally.

When I met Snazzy she was about to turn 3 years old. I was an occupational therapist for the public school system. The therapist she had in infancy taught me how to hold her safely, but it was many months before I had the confidence to lift her. She was very wary of strangers, and she spoke to me only rarely, in tiny whispered words. She was the size of an infant. It was clear, though, by her alert eyes and her comical expressions, that she had a sense of humor. One of the first responses she made to me was to imitate my raising and lowering my eyebrows quickly, à la Groucho Marx. Therapy time was spent in noncontact interactions designed to tempt her to lift her arms and reach with her hands for streamers, bubbles, or balloons, and with moving her feet and legs using dance music. Feeding time was difficult for her and the family: her position flat on her back made it hard for her to swallow soft food properly. Most of her nutrition was via liquids in a baby bottle.

Snazzy's first upright positioning came not from a small wooden chair like those designed by Sister Joanna, but from a vacuum mold, body conforming, bean-bag type of seat made by the children's hospital. It didn't last too long before it developed an air leak and slowly lost its shape, but in that short time it opened up possibilities. Snazzy could see pictures and letters right-side up, she could keep soft food in her mouth when fed, and the other foster children in the house could talk with her face to face.

When Snazzy was old enough to start kindergarten, at age 5 or 6, her family and the school took the brave step (and, as it turned out, the right step) to bring her to school. Snazzy was not much bigger than she had been when I had first seen her. Staff members came out to the house first to meet her. The teacher and a teaching assistant received supervised practice in lifting her to place her on a changing table for a diaper change (in a private bathroom) during the day. With much patience, a wheelchair was designed for her at the children's hospital, with a molded seat (using an improved technique). Her family (by now she was fully adopted) found a baby bottle that looked like a soda can, although with a nipple on top. The principal walked through Snazzy's daily path at school to be sure the chair could have a smooth ride. Then, with all those preparations completed, the wheelchair van came for her one September morning, just as it came for the other foster children in the house.

Once Snazzy was at school, her naturally gregarious personality began to shine. She knew the names of all her classmates and teachers within the first week. She loved music class and began to want her voice to be a bit more audible. It didn't seem hard to imagine that she could be eating by herself, drinking from a straw, and using the toilet for her bathroom needs. Each step of that process was unique to Snazzy. A friend of mine who does metal work in his basement made a bracket that held a curved-edge scooper bowl. With the bowl clamped sideways onto the edge of a table or desk, Snazzy could get close enough to reach it with her spoon. With a long-handled tiny spoon bent in two places, she could swing the spoon into and out of the bowl to feed herself. She could suck from a straw, but it was not until the teaching assistant found a cup that had a built-in straw and very narrow handle that she could hold it herself and drink. It took an adapted bedpan, combined with an infant car seat insert placed on the changing table, for Snazzy to achieve a good position for toileting. Once she was secure, she achieved consistent success in staying dry within a few weeks. Snazzy's teacher walked her through the process, using stickers of her favorite character, Barney (at which she would now blush!), and her own kind, matter-of-fact style to accomplish the change. By the end of kindergarten, Snazzy was wearing big-kid pants to school, eating and drinking with her classmates, and learning to read and write. Snazzy used the eraser of a nonsharpened pencil to push the keys of a computer. Her ease of forming words increased when the school system obtained a tiny keyboard that required no pressure to activate, as it worked by contact with a metal stylus. Snazzy turned out to be a committed, even dedicated, student, who never wanted to have a day off.

Snazzy had another good year in first grade, including attending a classmate's birthday party (which was accomplished by some ingenious planning on the part of the family). Her first grade teacher set up a metal music stand at Snazzy's place, and her work was positioned with magnets to allow her to see it at eye level. The next year, Snazzy's second grade teacher suggested a mirror be put over the teacher's desk at the front of the room to allow Snazzy to see the classroom and to know who was speaking. This was a great help in following the classroom discussions, and again I was reminded of that wonderful morning in Peru.

Unfortunately, during the second grade, Snazzy became short of breath. The doctor placed her on oxygen and prescribed home-bound education. Snazzy's occupational therapy continued at home, as did her school work and music therapy. She was taken off of her program of drinking and toileting and returned to use of a bottle and diapers, due to the increasing stress on her heart. Snazzy's tutor stayed in contact with the classroom teacher. Snazzy's friends (including teachers and the principal) visited from time to time, and Snazzy entertained a few "Ask Snazzy" advice letters from classmates.

(Question: "My little brother bothers me. What should I do?" "Answer: Just tell him, 'Scram.'")

Snazzy dictated her thoughts to her diary, with the help of the occupational therapist and tutor, and for the first time expressed the wish that she could grow to a bigger size and run.

Notwithstanding the second grade setbacks, there were more miracles to come. During the spring of Snazzy's third grade, the family and children's hospital decided she was mature enough to use a power wheelchair. After much fitting and trial use, she was placed in the power chair (with the oxygen tank strapped on her back) and given her license to drive. On the first day of this freedom, Snazzy motored into the largest open area at home—the kitchen. Looking around to be sure there were no children underfoot, she set the joystick to spin in place. "Joy" stick is no exaggeration—that was a new form of happiness!

At first, however, Snazzy was a bit of a menace. The front of the chair stuck out beyond the edge of Snazzy's feet and made it hard for her to see where to stop so that she wouldn't gouge out the corners of the door jambs when turning corners. I found two tall poles with pennants—bicycle flags! With these attached to the front corners of her wheelchair, her driving became much less violent. She did lose her license on two or three occasions for "traffic violations," but generally found success and a new measure of independence... as well as stamina and lung capacity.

When the summer drew to a close, the family asked the doctor for permission to let her go to school. And that's where Snazzy goes every day, the fourth grade. For 1 hour each day, Snazzy motors down the hall to her room, puts away her things, and learns with her old friends. Although I remained her "home therapist," her school therapist is Mary, my COTA friend. Mary visits the classroom regularly to position materials and to adapt the academic material so that Snazzy can participate in the same curriculum as her classmates. One day last week, Snazzy drew a picture in her journal to illustrate her story by using long, thin markers and reaching out to the paper, held on the music stand by magnets. She then held the book in one hand and motored up to the front to show and explain, in a very loud clear voice, exactly the point of the drawing. Then, driving responsibly, she brought the picture around to each desk to give her classmates a closer look. Did I mention that she is one of the most popular fourth graders in the school? Maybe it's the Groucho Marx trick with the eyebrows.

It is that sort of thing that makes me glad I met Sister Joanna so many years ago.

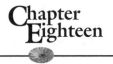

Silence Is Not Always Golden

Elizabeth J. Healey, OTR

He lifted his head as I spied those sparkling brown eyes and then he dropped to his knees, exuberantly but silently pushing the truck. I had not received any paperwork with directives to evaluate this lively new boy who was playing with the truck. He soundlessly moved among the other children and when I blocked his path, he quickly stopped, smiled up at me, but did not respond when I asked his name. With his happy demeanor he continued his truck pushing activity.

When I asked for information about him from his teacher she informed me that everyone thought that Keith's problems were related to his speech, or more precisely, his lack of it. She said there were no problems with his motor planning and that his fine motor skills were very age appropriate. Since these are the areas of expertise for me, the occupational therapist, she wasn't certain whether I would be involved with Keith at all. I asked, "Does he make any noises or vocalize at all?" She answered, "He sometimes cries when he is hurt or sick, according to his mom, but otherwise he is silent. I haven't heard any sounds as yet, but he does seem to understand."

She shared the reports concerning various testing done to rule out hearing or physical reasons for his mute behavior. Nothing significant was found. Neither family history nor birth history contained any reasons or prior causes to explain his lack of sound or speech. Indeed, his older sister was known to head up the seventh grade cheerleaders with her very apt vocal ability.

Flashing lights, bells, and whistles went off in my head as I thought of the research about sensory integration. I had just finished occupational therapy school the previous year and those books, chapters, and references were fresh in my mind. The vestibular system, the portion of the brain that controls our equilibrium or balance, was said to be connected, in ways that we don't quite understand, to the part of the brain that controls the making of sounds. Occupational therapists have found that stimulating the vestibular system by repetitive motion can have the side benefit of helping with speech problems. One of the best repetitive motion activities used for this purpose is swinging, particularly swinging done in the prone position, while lying on the stomach. Such swinging often triggered the brain chemistry involved in our producing sound.

Maybe, just maybe, this was the missing ingredient in this child's development. Maybe a steady dose of this type of stimulation was the needed link? I proposed the idea to his teacher and got permission from his parents to begin a daily 10 to 15 minute swing session in the therapy room.

This was implemented primarily by the teacher's aide. Within a few weeks, Keith began making sounds while on the swing. We were astonished, as was he! The sounds increased daily and then the teacher and parents reported vocalizations both at home and in the classroom. This was the third week and progress increased daily as all of our excitement mounted. He began repeating single syllable words over the next few weeks. His progress was slow but steady, and each day we witnessed this miracle of his speech unfurl. We gradually lessened the daily swing sessions and tapered them off toward the end of the school year.

The speech therapist worked successfully with Keith as he made rapid gains over the next year. I had not seen him for almost a year, and one day I spied him playing ball with some kids after school outside my room. My heart soared as I heard Keith's boisterous yell to one of his friends, and I remembered back to that silent, little boy with the big brown eyes on the swing.

Working With
What We Have
Kathy Swoboda, COTA/L

"Your son has MELAS," said Dr. Bay. I had rushed to her office after receiving a call from her saying that my son's test results had come back. I'd been searching for several years for a reason for my 6 year old's poor health. Now I had an answer, although I had no idea what MELAS was.

"MELAS is mitochondrial encephalopathy with lactic acidosis and stroke," she explained. "It is a rare disease that causes extreme fatigue and eventual inability to keep all the body's organs functioning. The body simply does not produce enough energy to run itself." I was still absorbing all of this new information, so I was not prepared for what she said next. "MELAS is almost always fatal once symptoms occur."

"What are the symptoms?"

"Joey is already exhibiting lactic acidosis," she said gently. "There is a good chance that he will experience strokes, deafness, visual field loss, seizures, learning disabilities, and lack of energy."

When Dr. Bay told me that there is no treatment for this disease, I simply wouldn't accept that. I pressed her until she told me about an experimental drug protocol. Clinical trials for the drug were starting at the University of Florida in Gainesville. If Joey could get into the study, we would have to travel from Ohio to

Florida every 3 months. It would be worth all the trouble if the drug proved helpful.

We were delighted that Joey was accepted into the experimental program. On June 13, 1995, Joey and I made our first of many trips to Florida. A wonderful group of pilots made sure we got there, free of charge, on their "Angel Flights."

I had no idea what was involved in human drug clinical trials. We began the drug trial immediately and were given a 1-liter bottle of something—we had no idea if we had the sought-after drug or a placebo. I decided not to question what it was; I had to believe that Joey had caught a break and had the real drug.

On July 21, 1995, Joey woke up very ill. That evening, he had his first of many seizures. Seven days later, Joey had a stroke. Our family was devastated. The months that followed were a blur as our 6 year old's health deteriorated. We prayed, asking God to let Joey stay with us, but we knew we had to prepare to let him go.

Dr. Bay suggested that physical rehabilitation might be of some help to Joey. He couldn't tolerate the gross motor movements of physical therapy because they depleted his energy. Instead, we turned to occupational therapy, and we met a new angel, Linda Ankerman, Joey's occupational therapist. She began the tedious process of helping him recover from the effects of MELAS.

When I asked Linda what her treatment plan for Joey was, she simply responded, "We'll work with what he has."

I wasn't sure what that meant, but I soon found out. Joey had five strokes; virtually every part of his body was ravaged. Our physicians told us to accept the disease's process. Yet Linda never gave up. She was cautious about improvement, knowing his diagnosis, but she encouraged us when we became discouraged, saying, "We'll work with what we have."

Somehow, Joey made it through the drug trials. When the trial ended, we were given the opportunity to purchase the experimental medicine—now we could be sure that Joey had the actual drug.

Joey's condition slowly improved, and Linda continued to work with what he had. She never gave up, never looked at him as a kid with a terminal illness, and always worked with what we had.

Through many dark hours, Linda was a shining light. She never wavered from her treatment plan. Because of her, our little boy's broken body became well again. His wheelchair sat unused in our garage. Linda continued to work with him every week, improving on what he had—almost a whole body. We are so thankful to Linda for believing in Joey. She has been a special friend to Joey. If ever there was an angel on earth, it would be Linda.

And our story has one more twist: I am now studying to become an occupational therapist. I plan to always work with what my patients have, never giving up, always believing.

Louie Talks
With His Nose

Amy B. Westerman, OTR/L

For a kid who couldn't talk, Louie sure knew how to communicate. I first met him when he was 8 and living at a state school in Massachusetts. Louie had been sent there because he had a form of cerebral palsy that left him unable to control most of his muscles or make them function. We made for a good match—I was a young occupational therapist and was working at the school as part of my training, so we were both a little inexperienced.

At first, like any 8 year old might be, Louie was homesick and cried a lot. He came from a big family, but he only got to see them on weekends. As we worked together, however, Louie began to show a strong independent streak.

Louie had a big heart, and after a while, he and I became very close. He was a small kid, but he had a smile and big brown eyes that had captured my heart immediately. Although he couldn't talk, he quickly learned to connect with me using his eyes, his gestures, and an occupational therapy-produced communication board that he operated by touching letters and words with his nose. Soon, Louie was spending lots of time with me in the occupational therapy department, working hard to control his trunk muscles to help him maintain sitting and standing balance and to learn to control his hands and arms.

Chapter Twenty

As Louie learned to communicate, he told me that what he wanted most was to be independent. So, back to the occupational therapy drawing board we went. At first, the staff set what we considered to be small goals for Louie that would lead to more independent living, though we knew that these goals were not such small goals to Louie. After months of work by Louie—exercising his throat, mouth, and facial muscles; learning how to eat and drink with control and without choking—he was finally able to do something the rest of us take for granted. Score one for independence.

Louie wasn't satisfied just with eating and drinking, however. Soon, he communicated to me that he wanted to increase his ability to move about independently with his wheelchair. Another occupational therapy goal was established. Before we started, I told Louie that he might not be able to do this and not to be disappointed if he couldn't, but Louie told me he was determined to succeed. So again, we worked for months figuring out what motions he could use in order to achieve that mobility. We settled on practicing the only motion he could control, extending his leg, which allowed him to push himself backwards in his wheelchair, and he soon mastered the strange technique (maybe the first time that moving backward could be counted as progress!). Score two for independence. It was not the last time that Louie would prove me wrong.

Even with all his limitations, Louie was a happy boy who had the rare ability to connect with people and bring happiness into the lives of everyone he met. Typical of Louie's ability to communicate and to achieve big things was his grand scheme to introduce me to one of the recreation therapists at the school; Louie plotted for weeks and finally accomplished his goal! Score three for perceptiveness: this great guy and I have been married for over 21 years!

I have so many wonderful memories of Louie, but this is the one that stands out in my mind. At the wedding, I saved a special dance for Louie, and as I held him in my arms and we whirled around the dance floor, there wasn't a dry eye in the room.

Not bad for a kid who couldn't talk.

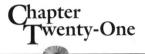

Chapter Twenty-One

Let Your Switch Do the Walking

Jan Johnson, OTR

When Trevor heads down the hall at school to work with the robot he is expectant. When he is behind the control switches operating the robot he is powerful. The power is precious because it has been earned. Trevor had to work hard to learn how to use the robot.

Hands are amazing parts of our bodies that give us control of our world. The infant begins by watching his or her hands. Then he begins to use them for a purpose: he holds an object such as a rattle, he moves it about in the air, he transfers it to his other hand, he puts it in his mouth, he picks it up, he drops it, he uses the rattle to explore yet another object: he hides the rattle in a box, he bangs it on his metal high chair tray, on the wooden floor, on the soft mattress of his bed. He uses his hands to experiment and discover what objects will do when put together, on top of each other, through and beside each other. He finds that round pegs fit best in round holes and square pegs in square holes. Several objects can form a new and different whole. The rings of many sizes become a stacked cone. The funny-shaped pieces of a puzzle become an image, a picture. The young child learns basic principles and awareness of the laws of physics by manipulating objects and through body movement. Exploration of the structure of his body and how that body works introduces him to basic anatomy and physiology.

But what of the child who is so bound inside his own body, because of a disability, that he cannot direct those most basic of hand movements. He cannot pick up and hold a block, a ball, a cookie. When he does manage to grasp an object to explore it more fully, he soon drops it involuntarily, or he squeezes it unmercifully tight in a hand that won't bend or twist to an angle to do something functional, like to put the cookie in his mouth. His most basic tools to act on his environment are his hands. Without the use of fully functioning hands his ability to work, learn, play, and take care of himself is so limited that he is dependent on others or, at best, must spend a great deal of energy and ingenuity adapting methods to perform the most basic of these activities.

Trevor is such a child. His hands do not function effectively. He cannot touch and explore his world. As his occupational therapist, I searched for a way to help Trevor experience the power and joy of manipulating something in his environment so that he would understand how things work, the principles of cause and effect, the excitement of controlling an object, and the thrill of mastering a part of his world. A device that used the concepts of a simple child's toy, but certainly did not look like one—a complex remote-control robot—would prove to be the way of unlocking all of these experiences, and more, for Trevor. The mechanical robot was the result of an elaborate research project aimed at helping children like Trevor learn to manipulate objects. The research team of engineers, computer programmers, psychologists, and occupational therapists had produced a "toy" with a computer monitor and a robotic arm attached to a work surface 3 feet wide by 5 feet long. The question was, "Can this 'toy' be useful to Trevor?" It was up to me to find out. But first, he had to learn to control it using the only tool he had—the ability to press a switch. It was a long, slow process.

"Trevor, look at the monitor."

"Which motor do you use to move the robot to the toy car?"

"Think, Trevor, show me on your communication board."

"Let the robot show you if that is the motor to use."

When Trevor first was introduced to the robot, he approached it with unfettered frenzy. He pressed switches aimlessly and constantly. There seemed to be no understanding of cause and effect. He liked watching the robot move, but was unable to command it to do a specific action.

"Knock over the toy duck, Trevor."

"On what color block is the duck sitting?"

"Look at the monitor, Trevor. Move to the blue square."

"Which switch do you use?"

And then, "You use this switch."

"Good, Trevor, you made the robot go to the blue square."

So much help he needed. To be successful he required each press of a switch to be guided so that only successes would result.

"Which color, Trevor?"

Trevor looked to me for direction... all right! He was wanting to make the correct move! We were on our way! Now the hints could be less direct.

"What color is the animal on? Move to that color." I waited to see if Trevor chose that color.

"Let the robot tell you if that is the right choice." Trevor activated the go button, and the robot swung to the position he selected.

"Is that where you wanted to go?" He shook his head no.

"What color do you want to choose?" He selected the correct color position on the menu shown on the monitor screen and looked to me for feedback.

"Let the robot tell you; make it go."

Yes! He selected the right position and the robot went where he, Trevor, directed it to go. He watched it incredulously and turned to me again for approval. My huge grin told him what he needed to know.

This process continued throughout the activity, and the next, and the next. He gradually learned how the specific motors of the robot moved. At first, I gave him enough hints to ensure success. Then Trevor had to learn how to use the robot without me. He needed to let the robot give the feedback, letting Trevor see if the robot went where he wanted it to go. All the while I needed to guide the selection just enough so he didn't mislearn an action.

It was like a dance, with me leading, Trevor following at first. It was so smooth; I almost didn't notice when the lead changed in mid-dance. He gave me direction, I gave him a hint. He took my cue, I caught his hesitation and gave another. Back and forth we went. Gradually the robot became the music. Trevor was responding to the robot! I was a partner, but he could move on his own. He was moving to the music of the robot. He was becoming at one with it. He was changing partners. The robot was his partner of choice. I was spending more time as a wallflower.

This was what we wanted, wasn't it? Trevor was using the robot to hold, pick up, move, and place objects, things that he was unable to do with his hands. He was learning to think, to sequence his movements, to judge the results, and to direct a moving object!

Today's activity is to rearrange the letters in his name that have been placed randomly on the work surface and correctly spell his name. One by one Trevor selects, picks up, and places a letter card in a row. When the final "R" is placed at the end of the row, he and I give a whoop, raising our arms in the air in exhaustion and the thrill of victory. Trevor is as big a winner as any Olympic champion.

Chapter Twenty-One

So why am I tired? Perhaps it is because occupational therapists are so used to doing "hands on" therapy that it is tough for me to keep my hands off so that Trevor's switch can do the walking that his own hands can't do.

Chapter Twenty-Two

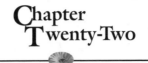

A Penny Saves the Day

Rhona Feldt-Stein,
BSc OT, OT Reg (Ont)

The crowd went wild when they saw who was accompanying Michael onto the court. With Penny's help, he stood tall, basketball in hand, with his eyes firmly fixed on the basket. What happened next was a miracle of cooperation between two arms, two heads, six legs, and a tail! Even without a uniform, Penny was a shoo-in for MV(C)P—Most Valuable (Canine) Player of the game!

Penny was 65 pounds of copper and white shaggy fur surrounding a Collie, a jewel in a rough untamed coat with a happy and playful disposition. Her brown eyes seemed to hold the wisdom and insight of an old woman with years of experience and kindness. She always seemed to have a sense of when to be exuberant and when to hold back. It was as though she could read the minds of those around her. Who could predict that these were the perfect credentials for becoming a four-legged occupational therapist!

Adopted by us as a tiny puppy, Penny went on to become a caring and gentle family member. She enjoyed outings to friends' homes, to parks with my children, and especially to the place in which I work as an occupational therapist and owner/director of a children's therapy clinic. She didn't even mind the two cats who live and work there. To Penny, they were just two more things for her to keep track of, something she liked to do with her herding instinct. She was also a patient learner during the obedience training classes we attended, always forgiving me for confusing her with mixed instructions and hand signals. I often wondered who was getting the most training. She especially enjoyed and was particularly gentle with the children who came to the clinic for therapy, and they in turn loved her companionship.

In addition to my clinic practice, I am also a consultant to a local district school board, helping children who have special needs meet their educational goals. One class contained children from grades one through three. The class had seven children, with three educational assistants and Mrs. Ritchie, their teacher.

Evan, Kyle, and Melissa were children with cerebral palsy. Evan, age 7, with his brown straight hair and eyes fringed by long dark lashes and keen sense of humor, and Kyle, age 7, with his blonde hair, blue eyes, and the determination of a mountain goat, were wheelchair users because of their inability to walk. Melissa, a petite young lady of 8, with a mass of brown shoulder-length curls and blue eyes, could walk independently but had a rather unstable gait so she was in danger of falling. These three children also had problems in their arm movements. Joe, a withdrawn young boy who looked older than his 8 years, with hair the color of coal and dark brown eyes that had the expression of a searching soul, had a traumatic brain injury causing both visual and hearing impairments and partial paralysis of his left side. Jason and Denise, both age 8, while being the most physically able students of the class, were unable to functionally communicate because developmental disabilities delayed their cognitive development, and autistic tendencies made it hard for them to relate well to others. These two could almost pass as brother and sister with their gangly builds, sandy brown hair, and green eyes, which unfortunately were only able to make fleeting contact with others. Last was Michael, 8 years old, with spina bifida, which caused his legs to be without feeling and made him unable to bear any weight on them. He was the most boisterous child of the group. There was nothing Michael wouldn't try or do to make others aware of him.

One day while I was with them, Mrs. Ritchie was talking about animals and how they help people and the environment. The discussion led to how animals provide food, clothing, medicine, and so on. The children in their own special ways communicated about their own pets and how they saw their own pets contributing to their lives. Melissa asked if they could have a classroom pet. The teacher discussed all the merits of having a class pet but also the responsibilities of its care, where it would stay on weekends, holidays, etc. It was clear to all that having a "live-in" class pet would not be possible. Nonetheless, she asked the children to think of how an animal in the class could benefit their learning.

Kyle wiggled enthusiastically in his wheelchair using all of his physical effort to raise his spastic uncontrolled arm in the air. In his halting voice, Kyle suggested that an animal that visited the class could help them with their chores and be a friend. The teacher explained that the visiting animal could be a "mascot," doing many of the things Kyle described. The children were elated. Evan and Melissa were quick to contribute their ideas how to use the mascot. Joe, Jason, and Denise either "signed" their thoughts or used picture boards or mechanical talking devices to give their suggestions. Michael seemed the most excited of all, but indicated merely that he could think of a "secret use" for a mascot. I had never in my 3 years of coming into this class-room seen such enthusiasm and excitement or so much voluntary physical activity.

I suggested to the class that a mascot did not have to be in the class all the time, but could be like a volunteer who comes in on a regular basis, helps them out, and can also be with them for special events. The children loved the idea, and the teacher asked that the children either draw, write, or tell one of the classroom assistants what kind of animal they would like as their mascot.

On my return visit to the class the next week, the students were excited to tell me they had decided that a dog would be the perfect mascot. What they could not decide was whose dog it should be. Naturally everyone want-ed to have his or her dog be the "chosen one." Mrs. Ritchie, in her wonder-ful wisdom, suggested that it be a dog from outside the classroom, so no one would be hurt if his or her dog wasn't chosen. I immediately thought of Penny. She had shown herself to be a very gentle dog with my own children and loved herding them away from the street when she felt they got too close. She enjoyed being with other children and animals at the park, and she was excellent with the children in her regular visits to the OT clinic. I described Penny to the class and teacher. They were very enthusiastic, and we immedi-ately arranged an introductory visit.

Penny sauntered into the classroom the next week like a large bear with a distinct waddle, her long fur swaying with every movement. She sat waiting at the door as if anticipating their response, looking around at the wide-eyed gazes that confronted her. The children were restless and wriggled with excitement. Upon the teacher's signal, Penny wandered unleashed over to her desk and sat waiting for some directions. Under my instructions, as if to introduce herself, Penny approached each child and either put her face into the lap of every child strapped into a wheelchair or gave a paw to those wait-ing patiently at their desks. Everyone eagerly wanted to give her a piece of cheese or biscuit. Tremulous hands, fisted grasps, or open laps were the providers of snacks that day. The classroom finally had a mascot, and her name was Penny.

Our regular Tuesday visits every second week were highlights for the class. Other children in the school decided they, too, wanted a mascot. Mrs. Ritchie's class however, retained its "special" title, as they were the only ones to have a living mascot. The children were always thinking of things for Penny to do. Evan asked if Penny could help him with his walking exercises. He thought that if he could hold onto Penny when she walked, it would help him with his balance. Penny stood patiently while Evan slid out of his wheelchair and took hold of the long fur on her back. As he took a step, Penny gingerly took a step and waited as Evan regained his posture and balance. The two of them lumbered down the hallway until Evan stopped and exclaimed, "She's the best therapist I've ever had!"

Reading also became a great group activity with Penny. She would lie down in the middle of the classroom, and a few of the children who had poor sitting balance would lie down, resting their heads on her firm shaggy body. The children thought this was the best way to read or listen to a book. Penny didn't seem to mind either.

For some of the children, Joe and Denise in particular, who had been rather afraid of having such a beast enter their classroom, Penny's visits were an education in respect and tolerance. For Joe and Denise, the sensation of touching Penny's fur was especially fearful. Their hypersensitivity to touch had already made it difficult for them to tolerate many of the sensory activities often used within the classroom program. To help Joe and Denise, the assistants and I would first use a special brush to firmly brush Joe's and Denise's arms and hands. This helped to desensitize their skin to the initial light touch of the fur. At first, we had Penny sit near the children and we had their hands push down on the fur with hand-over-hand assistance. Penny sat patiently, seeming to know that this was all that was required of her. Gradually, as the weeks went on, simple and firm patting replaced the pushing, until after a few months, both children were able to touch Penny's head and back on their own. Denise in particular was actually going over to Penny on her own and would stroke Penny's back and then jump up and down clapping her hands, smiling from ear to ear about her accomplishment.

Penny also became special to the other children in the school. She would accompany "Mrs. Ritchie's children" (as they were often known) outside at recess, always unleashed but faithfully by their side. These often forgotten children were suddenly everyone's best friends because of "their mascot." Penny's presence with them seemed to encourage the other children to see her charges in a new light, without their wheels and restrictions. Suddenly, these "special children" had something truly special and were the envy of all the rest.

For all of the children, having Penny visiting the classroom was a new experience in being attentive and sensitive to another creature besides themselves. Most of the children had always had things done for them or to them. Now, they were responsible for something else. Suddenly, they had to think of how they could help Penny or respond appropriately to the needs of another living being.

One day, Michael hesitatingly revealed his "secret idea" about how to use Penny. He suggested that Penny could help him during gym class when they played basketball. Michael was integrated into another grade three class for his physical education program. Up until now, he had been relegated to being the referee during basketball, as he could not reach the fixed height of the basketball hoop from his wheelchair. Michael desperately wanted to play basketball himself. Michael thought that if we placed him in his standing frame, which had wheels, he could get Penny to pull him down the court and he could then take shots at the basket.

There were weeks of practice, with special ropes and a leash tying Penny to Michael's standing frame, and Penny's pulling him around the gym with lots of encouragement. Finally, the last day of the season came. During gym class, as prearranged with the teacher, the whistle blew and in came Penny, with Michael in tow, for the free throw. The other children watching the game stood with their mouths open, looking from one to another in bewilderment.

Penny was positioned with Michael standing just in front of the basket. Michael took two shots and missed. Penny sat like a statue. With the third shot, Michael made the dunk and the class went wild. Penny barked and jumped with enthusiasm, almost pulling Michael into the bleachers!

The lessons that Penny taught the class and the teaching staff could not have been learned by the children in a more caring and understanding manner. She asked for nothing, yet gave and got so much in return. The children, on the other hand, got even more than they bargained for. They not only got a mascot, but the experience of love and devotion from a patient friend. Michael will never forget the thrill of making that basket during that special game when Penny saved the day.

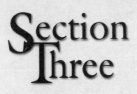

Section Three

Teens

Avoiding Hazards on the Path

Avoiding Hazards on the Path

Here are stories of nine pre-teens and teenagers who deal with the ordinary changes of the tumultuous teen years while growing up with disabilities or dealing with sudden accidents or illnesses that make coping especially difficult.

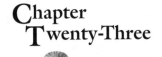

Steven's Box

Ronda Christopher, OTR/L, MEd,
LNHA and
Rebecca Rogers, MEd, OTR/L

The sight of Steven with a hammer in his hand meant only one thing to the hospital staff in the adolescent psychiatric unit: Duck before a flying hammer found its mark in your head! Everyone agreed, Steven was hopeless, an out-of-control and aggressive teenager who could never be trusted with anything, especially not with such an attractive potential weapon.

Here we were, two occupational therapy students just out of school, on our first day of our full-time fieldwork internship in a long-term center for psychologically challenged children. To make matters even more daunting, we were going to be the first full-time occupational therapists with which the staff had ever worked, so we felt some pressure to do a great job. During our orientation and training and throughout our first week, just about every staff member, from maintenance workers to resident assistants, warned us about Steven.

By all accounts, Steven was a cunning, angry, and extremely aggressive young man who had managed to have himself removed from the last 2 weeks of his public school due to his violent behavior toward classmates and staff. We were told that he would be our biggest challenge, and that he was not capable of the emotion remorse, so beware! We were already afraid of Steven, and we hadn't even met him yet.

Chapter Twenty-Three

We were told that Steven would bite, kick, and scream at staff. He would become so provoked at times that he would throw anything he could get his hands on toward staff or a resident's head, and he would readily admit to wanting to cause them harm. His deprived background and terrible social history could make an unbelievable Hollywood storyline. He had been living at the center for more than 6 months, and there was little hope of foster care placement or a family reunion with his mother. Steven's future looked grim, and ours, having to eventually deal with him in occupational therapy, looked scary.

We knew that the day would soon come to meet Steven and begin his OT treatment. We were armed with our occupational therapy theories about the positive power of purposeful activities—things that have personal meaning for each person—and the potential good results obtained by creating a sense of mastery and competence for people. This seemed like the perfect situation to test those theories and hope that they were correct! We decided that the best way to survive this experience would be to try to get Steven to pick for himself various craft projects that he wanted to do.

Using this approach, we began by offering Steven the chance to do projects he liked and considered important. We found to our delight that, in fact, Steven was a textbook example of how purposeful activity can truly bring out the best in any person. When he attended our daily craft groups, he was methodical and committed to completing projects. He showed signs of creativity and an understanding of how to execute and complete a project. Then, the moment came when we saw an unbelievable human example of all that we read about in OT school. Steven showed us just how true were those theories about the use of meaningful purposeful activities and the use of occupation for the achievement of potential. Here's how it happened.

During our last 2 weeks, we asked Steven to plan a project he would like to make, anything he wanted, within reason. He chose a wooden box. He made blueprint drawings on paper of several designs, and when he chose one, we supplied the necessary equipment to begin. He needed four pieces of wood, sandpaper, a handle, stain, and what to others was considered unthinkable—nails and a hammer. If we had told anyone on the staff that we were about to put nails and a hammer in Steven's hands, they would have told us we were crazy and that we could not do it. So we took a chance and didn't say anything to anyone.

The day was sunny with a nice breeze. Steven took his supplies outside on a picnic table and began what was the most beautiful OT moment of our lives. With a passion that came from deep within him, Steven started sanding and hammering and building his box. At one point, Steven found that the hammer was too small. On any other day, Steven would probably have angrily demanded another one, while quite possibly heaving the too-small one at the head of the nearest person. On this day, while engrossed in his project, Steven simply asked for another larger one.

Several staff members passed Steven while he worked. They were all amazed at his determination and apparent desire to complete his box. The best testament to what we were seeing came from our biggest critic, the director of resident assistants, who said, "It's about time we gave him something to put together." Steven hammered his heart out, and when he was done, he had produced a perfect 2-foot square box that he displayed with pride.

The summer of 1996 seems very long ago, but the vision of Steven hammering and creating his box is as present in our minds today as it was then. Steven's ability to control his aggression and pour his energies into creating something with the hammer rather than using it as a weapon was a milestone for him and for the staff, who still marvel at what can be accomplished when the activity is meaningful to the person. It certainly showed us that like Steven's hammer, those occupational therapy theories have really "hit the nail on the head!"

Chapter
Twenty-Four

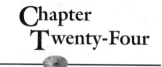

Struggling
to Get By

Joshua M. Eisenstein, MA, BS

As a child, school was always difficult for me. It seemed to take me forever to finish my work. While other kids had already left for recess, I would still be writing. For a child with a learning disability, that's just the way things are in a mainstream classroom. No matter how smart you may be, school is one big frustration.

This went on with me for many years, even after I was diagnosed with dysgraphia, extreme difficulty in writing, accompanied by a perceptual impairment that affected my eye-hand coordination. To compensate for my problems, I devised all kinds of strategies.

I did massive amounts of work in my head to avoid having to write. I started tests while the other students were still listening to the teacher's instructions. I invented rhymes and alliterations to help me stay focused on my homework. I struggled terribly, but because I "got by," my schools would not give me any special education services. You see, there is an ironic twist to the law about guaranteeing all children the opportunity to get the help they need to succeed in school, which works to the disadvantage of the most intelligent students with learning disabilities. The law doesn't offer learning-disabled students special help if they are able to pass most of their classes and can read at a grade level within 2 years of the norm. Because of this, a learning-disabled student's intelligence, creativity, and excruciating efforts are often rewarded with inevitable failure.

Consider what my sixth-grade guidance counselor said: "He's pretty smart, but he daydreams too much, and he's lazy about assignments. Maybe he should switch to a lower grade level, where the workload won't be so tough." This is a typical reaction that teachers and administrators often have to children with learning disabilities. Because we don't use hearing aids or canes or have a physical deformity, students with learning disabilities appear to be normal. The schools, rather than doing what's best for these struggling students, often try to get by with doing what's easiest for themselves and their staff by denying that there is a special need. Parents and children, too, sometimes deny that there is a special need. They deny that there is a problem because it is hard for them to admit that the child may have a disability. After all, who wants to be "abnormal"?

Luckily for me, my parents didn't rely on the schools to help me. Instead, they insisted that I stay at the appropriate grade level for my age, and they decided to hire an occupational therapist to help me combat the difficulties presented by my disability.

Dr. Lila Silverman, an occupational therapist and specialist in learning disabilities, came to work with me at our house. In me, she saw a highly intelligent pre-teen with low self-efficacy, inadequate people skills, and monumental difficulties in writing and processing information. But before we even sat down at the dining room table for our first session, I was already resisting help. I was depressed about my troubles in school and my difficulties in socializing with other children. All I wanted to do was watch television.

When Lila finally convinced me to join her, she reached into her bag and pulled out a blue box. Inside was Boggle, a game that I'd played before with my friends. Boggle consists of a plastic box containing 16 cubes. On each side of each cube is a letter. Players shake the box until each cube has settled in one of 16 available slots. The goal is to form as many words as possible in a limited time using the letters facing up in the slots. Learning to write quickly and correctly is the key to getting a high score.

This game became very important to me in the following weeks. Lila observed the way I wrote while we played and gave me encouragement and helpful suggestions. Her input was so subtle that I barely noticed I was being tutored. When I sometimes became frustrated, Lila always kept me on task and reinforced appropriate social responses.

Lila had her work cut out for her, and helping me was not all fun and games. I was a troubled child, as many children with learning disabilities are. Having a disability can be very difficult emotionally. But all of us, regardless of our limitations, have to learn how to act appropriately. Lila modeled the kind of behavior she expected of me, and she made her expectations clear: I was responsible for acting in a way that fit my situation. I had to listen, pay attention, speak politely, and stay focused. When I fulfilled these responsibilities, she smiled and spoke warmly. When I did not act appropriately, she withdrew her support and stopped playing games with me. Regardless, she was always upbeat and positive.

Throughout, she believed in my ability to do well in school, and she helped me develop the skills necessary to achieve this. My writing and vocabulary slowly improved, as did my temper and my enjoyment. Lila also helped me with my organizational skills, using strategies like daily and monthly calendars, color-coded subject folders, and regularly emptying and organizing my notebooks. Our family had a personal computer, and Lila encouraged me to type my assignments instead of writing them by hand.

Meanwhile, my mother, a university professor of special education, educated my teachers and counselors so they would better understand my situation; Lila encouraged me to be open about my disability instead of embarrassed by it. By our last session, I was beginning to have positive academic experiences. By the time I reached the 10th grade, my mother had convinced the school system to finally classify my disability and give me the accommodations I needed to succeed.

What Lila did with me really worked! I have almost completed my doctorate in educational psychology and hold a fellowship to conduct cross-national research on attitudes toward corporal punishment of children. I am currently working at Temple University in Philadelphia, teaching and practicing clinical school psychology. To accomplish this, I earned my bachelor's and master's degrees in educational psychology at New York University, where I graduated cum laude.

I still write much more slowly than the average person, but my script is readable and I have the skills I need to accomplish my life goals. Without Lila to help with my writing, who knows where I'd be? I know that some people believe that regular occupational therapy for students with learning disabilities is expensive and doesn't make a difference. But for me, it made all the difference in the world. Looking back now, I cannot imagine what my life would have been like without Lila. Just thinking about how I might have been left behind to fend for myself boggles my mind!

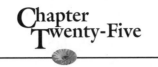

Chapter Twenty-Five

Can You Stick Out Your Tongue?

Anitta Boyko Fox, BS, MA, OTR

"You're the therapist?!" That was the question that greeted me when I walked into the room of my newest patient, a teenage girl who'd always wanted to be a dancer, but whose major achievement now was that she had survived polio. The year was 1952. Both her parents and grandparents had come to her first occupational therapy session.

"We expected a man," her parents stated in unison.

"A man," agreed her grandparents.

The bombardment began: "Can you handle this case? What's your background? What kind of training do you have?"

I patiently recited my education and experience for them: a bachelor's degree in occupational therapy from New York University; a master's degree in vocational guidance and rehabilitation, with a major in psychology; certification with the American Occupational Therapy Association; and certification in rehabilitation of the severely handicapped and homebound. I explained that Karen's physician had asked me to take her case because of my diverse background. I may have bolstered their confidence in me, but from their next question, it was clear the family had no confidence in Karen. "What can you do for Karen? She can't do anything," her father said.

Chapter Twenty-Five

"Nothing," came the agreement all around, followed by a long recitation of all the things that Karen couldn't do. Karen sat in her wheelchair, quietly sobbing into her hands.

I waited for her family to finish, then I turned to my patient. "Karen," I said, "I am really more interested in the things you can do. Please tell me what they are."

"Nothing, nothing, can't you see?" she wailed. "I'd like to die, right now!"

I had seen similar despair in patients before. I knew it was up to me to prove to Karen she was wrong. There were many things she was capable of doing. "You can certainly speak," I pointed out. Her crying began to subside. "Can you blink your eyes?"

"Of course," she said.

"Can you open and close your mouth?" I continued. "Can you stick out your tongue?"

"Yes," she said, trying to hide a smile.

"You can smile! That's wonderful! Can you blow your nose?" I handed her a tissue. "Can you eat by yourself? Hold a cup? Brush your teeth? Button a blouse? Shake my hand?" We soon had a long list of all the things Karen could do. "And I'm sure there are many more," I said. "Now, let me ask you an important question: What is the one thing you would most like to do that you can't do right now?"

We had the attention of the entire family. Karen hesitated, and her face flushed. "If only... if only I could get to the bathroom by myself! Do you think... maybe?" she finished with a whisper.

It had been easier than I'd anticipated. Karen had chosen a goal! She seemed motivated. Now, my challenge would be to help her reach that goal. "Okay, young lady," I said. "If that is what you want, we have a lot of work to do. And we'll need your mom, dad, grandma, and grandpa to help."

We drew up a list of activities that Karen would have to master to achieve her goal: Learning to put on her underwear and leg braces while in bed. Learning to safely use a "transfer board," a special device for sliding from bed to wheelchair. Our biggest obstacle seemed to be how to enter the bathroom from the wheelchair (these were the days before the Americans with Disabilities Act, when most public restrooms—and certainly private homes—did not have wide doorways or wheelchair-accessible stalls with handrails). However, we did have two important allies: time and Karen's increasing motivation, both of which would be instrumental in the recovery of muscle strength and skill in managing her body and activities of daily living.

Meanwhile, Karen developed an interest in planning meals appropriate for herself and her family to keep everyone's waistline under control. She took over some of the kitchen responsibilities. She began to take care of her clothes and take pride in her appearance. Her attitude, as well as those of her family members, became more positive. Her family learned to lend a helping hand only when asked, and they were calmer and more confident in Karen's abilities. Everyone believed that Karen would achieve her goal.

This was incredibly encouraging to her. As the weeks went by, she continued to progress noticeably and became more daring. After 1 year of rehabilitation, Karen wanted to walk. Her arms had gained strength, her general physical condition had improved considerably, and, most importantly, she wanted to try.

At her first walking session, though, she refused to use crutches. She was ashamed of them, and instead insisted on using two canes for mobility. She had great difficulty supporting her body on the two unstable canes. She laboriously dragged her legs one at a time a few steps, then fell.

For the next session, I brought the crutches and my home movie camera. Karen agreed to dress up for the movie and, just to please me, to try the crutches. We first filmed Karen struggling to walk with the canes. Then she took the crutches. She agreed that she felt much safer with the crutches while standing against a wall. Soon, she realized that she could also move much more easily with them.

The home movie confirmed what she'd felt. Her struggle with the canes was a discouraging sight. But with the crutches, Karen saw herself standing straight, her head high, looking very attractive. She chose to use crutches after that. Getting into the bathroom was now no longer a problem. Karen had achieved her seemingly unreachable goal and learned many other necessary activities at the same time. She was completely free of the wheelchair soon after.

Karen also discovered a career goal: to become a rehabilitation therapist of some kind. Before polio, Karen had aspired to be a dancer. After polio, it seemed as though her dream of a performing arts career was shattered. Now, her victories convinced her that her old goals were not impossible. Although she now wanted to be a therapist, the thought of attempting a simple dance routine, which could lead to a satisfying creative outlet as a leisure pursuit, was an exciting challenge. It was time for more occupational therapy.

Karen found that if she held onto a coil spring attached to a doorknob, she could balance enough to slowly move her pelvis and rotate her torso. After several months of practice, she needed only one hand to hold on, performing graceful arm movements with her free hand. I filmed her dancing, and we shared a tremendous sense of accomplishment and delight when Karen liked what she saw on the home movie.

Next, she wanted to dance for an audience. She choreographed a dance for herself and her former classmates from dance school. Karen took center stage, while the other dancers moved around her. She had sewn her own costume, a flower, for the performance. No one in the audience was aware of Karen's coil spring fastened to the floor, as she stretched and contracted in graceful movements, swaying gently in time with the music and an imaginary breeze.

Karen was well on her way to achieving a full, enriched life. She was well-groomed, beautifully dressed, and self-confident. As the years passed, the girl who had wanted only to be able to get to the bathroom without help finished high school, learned to drive a car with hand controls, graduated from college, became a speech-language pathologist, married, and gave birth to a daughter.

Karen is now a proud, capable, successful wife, mother, homemaker, and rehabilitation professional. I will never forget her determination or her courage. Needless to say, her parents and grandparents are delighted.

Chapter Twenty-Six

A Debt Repaid
Laura Faye Clubok, OTR/L

"Mommy, why are you crying?" asked 3-year-old Emily, as I sat with her and her mother in my occupational therapy clinic. Her mother was crying as she watched her only daughter pick up marbles for the first time ever with her left hand, her "little hand." Emily knew that there was a difference between her right and left hands, that is, her "big hand" and her "little hand." But she didn't grasp how or why this difference could drive her mother to tears.

"Mommy's happy to see you holding those marbles," Emily's mother replied carefully, dabbing her eyes with a tissue. But I knew that her explanation was incomplete. I understood why Emily's mom would cry, both from pleasure at the success of the therapy and from regret that such therapy was needed. Today's tears of thanks for Emily's accomplishment were also a continuation of 3 years of sadness that her beautiful daughter, Emily, had been born with an unusual left hand.

How do you explain to a 3 year old that the shape of her hand has turned your life upside down? How do you explain this to your daughter without making her feel that it's her fault? As I watched this interplay between mother and daughter, I found it increasingly difficult to maintain my professional composure because 25 years ago, I was the small girl who couldn't understand why the absence of fingers on my own left hand had turned my family's world upside down.

Like most small children, I learned by trial and error to use the tools that I was given at birth. Grasping, gripping, pinching, pulling, holding, releasing —these were the activities of an inquisitive little girl busily exploring her world. It just so happened that the tools on my left hand—a palm with a thumb and nubs of the other fingers—were packaged differently than those of my peers, and they came without a "use and care" guide.

As I was growing up, no one taught me preferred grip patterns. No one analyzed my use of thumb and partial index finger to grasp toys. No one worried that this unusual grip pattern might cause strain in overworked tendons. So when I began to experience pain in my left hand at age 9, my doctor explained to me and my parents something about "nerve injury" and referred me to an occupational therapist who crafted me a little girl-sized splint to rest the tendons. At that time, all I wanted from my first exposure to occupational therapy was to resume the life of a normal third grader, pain-free.

As I grew, I recoiled from drawing attention to my difference, preferring, as did my peers, independence in my activities. However, the adaptations that my youthful ingenuity had devised to perform everyday tasks independently— open a jar, tie my shoes, hold a necklace—began to cause me problems. It never occurred to me or to anyone else that the resting hand splints might temporarily diminish the pain, but that they would not eliminate the source of the pain completely. So I became a regular visitor to the occupational therapy treatment room at a local hospital, returning annually for a bigger resting splint for my left hand. At first glance, this room might have seemed like any other 1970s hospital room, impersonal and uninviting. To me, it seemed a magical place. Under my occupational therapist's expert touch, once-inflexible plastic sheeting dipped in scalding water grew soft and supple, enveloped my hand, and then rehardened, forming a custom-protective cradle. Snug Velcro straps cut to size held the splint in place. I marveled at the splint fabrication process and imagined someday making my own splint, which I then would proudly wear to school, Girl Scouts, and soccer practice.

I visited that occupational therapy treatment room frequently for portions of my childhood. I vividly recall images of wooden peg boards; containers of blue, brown, and green putty; and hard plastic sheeting. The different materials in the room fascinated me; I longed to explore the cabinets and play with what I found. The occupational therapist showed me how the putty could help me strengthen my unaffected strong right hand. Indeed, during those years I learned many occupational therapy strategies that enabled me to rely on my strong right arm and hand to do activities, with my left hand assisting.

An automobile accident during my senior year of high school dealt my body a terrible reversal of fortune, as I received a fractured collarbone with whiplash injuries to my neck on my right side. When the injuries healed incompletely, my right hand was too weak and painful to do much of anything, including brushing my teeth, opening doors, and carrying textbooks. When I started college 9 months later, my right hand and arm just couldn't withstand the added strain of undergraduate life. Just 6 weeks into my first year of college, I began to awaken with pain surging throughout my right arm and hand. Getting through each day was an overwhelming challenge, as I struggled to perform formerly simple tasks like getting dressed and eating. Buttoning my shirt and zipping my jacket were painful. Cutting meat and peeling oranges were fatiguing. Within several months, one-handed typing and ultimately even writing were too strenuous. I initially assumed that the situation would be temporary, that my right hand would heal completely and that I would return to life as it had been before the automobile accident. But 8 weeks of immobilization failed to rest my right arm sufficiently to avoid pain.

When I returned for my second year of college, a pervasive, chronic muscle pain syndrome further limited me from normal college activities like attending lectures and turning pages in my texts. It became clear that because of my earlier over-dependence on my injured but healing right arm and hand, I had not been able to give that side the rest it needed to recuperate fully. Over the next 2 years, pain from muscles that were wasting away, muscles that were overused, and pressure on multiple nerves became a permanent facet of my increasingly difficult daily life. Gradually, I began to lose hope of ever climbing out of the morass in which I found myself.

This meant that I needed a lot of help. During the long and difficult phase of my recovery, miraculously, family, roommates, friends, peers, and even strangers showered assistance upon me. My mother bathed me, roommates did my laundry, peers shared their lecture notes and typed my term papers, and dining hall staff and friends carried my tray in the cafeteria. (I had no clue at the time, but I was destined to marry one of those helpers many years later.) Although these acts helped me physically, they made me despair of ever being more than a burden to those around me. With each gesture of kindness, I felt an ever-expanding emptiness inside, as I ached to repay the "debt" I was rapidly accumulating.

As I consulted physician after physician during the 2 years in which my condition worsened, occupational therapy once again was my one mainstay of support. The therapists guided me throughout my difficulties. They fashioned several hand splints that I wore constantly to relieve the burning sensation in my right hand. In fact, the splints were so integral to my daily attire that I replaced the muted, boring, tan industrial Velcro straps with ones that matched my clothes each day.

Suddenly, I was forced to rely upon my left hand for daily tasks, which had never before served as more than a "helper" to my right hand. To break out of the cycle of right hand overuse and weakness, I needed nothing short of a complete lifestyle overhaul. I urgently needed to acquire new skills, so I could depend on my fingerless left hand while restricting my formerly strong right hand to the unaccustomed helper role. Only when my right hand was fully rested would it be ready for restorative strengthening exercises. The recovery process would be long and difficult; I needed information and strategies, and most importantly, someone to guide me. Again I turned to occupational therapy. This time my experiences were much more diverse. In addition to splints, my occupational therapists introduced me to strengthening activities, gadgets that made life easier, and principles of building a balanced body.

The occupational therapists problem-solved with me, helping me to figure out how to pursue the activities that were important to me. They introduced me to catalogs filled with products that could facilitate activities that I could no longer perform. Between OT appointments, I spent hours poring over these catalogs, fascinated by the gadgets that simplified cutting vegetables, opening twist-off jars, stabilizing a dinner plate, and tying shoelaces. When I returned for my next visit, they would discuss the pros and cons of the various items on my list, allowing me to experiment with the ones they kept in the clinic as demonstration aids. They taught me how to incorporate these new tools into my daily routine; simultaneously, they taught me exercises to strengthen my now rested but very weak right side.

As I began to see signs of real improvement, occupational therapy gave me an even greater gift: a potential outlet for repaying my debt of gratitude. My early experiences with occupational therapy, reinforced by my more recent ones, had shown me how one caring therapist could ease another's suffering, transforming another's life. Now my fascination with the gadgetry of OT could be put to practical use. When I casually told friends that I was considering a career in occupational therapy, they cheered that I had found a calling that would allow me to channel my life experiences.

Since earning a master's of science degree from the Boston School of Occupational Therapy at Tufts University, I have been treating children with developmental disabilities in Ohio. This work gives me ample opportunity to make my contribution to society. From my perspective, as I help an autistic child to use the toilet independently, as I assist a schoolteacher to accommodate a child with Down syndrome in her regular third grade class, or as I help a teenage girl with limited hand dexterity to manipulate a hairbrush, I'm whittling away at that debt amassed so many years ago. Sometimes the work is difficult. Sometimes my clients don't want to do the therapy activities. Sometimes I emerge from a treatment session frustrated by our lack of progress.

All of my work, everything I went through, is made worthwhile when I see the smile of success on a little girl's face as she picks up marbles for the first time ever with her "little" hand, and we both see her mother's bittersweet tears of joy.

Soon to Be a Butterfly

Beth Larson, PhD, OTR

"*Dear Elizabeth, Someday when I have enough time, we'll go and find one... a real, live, honest-to-goodness caterpillar... the type of which spins a cocoon about itself and then waits... for this process to happen, not unlike making a cake from a mix, and where the one-time worm just unravels itself and flutters away.*

"*When it gets out, it seems to know where to fly. Nature seems to point a way for it. Its old tomb or bed or whatever dries up and disappears. It is gone, honey. It is the way of life.*"

This father's letter to his daughter brought me to tears the first time I read it. This poem was part of a father-daughter piece of art. Next to her father's life-like butterflies were Elizabeth's child-like butterflies and caterpillars, and in large gridded blocks at the beginning of the poem were Elizabeth's large printed letters. Elizabeth and I had been working together since she was 10, and writing her name was one of her first goals. Not only was I touched by her artwork, something I had a hand in, but also by the profound poem penned by her father.

When I first met Elizabeth, she was nearly as tall as I was; she seemed like a puppy, ambling and still "growing into her feet." One of her mother's concerns was Elizabeth's deportment.

Elizabeth's tall stature belied her child-like wonder and bounding movement. She wanted to be a paleontologist when she grew up; her vocabulary was stunning and her strongest asset. Yet Elizabeth often seemed "lost" in space and in social circles. Later, when she started middle school, she frequently lost her way going between classes, forgetting to look for markers that would guide her.

In the first year of treatment, Elizabeth participated in a therapy group in which she worked on both gross motor and fine motor skills. She chased with other children down the school halls on scooter boards playing tag, lined up for rides on a scooter board train, played catch and kickball. The children learned writing in the Rainbow writer's program, practicing rows of letters each in a different color. At the end of a session, children earned stars that they could cash in for their favorite activity on Fridays. However, skill in printing, drawing, art work, and game playing came slowly for Elizabeth.

In seventh grade, her parents and I decided to take a new track in her therapy services. Together we designed a community-based instruction program that would develop the skills that Elizabeth would need for adult life. We recognized that Elizabeth's education needed to prepare her to be a member of the community. This type of program was new in the school district, and the special education director allowed me to implement it and even provided some stipends and travel expenses. While Elizabeth continued to work on basic academics such as writing simple sentences and adding single digit numbers in the class for learning disabled students, she and I employed these skills by writing out an address book complete with friends, family, and emergency numbers. We practiced using her new address book and the phone book to call for information, to report an emergency, or get directions. Having gained this skill, we ventured further out into the community on buses and in taxis.

Elizabeth's comrade in this adventure was her best friend, Shaughnessy, who was in the same class. The two had become best friends in the occupational therapy group. While Elizabeth was expressive with a silly sense of humor, Shaughnessy's words came in fits and starts and were difficult to understand. But Shaughnessy had the common sense that Elizabeth lacked. In many ways they complemented each other.

In the fall, we began taking the bus to local recreation spots and the local mall. Making sense of bus schedules, learning where to stand to board the bus, and going to the correct destination became part of the challenges of our weekly treks. Slowly Elizabeth and Shaughnessy gained confidence in depositing the bus tokens and asking for help when they needed it. Shaughnessy, though less articulate because of her disability, had the cooler head and was more logical. She often coached Elizabeth on how to behave when she got flustered.

At Christmas time, the pair shopped for their families' presents. They made lists, budgeted their money, and planned the adventure. In public, Elizabeth sometimes panicked. Afraid to speak to clerks, she was impulsive in her conversation and often took flight before completing her purchase. Before this Christmas shopping adventure, we practiced how to ask for help and how to pay for purchases. I taught her the dollar method, so that she was confident enough to pay for her purchases. Elizabeth learned to give the number of dollars that the cashier told her plus one more for any change required; that way she didn't need to count out the appropriate change.

This tiny strategy allowed Elizabeth to successfully make a purchase on her own. Although the girls bought only small tokens for their families, it meant so much to them and to their families. They were growing up.

Over the weeks of the school year, we walked to nearby stores and grocery stores; we traveled to the local church, where we cooked; and to Elizabeth's family home, where we cleaned. Although I sometimes feared Elizabeth's crossing the street on her own or using a knife to slice food, she became confident in herself. The end of the year celebration was a pizza dinner prepared for their families. Elizabeth and Shaughnessy planned the entire menu. (I suggested some "healthy" additions like a salad.) That day they shopped for the ingredients, and later that afternoon they read directions, sliced and measured, and prepared the perfect pepperoni pizza dinner complete with salad and warm rolls. I faded into the background while they rose to the occasion. Though Shaughnessy was certainly more adept at using a knife, Elizabeth insisted on slicing the tomatoes for the salad. Despite her preoccupation with conversing and her intermittent gazing away, Elizabeth safely sliced the tomatoes for the salad. It seems a simple thing, but I was never more proud of her and it really made me believe that she would someday take her place in the adult community. Together, she and Shaughnessy managed to serve a successful dinner to their appreciative families. It gave us all such pleasure to see them proudly serve their dinner.

The following fall, I left the school district to study for my PhD. Before I left, I invited all the children and their families to my home. Again I was brought to tears by something that Elizabeth's father wrote. He read this to the gathering that day:

"To Beth on Her Departure:
Who's that young-looking girl trying to teach my child?
'Touch your toes, kids, touch your heads,
Let's cruise the halls on roller sleds.'
Does she have a plan, some hidden design?
'Throw these balls, children, then catch them to your heart, then place gold stars on your progress chart.'

She doesn't deal in miracles, but at least she seems to care.
'Just make these loops in rows of ten, then lines once and twice and again and again.'
So what now? Beth is leaving? Was it something I said?
A woman with sensitivities must somehow see that she's now an official caring aunt, a part of the family!
Your genius, Beth, is something already proven.
Here, we give you that title by mutual decree.
So what's this genteel business; Doctor of Philosophy?
Oh, I know. You have ambitions; things to be proven.
Oh, and I know we'll be in touch, we'll see you around, you'll never go away.
So let's keep our eyes dry and believe that for today.
Do you somehow think that you can be replaced...?
Oh pardon, pardon me if I, perplexed, throw out the net of guilt...
On such base things are enduring friendships built."

Elizabeth became a butterfly through our years together, and as nature pointed the way for both of us, we fluttered away, on different paths. But she and her family were changed by the process and so was I. Working with families such as Elizabeth's permanently imprinted my life. It made me realize that as health professionals we do become part of the family, stepping into a very private sphere of family life. In doing that, we have a responsibility to care, as an unofficial "aunt," to foster and further the family's hopes and dreams.

Postscript: The piece of artwork referred to in the beginning of the story still hangs in my home and reminds me daily of my life before graduate school. In the years since I have left the community in which Elizabeth and her family reside, I have earned my PhD and taken a position as an assistant professor, teaching future occupational therapists and doing research on families' management of daily life activities when parenting children with disabilities.

Chapter Twenty-Eight

Jessica's Dream

Peggy Lee Gurock, OTR

Jessica had a dream. She dreamed of doing something that most of us consider a very routine part of our lives—to bend over and tie her own shoelaces. For so many months, it was just that—a dream—but it was a dream that kept Jessica going.

The ability to tie her own shoelaces was a dream because Jessica had lived her entire young life with spastic cerebral palsy. Cerebral palsy causes loss of muscle power and coordination due to a problem in the brain. Her specific type of cerebral palsy includes increased muscle tightness and exaggerated reflexes resulting in sudden and involuntary tightening of those muscles.

When I first met her at her public school, Jessica was a bright girl of 12 with an infectious smile that showed she had dreams and desires. When I evaluated her for occupational therapy services, I found that she was in need of fine motor hand skills associated with classroom tasks such as handwriting and using a calculator or computer. I also determined that although she was pretty independent, she needed to further develop her self-care skills such as dressing, feeding, and grooming herself, as well as the gross motor skills of trunk rotation and hip and knee flexion. Tying her own shoelaces was something that she just could not accomplish at the time. That's when I learned about Jessica's dream, to put on her socks and shoes and to tie her shoelaces by herself.

Jessica made her way around school and home with the assistance of a rolling walker for support because of the difficulty she had with her trunk rotation, as well as with hip and knee flexion. She had enough hip and knee flexion, though, to climb up steps by holding onto rails on both sides. But in order to put on her socks and shoes, as well as tie her shoelaces, she needed to use trunk rotation as well as hip and knee flexion. So, the inability to rotate her trunk was now the biggest obstacle we had to overcome to realize her dream.

The results of Jessica's evaluation also showed me that she did have the necessary finger isolation movement and hand strength to fulfill her dream. She enjoyed playing finger games with me such as "Tricky Fingers," which requires moving the fingers separately from one another along with motor planning and speed to see who could copy the other person's finger movement pattern first. These games also helped Jessica with her handwriting issues. She had learned to manipulate buttons to fasten her blouse, but her big frustration was still her inability to tie her own shoelaces. Since she had never mastered the technique for tying a knot and bow, and due to her lack of flexibility, previous therapists may not have considered it important to help her learn these skills.

I was convinced that with the proper therapy, both occupational and physical, coupled with Jessica's personal desire to master this task, she would be able to learn to tie her shoelaces by the end of the school year. She was delighted. We started immediately in the fall.

We began by working on trunk control, as well as hip, knee, and ankle flexion, in preparation for her being able to sustain her reach to her shoes long enough to tie the laces. Slowly at first, we worked on the activities on an obstacle course, with Jessica lying prone on her stomach on a scooter board. We built up her hand strength as well as her trunk stability. We also worked on activities like putting clothes pins on her and on me. I also had her put them on or take them off while straddled over a bolster. I had her pick up objects from the one side of the bolster and place them on the other side or in front of her in order to develop the necessary torso muscles as well as having her keep her hips and knees in proper alignment.

It was a slow process, and Jessica was not always happy performing activities that were hard for her. But by linking these activities to tying her shoes, I was able to get her to stick with the program and even to do these activities as her homework, since she was only being seen once a week for occupational therapy treatments.

At the same time, while we were teaching her body how to bend over and move, I had Jessica working on a lacing board, so her fingers could learn the "X" pattern of crossing her midline for lacing her shoes and for tying the knots and bows on her shoes.

Chapter Twenty-Eight

When I began her therapy at the beginning of the school year, Jessica was able to bend over but needed to hold onto anything near her for support. By February, she was able to sit upright on a bolster unsupported and participate in a game of "Tricky Fingers." This was a big accomplishment by itself because it demonstrated that she was beginning to develop the necessary trunk flexibility for getting her hands down to her toes. This increased Jessica's feelings of independence, and it showed her that her perseverance was paying off.

The next step was to get her to put on her socks, then the shoes. We accomplished this task by assigning Jessica the homework of pulling her shoes and socks off every night and putting them on as best she could every morning. Although I was still only seeing her once a week, I could see her progressing.

By the end of spring break in April, Jessica was really excited. She had been practicing her activities over the break and had maintained her gains rather than losing her skills. She had succeeded in learning to tie a bow not only on the lacing board, but also on her wrist. She was now getting close to her goal.

The big day came at the end of May. Jessica was ready and able to try to tie the laces on her shoes with the shoe on the table in front of her, demonstrating the ability to transfer the techniques she learned from the lacing board to her shoes. She continued to practice this technique at home as homework, all the while still continuing to work on her lower body flexibility. At each therapy session I monitored her progress, and several weeks later I realized it was time to pull it all together. She put her shoes on her feet and bent over to tie the laces.

After she finished tying that first bow on her shoe, she then moved on to the other shoe, and tied it just a little quicker. This was still no easy task for her, her legs were still tight, but she had a window of flexibility to get her hand to the tips of her shoes long enough to tie her laces. You had to see her reaction! Her sense of accomplishment could be seen all over her face.

For me, as an occupational therapist, it was also an exciting day. I shared in her accomplishment, taking pride in realizing that not only had Jessica succeeded in making her dream a reality, but had done so in time for the end of the school year. I knew that she could now handle what was ahead. So bring on the summer sneaker season, Jessica's ready!

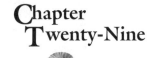

Think Right Hand

Irene Phillips, MPA, MA, OTR/L

"This is it," said 16-year-old Richard, as he held the fingers of his right hand straight out. "I can't bend my fingers and make a fist like you want me to." I tried to refrain from laughing at this defiant teenager, but lost control, and to my surprise, Richard and the family laughed with me.

Richard has sickle cell anemia and is HIV positive resulting from a blood transfusion he received when he was 2 years old. Sickle cell anemia is a painful disease. The pain, called a "crisis," can strike anywhere in the body and render the person debilitated for long periods of time. So when Richard got a crisis in the muscles of his right forearm, he decided that it was too painful to use his hand at all. Instead, Richard kept his fingers extended during the 4 weeks of crisis, which resulted in an extension contracture of his four fingers. Those fingers were stiff and "locked" in the stuck-straight-out position, and nothing, he was certain, would ever change them.

Richard was motivated but also a little dramatic. He made sure I knew that he was ready for me to do whatever it took to get his right hand working again so that he could reach his two goals of returning to normal school life and getting a driver's permit so that he could drive the family car. Richard's family was very involved in his treatment and were all for Richard's going back to school. But like most parents of 16-year-olds, they were not so keen on the driver's permit.

The insurance company paying for Richard's occupational therapy treatment gave me 6 weeks to meet this challenge of getting Richard's hand back to full use. We went to work. I got Richard to show me every task he does from the time he gets up in the morning to the time he goes to bed. The idea was to see just what he could do with his right hand or how we could use the tasks as treatment activities between my weekly visits. From this point on, we began to "think right hand." Richard was to "think right hand" in all his activities.

I left Richard on the first visit with exercises to do for his hand when he was in the shower. We used the shower as moist heat to relax and loosen up the hand so that the exercises would be easier. We used the wringing out of the washcloth as a beginning step to get closure of the hand and to increase muscle strength as much as we could at this point in treatment.

When I came for the second visit, I brought Richard a "finger flexion glove" to wear according to a schedule I set up. The glove passively pulled his fingers into flexion, providing a static stretch. Although it was clearly beneficial to Richard's therapy, I had to pay for the glove myself because the insurance company would not guarantee reimbursement, and prior approval would take more than the 6 weeks I was given to complete this case.

I looked forward to my weekly visits with Richard as much as he did because each time I came, we were able to measure the progress Richard had made for each finger between my visits. Richard was proud of his steady progress and was eager to demonstrate the gains in the tasks he does.

Periodically I would vary the exercises for Richard to prevent him from getting bored and to be more aggressive with his treatment. Whatever activities I gave Richard for his hand included things that were already in the home. For example, a large bowl filled with rice with coins dispersed throughout was used for increasing pinch, opposition, grasp-release skills, and strength. He was shown how to use the doorknob to increase closing and strengthening of the hand.

At the same time, Richard was using a built-up handle on his toothbrush for brushing his teeth, a built-up handle on his knife and his fork for eating, and a built-up pen for writing. Richard was happy that the therapy was becoming more aggressive because the faster he was increasing the range and strength in his hand, the faster he could, as he said, "dump the gadgets."

The difference in Richard's goals and those of his mother were clear. Richard's mother asked how soon could he start doing some of the chores around the house. Needless to say, Richard was given the chore of sorting and folding clothes and the chore of washing dishes, both of which also exercised his fingers. But Richard had his mind set on a different goal—getting his hands wrapped around the steering wheel of the car!

Did Richard return to the full use of his right hand in 6 weeks? Did Richard return to school? Did Richard get his driver's permit? I can say yes to two of the three. As for the permit, you'll have to ask Richard and his parents. Rather than get in between parents and a potential teenaged driver, I decided that in this family issue; discretion was the better part of valor.

Chapter
Thirty

———————⬮———————

Ten
Finger Exercise

Nina Paris, OT/L

For most teenaged girls, checking the color of their fingernails several times a day means they want to know how the
current nail polish they are experimenting with looks in different lights or with different outfits. But for Mary, fingernail
color was not a matter of vanity, nor did it involve nail polish at
all. Frequent daily checking of the color of her unpolished fingernails and being aware of how her fingertips felt told her
whether or not she would be able to use her hands to type or to
write out her homework. Mary's natural fingernail color was the
indicator of the temperature of her hands and reflected whether
she had enough blood circulation to allow her to use her fingers
at all. And so for Mary, mastering occupational therapy relaxation techniques to increase blood circulation and change her
fingernail color meant the difference between success and failure
in her exams at school.

Mary had experienced a brain injury at birth, which made her
right dominant side weaker than her left side, much like someone
who has had a stroke. As a young child, she had had significant
problems with coordination. Her caring and attentive parents
made sure she had occupational therapy as early as possible, and
with that help she overcame most of her problems and did very
well in school as she was growing up. She still had a few remain-

ing difficulties in using her fingers, but none of these seriously bothered her during those years.

As Mary got older, however, she began having more trouble with certain activities and particularly with typing. But because she was by then a young teenager in junior high school, she did not want to be separated from her classmates to get the special help she needed at her school. She also didn't want her mother to interfere in her relationships with her teachers by arranging any changes in the requirements applied to other students in order to accommodate her inability to write and type. Remembering the success of her previous experiences, however, she did agree to have occupational therapy again, but only if it could be provided at her home.

Mary had also recently been diagnosed with Raynaud's disease, a circulatory disturbance that during an attack causes the blood vessels in the fingertips to constrict, or tighten, too much, leaving the fingertips icy cold, blue in color, and extremely painful. In addition to physician-prescribed medication for this condition, which Mary and her mother wanted to avoid if possible, some occupational therapists use biofeedback training, specifically including techniques for temperature feedback, to relieve the incapacitating symptoms.

I began seeing Mary at her home and spent several weeks teaching her finger coordination exercises and designing ways for her to use the homework assigned in her typing class as additional finger coordination exercises. At the same time, I taught her some relaxation techniques and imagery that she used while "attached" by wires to a biofeedback temperature monitor that I supplied. During this time, she would listen to a beeping sound that changed with the changes in the temperature in her fingers. If the temperature went up, the beeping tone went up as well. Although she learned quickly, it still took Mary quite a long time to learn to use the relaxation techniques to raise the temperature in her fingertips even one degree.

Mary was astute enough to realize that she often experienced the worst Raynaud's attacks right before she had to take a test at school and correctly assumed that the stress she felt about taking the test was probably triggering the attack. That attack, of course, made it even more difficult for her to type or write because of the extreme pain in her fingertips, so it caused her to have even more trouble taking and completing the tests. It seemed logical to her that the relaxation techniques she was learning to raise the temperature in her fingertips could also reduce the stress she felt before taking tests. Perhaps if she could control the pretest stress, she could stave off the impending Raynaud's attack and possibly prevent it altogether. Doubly motivated, Mary and I worked hard to improve her relaxation response so that it was quicker and easier to warm her fingers while she was still using the biofeedback machine. Little by little, and with lots of practice, the relaxation techniques began to feel like second nature to her.

Chapter Thirty

An otherwise typical teenager, Mary did not want to appear different from her classmates at school. Who wanted to stay hooked to a machine in school all day! That meant leaving the biofeedback machine at home, so Mary knew that in order for this kind of occupational therapy to be useful to her she had to learn to use the relaxation response without the biofeedback unit. She practiced diligently, and soon she could warm her fingertips without using the biofeedback machine.

Her stress-reduction theory worked! Within several weeks she was able to stop an impending Raynaud's attack at school using the relaxation training for fingertip temperature adjustment that she had practiced with me. She now no longer needed the feedback machine either. She could always confirm to herself that she was using the proper technique by looking at the color of her unpolished fingernails and being aware of how her fingertips felt.

An added benefit that neither she nor I had anticipated was that by learning to relax and thereby stopping attacks of Raynaud's disease before her tests, she was also experiencing a more total body relaxation before and during the exams. To her delight and that of her parents, her school grades improved dramatically. This was indeed a most unexpected but very welcome result of her occupational therapy.

Mary never did experiment with nail polish the way her friends did. She didn't need to. She didn't need bottles of polish to change the color of her nails; she didn't need to be in her bedroom at home or at the beauty parlor to do so. She could do something with the color of her nails that none of her friends could do—change it on her own. She could change the color of her nails with her mind and her breathing, at home or in school, whenever she needed to, and by connecting her brain to her fingernails, get the added benefit of improving her grades at school, something that no nail polish advertisement ever promised.

Chapter
Thirty-One

A Letter
to Remember

*Bethany S. Walls, MA and
Rhona Gorsky Reiss, PhD, OTR/L,
FAOTA*

Imagine being unable to communicate with anyone for 11 years. Unable to write, to talk, to type. Unable to express a thought out loud, even to yourself. The year was 1970, before the age of widely available personal computers, hand held organizers, wireless e-mail, and adapted communication devices. In 1970, this was the reality for Rhona Gorsky Reiss's students with disabilities at the Widener Memorial School in Philadelphia.

As an occupational therapist at the school, Rhona treated children who had severe movement and speech impairments because of cerebral palsy. But the cerebral palsy did not affect their minds, because in 1970, children with special needs could not go to school at all, even to specialized schools for those with disabilities, unless they were "educable." That meant that they had to have an IQ of 50 or more, which meant that the Widener School had a group of bright but very physically handicapped special education kids. Brett was one of the very brightest of the entire bunch, but the only part of his body that he could control was his left foot.

Few people outside of the school knew what these children were capable of achieving, locked as they were in bodies that didn't work. Without speech and movement, the children missed out on the typical experiences of most schoolchildren, such as presenting their parents with an "A" paper or a finger painting. They couldn't tell their families about or show them what they were doing in school. They certainly couldn't communicate at all with people in the wider world.

Rhona attended the annual conference of the American Occupational Therapy Association in New York that year with her students' needs in mind. She strolled through the exhibit hall, where new products were introduced and demonstrated, examining the products being offered, and she stopped short when she saw the CyberType. "Here," she thought, "is something that could radically change the way my students participate in school."

CyberType was a precursor to the computer, almost like an electric typewriter, that could be adapted for people with severe mobility impairments. Instead of tiny keys with letters of the alphabet, it had an enlarged keyboard with fewer keys. Combinations of keys produced letters on a paper printout. The exhibitor was looking for occupational therapists to try out the device with their patients and to report on its success or failure. Rhona immediately volunteered.

"In 1970, this was very innovative," Rhona recalls, "an early stage of computer technology at a time when mainframe computers took up the space of an entire building." Some of the students at Widener had tried to use electric typewriters with Rhona's specially built adaptive keyboard shields that protected the keys from being struck at the wrong times by hands that could not control their random movements, but most of the students could still not control their fingers enough to produce any meaningful typewritten pages. For them, there were no types of alternative communication systems other than language boards. Language boards were large, awkward, limiting in what could be expressed, and required much patience on the part of the communicator and the recipient of that communication. It was a tedious process: the language board had to be placed on the wheelchair lapboard or footboard, and it had pictures or words to which the kids pointed. But someone had to stand and look at them while they pointed, and they could not produce anything lasting.

By contrast, the CyberType appeared to offer a breakthrough in communication systems for people with disabilities. Rhona was very eager to try it out. She envisioned the CyberType giving her students opportunities they never had before. For the first time, these children would be able to answer essay test questions or write poetry. Kids who had never before been able to show their parents a spelling test that had earned a gold star or bring home work to be displayed proudly on the refrigerator would now be showering their families with such samples of their accomplishments. But she never envisioned quite how far-reaching one student's work would turn out to be.

Back at the Widener School, Rhona set up the CyberType equipment in her occupational therapy treatment room and began designing individual methods for each student to use the equipment. Some had to use head pointers to press the keys, others needed mouth sticks, a few could use their hands with specially designed stabilizing pointers or other devices.

But one student, Brett, could only use his left foot. Although she has treated hundreds of patients throughout her career, Rhona will always remember Brett. Maybe it is because he was so severely physically impaired or because designing his interface method with the CyberType was such a special challenge. Probably it is because the CyberType gave her an opportunity to meet the child she suspected existed behind the bright eyes, engaging smile, and determined foot. Rhona came to know Brett as sharp, curious, and funny.

At home one night soon after learning how to use the CyberType, Brett watched a late night movie "A Night To Remember," the 1958 film about the sinking of the Titanic. At the end of the film, the producers ran a list of the names of all the people who had died on the ship. Brett saw a name he recognized: Widener. He knew that the Widener School was named for a very wealthy Philadelphia family who had donated money to have it built. He came to school the next day, and in his occupational therapy session decided to write a letter with his foot to the Widener family.

Brett's letter went something like this: "My name is Brett. I am 11 years old. I go to the Widener Memorial School. Did Old Man Widener go down on the Titanic?" Then he added, "This is the first letter I have ever written in my life." Rhona dutifully mailed the letter, never expecting a reply for Brett's first effort at communicating with the outside world.

A member of the Widener family wrote a reply to Brett that, yes, Mr. George Dunton Widener, the family patriarch, and his son, Harry Elkins Widener, had indeed died in the Titanic sinking. Mrs. Eleanor Widener, George's wife, survived and devoted herself to charitable work for the rest of her life. She was devastated by the loss of her son, who was a collector of books and a talented student who attended Harvard University. She established several buildings, including Brett's school, in Philadelphia and Boston in memory of Harry. Brett's class buzzed with excitement for weeks after he received the letter.

"We were so thrilled," Rhona remembers. "It seems like such a small thing, but to a child who is very bright and couldn't talk or write, to be able to use that piece of equipment and in some way reach the outside world—it was such a miracle! And it was because of occupational therapy that he was able to make that connection," she recalls proudly. "Had I not gone to that conference, I probably never would have known about the CyberType."

Rhona lost contact with Brett after she left her job at the Widener School. He would be over 40 years old now. "Wouldn't it be something," she muses, "if Brett went on to become a writer?"

Chapter Thirty-One

Today the CyberType would not impress anyone who owns a computer. We are surrounded by monitors, adapted keyboards, and special software that enable people with just about any physical impairment to use those computers to do just about anything in the communication arena. Most of us these days take such technology for granted and have never even used some older forms of technology such as record players or manual typewriters.

But Rhona Gorsky Reiss's students at the Widener Memorial School will never forget the year she brought them the CyberType. It was the year they began to speak.

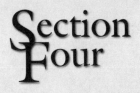

Section Four

Adults

Navigating the Perils of Illness and Injury

Navigating the Perils of Illness and Injury

Meet 14 adults coping with illnesses, injuries, progressive diseases, and life stresses with the help of therapists who showed them ways to redirect their energies, build skills for their jobs of living, and redesign satisfying lives.

Chapter Thirty-Two

An Apple a Day
Ann Burkhardt,
MA, OTR/L, BCN, FAOTA

One day in May 1994, the phone rang in my occupational therapy office. The voice on the other end was hesitant and anxious, but picked up speed as her story spilled out of her. "Hi Ann, my name is Dorothy. I am a cancer survivor, but as a result of surgery I have lymphedema, and it involves the palm of my hand. I'm a medical writer, and I need to use my hand. I'm just so upset. Do you think you can help me?" Dorothy went on to describe how her fluid-filled enlarged lymph nodes under her armpits caused swelling in her arms and hands that kept her from using her computer or doing anything that involved fine finger movements. We arranged our first appointment together at her apartment for soon after.

Dorothy and her husband, Jim, a freelance artist for a publisher in Connecticut, were both anxious to discuss treatment options that would most benefit Dorothy. They were aware that there were many potential treatment modalities. At this point, however, that knowledge was not necessarily comforting. Dorothy and Jim were somewhat overwhelmed by the multiple therapies available. They were confused, unsure who to believe and what was safe to try. So their concerns and problems were more complicated than merely the physical aspects involved in relieving her swollen arm and hand and her overall desire to find balance in life and seek wellness again. They previously had seen a doctor in Cleveland, where Dorothy was originally from, as well as two doctors in New York City—one who specialized in the treatment of lymphedema, and the other who was a physical medicine and rehabilitation specialist. Throughout, Dorothy had been under the treatment of a massage therapist for manual lymph therapy to reduce the swelling. The physiatrist had prescribed a sequential pneumatic pump to reduce swelling, which she used for an hour each day. But none of these seemed to be working. The massage therapist suggested that she call me, an occupational therapist.

On that first visit, I evaluated her and measured her range of motion (her ability to move her shoulders, arms, and hands in all directions) and how well she could do various daily living activities. After we reviewed her program together, all three of us agreed to try, as her primary therapy, compression wrapping for her arm, which included the use of a pressure insert for the palm of Dorothy's left, nondominant hand.

The compression wrapping addressed Dorothy's immediate physical problems. But along with those problems came some emotional issues. After her initial treatment for cancer, the lymphedema made her fearful of regression. She didn't want the lymphedema to interfere with her regular activities or to become an excuse for other shortcomings in her life. She was surviving the disease and trying to maintain a normal life, so her main goal was to find a balance between handling her health concerns and her enjoyment of life. Dorothy listened to guided imagery tapes, which helped her maintain some of this balance. Even so, she longed to spend time outdoors pursuing one of her favorite activities—picking apples, pears, and raspberries in the countryside. But as a city dweller without a car, at that time, she wasn't able to fulfill this wish.

During my weekly visits, my treatment focused on observation, listening, and intervention. Each week, Dorothy would share her personal handwritten notes and questions about her condition. In our sessions, I explained the workings of the lymph system, wrote directions to fine tune her home exercise program, and offered her contacts for community-based resources. In addition to working to control her edema and improve her range of motion, hand function, and the physical aspects of her health, Dorothy seemed to appreciate most my advice on how to make her treatment part of the background of her life, more of an ongoing habit than a primary focus of her activities. She wanted treatment of her lymphedema and her arm to become second nature, while she made enjoying life her top priority.

Over time, Dorothy became very proficient at her own treatment. Jim assisted whenever she needed his help. For a period of a year, I continued to follow Dorothy's progress on an "as-needed" basis whenever she would call.

One day in the winter of 1995, Dorothy called, sounding very upset. "Can I please see you as soon as possible? I've had a recurrence of the cancer. I'm so scared." Later that day, I found Dorothy with her sister who was visiting from Cleveland. A routine mammogram had shown irregular calcifications in her left breast. It seemed that Dorothy's lymphedema was the first sign of breast cancer. From a surgical perspective, she had been conservatively treated; aggressive chemotherapy would perhaps have been the treatment of choice. Now she was terrified. "I keep wondering that if I had seen a different doctor, if I had chosen a different treatment, maybe I'd be all right now."

Anxiety is common and natural at moments like these. I thought to myself, "What can I possibly say to this woman or do for her that will make a difference in her ability to cope with this news and the inevitability of further treatment?" At that moment, the goals and focus of occupational therapy changed from long-term goals to her immediate worries. I listened to her concerns that day. I offered as much information as I could to help put an end to some of her irrational fears, the kind that often feed anxiety. I helped her problem solve how to choose a plan of action, to keep doctors she knew and respected, and to choose some new doctors who were experts in treating her cancer recurrence. I was there to help comfort her and ease some of her fears, and this is what mattered most at that moment. The road ahead for Dorothy would be difficult, but not insurmountable.

Her doctors recommended that she have surgery to remove the tumors, and then undergo both radiation treatment and chemotherapy. Dorothy was most concerned about the radiation therapy, because she knew from her own research that it could worsen her lymphedema. While her radiologist downplayed this concern, Dorothy wanted to be vigilant about keeping her lymphedema at bay. The surgery revealed that the cancer was contained in one area. However, her pathology also revealed that the cancer cells had become resistant to the medications used the first time, so that chemotherapy would not be as effective at combating the remaining tumor cells. Radiation therapy soon became her greatest hope as well as her greatest fear.

As Dorothy received her radiation treatment, she had some stiffness and tightening in her shoulder joint. Additionally, the chemotherapy gave her an itchy rash, which she feared would spread to her left arm. Most significantly, her lymphedema also became more active, making her nondominant hand function even more difficult. Dorothy knew the signs of recurring lymphedema, and she was well prepared with all the medical self-treatment tools she needed. Even so, Dorothy had difficulty reaching for objects in the cupboard, cooking, and washing her hair using two hands. Finally, her time typing at the computer also had to be limited to brief sessions. In the midst of her recovery, not knowing what her future would hold, Dorothy moved from New York City to Connecticut to be with her husband.

After many months, her perseverance with radiation therapy paid off, and her cancer went into remission by the fall of 1996. Her perseverance with continuing her purposeful activities as therapy also paid off, and her lymphedema became controllable as well.

It was that same autumn that Dorothy told me again about her desire to get out to pick apples. I knew of an orchard nearby in Connecticut, and I suggested that this activity would be good for her at this point in her recovery. She invited me to participate, and I was glad to accept. So the three of us—Dorothy, her husband, and I—drove to the orchard and made our way up into the hilly peaks of the orchard where the apples were most ripe and ready for picking. We used a tall picking pole to reach the tops of the apple-laden trees. Dorothy was delighted to find that she had no trouble reaching up over her head and pulling off the apples from the tree branches, something she wasn't able to do previously because of the after effects of the surgery for her breast cancer. However, her motivation to resumer her role as a weekend harvester had kept her focused on continuing her daily activities—even when painful—so that she was able to regain her apple picking ability, something she could not do through exercise alone. "I guess it's true what they say: 'An apple a day keeps the doctor away!'" Dorothy said with a smile.

Dorothy is still enjoying country life. She occasionally ventures into the city, and we still touch base regularly on the telephone about her condition.

To this day, apple picking continues to be an annual outing for Dorothy, her husband, and me. Picking apples in the open air of the Connecticut hills will always be a celebration of life and good health for each of us, especially Dorothy, who does not miss her doctors at all.

Dorothy is proud of her success, but without hesitation, she identifies the source of her strength in conquering her health issues. She credits the value of occupational therapy in her life. "The information and intervention you gave me have been the single most important aspects of my cancer care. You were the missing link in my care," Dorothy told me. "I hope other people will be fortunate enough to find an occupational therapist to assist them as well. More people need to know the value of occupational therapy."

Chapter Thirty-Three

What Are You Going to Do Next? Go to Disney World

Michelle Anne Blackburn, OTR/L and Bobbie Andrews

My goal is to get myself to church and to go to Disney World, and I intend to do both. But I wasn't always so sure I could. It has taken a lot of faith and a wonderful, caring occupational therapist to convince me that my power wheelchair and I can successfully make the trip.

I was just 40 years old. I had three children and a beautiful, loving husband, Earl. I was so happy working as a hairdresser, putting on fashion shows, shopping, and enjoying my family and my home. Without warning, I began struggling at work; I was becoming clumsy, I began dropping things, and my bladder wasn't working properly. With the support of my husband, I got up the courage to go to a doctor. I was diagnosed with multiple sclerosis. I didn't want to believe it. I thought that African American people like me just don't get MS! Despite a second opinion that confirmed the diagnosis, I refused to give up. I continued to work and shop, until I started to feel even clumsier and stumble more. That was when I was told to use a cane. Me, use a cane? Even so, I ached from fatigue.

But that wasn't the end. Next came the wheelchair. I still wanted to continue shopping, so my husband pushed me in and out of stores and never complained. My MS progressed quickly, and the wheelchair became part of my life. I was so mad and angry. This just wasn't supposed to happen. I was destined to work and to care for my family. So, even from my wheelchair and later from an electric scooter, I insisted on mopping the floors and even vacuuming the rugs in my home.

After several extended hospital stays, I returned home, but I was confined to bed and could no longer sit safely without falling out of my chair. Now I could not do even the most personal things for myself, and I needed my husband to care for me full time, including helping me with my most private needs. My sons pitched in as well. They knew how much I cared about my personal appearance, and they quickly learned how to expertly apply my lipstick. But even this was not enough. I needed extra care in the house and now I even had to be lifted into bed, but my family never gave up.

After more bouts with my illness, including a serious drug reaction, a diagnosis of diabetes, and many more trips to the hospital, my husband and I faced the most painful decision we had ever had to make in all the years we were married. I would need to leave my family and home behind and become part of a new assisted living community where my growing health care needs could be taken care of. So I moved to Heritage Hall East, a nursing center in Agawam, Massachusetts. Do you realize how painful and difficult it is for a married woman to leave her husband? It was 1991, and I was not even 50 years old!

That's where I met Michelle Blackburn, my occupational therapist. She is part of my miracle. Without her, I wouldn't be able to use my electric wheelchair to leave my room every day. I wouldn't be able to paint. And I wouldn't be working toward my twin goals of driving my power wheelchair to church someday and making it to Disney World. For now, I am sitting on top of the world! Because this is her story as well as mine, I'll let her take over now.

Bobbie is a 55-year-old African-American woman whom I first met 3½ years ago. I knew she had been diagnosed with multiple sclerosis. MS is a disease of the central nervous system with no known cause that is usually characterized by attacks that can last for weeks or months, separated by long or short periods of relative disappearance of symptoms, known as remissions. MS has a variety of symptoms because of the spotty way in which it attacks the nervous system; these include loss of muscle coordination, strength, and feeling; lack of energy; and the progressively worsening nature of the condition, which has no cure. It wasn't a very hopeful outlook, but Bobbie wasn't your typical person, and she was determined to make the best of things in her new home.

I had learned many years ago in occupational therapy school the value of looking at the whole person and the importance of setting realistic goals with full participation of the patient. I tried to apply that training to Bobbie. But she really put me to the test. Notwithstanding the MS, the first thing I saw was a beautiful woman, her lipstick perfect and her hair with not a strand out of place. Her goals were very straightforward—Could she feed herself? Could she resume painting, one of her favorite hobbies? Could she learn to use an electric wheelchair? We both knew, although she wouldn't always admit it, that she had very little use of or function in her dominant right hand and could expect few appreciable gains in the use of her arm and hand. And things would probably get worse.

After experimenting with commercially available devices and equipment, and doing a lot of reality testing, Bobbie and I had to agree that total self-feeding was not a realistic goal. But there was something we could do. Bobbie loved eating in the main dining room with her friends. So our goal became to find a way that she could manage to drink on her own in a group setting. We tested a whole variety of cup holders and long straws, but none seemed to work. Then one night, I had an idea. I visualized a gooseneck-like attachment with a special holder on the end that we could attach to her wheelchair. I went to work creating it the next day. I was confident it would work—it had to work—and once created, it did. The adaptation was completed, and Bobbie has been using the special cup and straw to control her drinking independently in the dining room and in her own room for more than a year.

That moved oil painting to the top of Bobbie's list of goals. Her room gleamed with portraits and other works she had done in the past. Once more we had to ask ourselves the question—was oil painting again a realistic goal? After all, her arm was so weak that it needed to be supported, and only a few of her fingers moved on her dominant hand. I thought about using splints, thermoplastic material, and special tools for writing and feeding, and I began experimenting. What worked the best was a writing tool with strapping to hold a paintbrush with a built-up handle. This allowed her to paint once again. Even with this device, however, in order to paint Bobbie still needed a special set-up and guidance from the art class instructor. She had to work slowly, and it took her twice as long as it had before, but that never took away from her pride in her accomplishment, which was evident in the broad smile on her face as she showed off her paintings.

With two goals successfully accomplished, she was now eager to try to get around on her own. When it came to the idea of an electric wheelchair, at first I was skeptical. My first reaction was, "This is impossible." At the time, Bobbie was seated in a custom-designed, special, beautiful, hot pink "tilt-in-space" manual recline chair. And because she did not have torso or leg control and she could not change her position by herself, she was completely dependent on the staff for all her needs and movements in that chair. But with Bobbie, "impossible" just wasn't an acceptable answer.

Chapter Thirty-Three

I borrowed a standard electric power chair for a trial for a few hours. I knew I had to do it for Bobbie, but I worried that I was setting her up for a devastating failure. Was I wrong. Bobbie was able to tolerate and partially manage this trial power chair. She had every confidence that I could find a permanent chair for her and adapt it to her needs. But this was a major challenge for me. First, where was I going to get a chair? Her chair would need many adaptations. Custom chairs are very costly. Where would the funding come from? On the other hand, I knew that Bobbie really needed this "dream" power chair to keep her going in more ways than one.

The answer came from an unexpected place. Bobbie's husband had been told of the success with the trial chair and that he would be provided with more details at a future meeting. When I arrived at work the next day, Bobbie was elated. Her husband had rushed out and bought a used power chair for her. As for me, my heart sank. Because I had not even provided him with any of the recommendations from our OT evaluation after the experiment with the test chair, now I was faced with the challenge of taking someone else's customized used power chair and adapting it to make it work for Bobbie. I knew, though, how important it was to both of them. I had always hoped that someday the creative skills that my mother taught me and the technical skills I learned by watching my dad in his woodshop would pay off. If there ever was such a time, this was it.

It took many months, working with a representative from Neighborcare, Bobbie, her husband Earl, my occupational therapy colleagues, and my fellow team members from other professions to finally develop a finished product. I had spent hours at home working on it, and my table saw and staple gun had never had such a workout.

For Bobbie, her Christmas present came early that year. In November, her customized power wheelchair was ready for use. Everything on it that could be changed was changed. It was fitted with a different back and seat. Her left arm is supported on a tray. She has a special armrest that holds up her right arm. In addition, Bobbie wears a soft splint to support her right wrist. Her joystick has been modified with a special putty that is molded for her to make it larger in size. She has a doorbell at her head that she can activate by her head motions to warn people she is coming. Bobbie also has a specially adapted rear-view mirror that clamps on to her tray.

Even with all of these adaptations, we all thought that Bobbie might be able to tolerate only 1 to 2 hours a day in her chair due to anticipated fatigue. Wrong again. In fact, she is able to use her chair for over 5 hours each day. Bobbie has really persevered. She now can turn the chair on and off herself, and she uses it to leave her room whenever she wishes for dining and other activities. She visits fellow residents and has resumed her active participation in Bible study, in resident council meetings, and is looking forward to taking group trips outdoors and into the community.

Bobbie still intends to drive her chair to church someday and to take it with her to Disney World. With her drive, spirit, and determination, I have no doubt that she will succeed at doing both. Then who knows what even loftier goals she will set for herself? As Bobbie herself put it at the end of her part of this story, "For now I am sitting on top of the world!"

Chapter
Thirty-Four

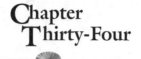

Clumsy Bob

Mary V. Donohue, PhD, OT, FAOTA

B ob was clumsy. His occupational therapy assessment confirmed it, but really there was no doubt about it as far as
those around him were concerned. Bob was totally inept at
anything requiring the manipulation of objects. In fact, he could
do nothing successfully with his hands. He couldn't play sports or
even participate in arts and crafts activities. Bob needed help.

At the time, Bob was 22 and still living at home with his parents.
They wouldn't permit him to touch anything in the house, fearing
he would break whatever he touched. It was unclear which came
first, their restrictions or his ineptitude. Sadly, Bob became trapped
in a vicious cycle of inactivity: he wouldn't try to touch anything in
the house, and his parents forbade him from doing so. It got so bad
that he felt he couldn't even turn on the television because his parents wouldn't allow it. His favorite activity became spending
lengthy periods of time standing in the shower, listening to Bob
Dylan music. Nothing could get broken there.

Bob was diagnosed with paranoid schizophrenia, a mental
health problem characterized by high levels of agitation or anxiety. At times, it also seemed that Bob showed signs of narcissistic
personality disorder because he would constantly check his
appearance, asking everyone around him, "How do I look?" Thus,
he looked better cared for than the average psychiatric patient

because of his constant checking and preening. He was being treated with appropriate medicines and receiving occupational therapy at a day hospital in a suburban environment.

At the day center, Bob was placed for treatment with other patients in an occupational therapy activities group that was organized to provide opportunities for them to explore various activities and to deal with issues of behavior control. On his first day, Bob wandered among the activity tables looking at what other patients were doing. He expressed no interest in their activities, saying aloud that he probably wouldn't be allowed to touch anything anyway. His resistance to participate in activities lasted for several days.

It was during a weekly field trip away from the hospital that for the first time Bob expressed interest in something: cars, which he spoke about constantly during the trip. Back at the hospital, the group was working on decoupage projects, a craft in which pictures are artfully glued to the outside of various objects and then covered with clear polyurethane to produce a decorative effect. We suggested that Bob find photos of cars he liked in magazines so he could participate in the project. Despite his customary view of himself as unable to do such things with his hands, he became highly motivated and worked steadily, even though every step required staff help to clarify the procedures for Bob and to assist him in sustaining his performance.

We guided Bob in tearing his picture of a red sports car around the edges in an artistic way to create the decoupage effect. We suggested to Bob that he mount the photo on a piece of wood that he could prepare as the background. On his own, he selected wood with an interesting grain, but then needed help sanding the wood to smooth the edges. We pointed out to him that he could speak with others in the group about some of his favorite topics while he was sanding.

Talking about cars, Bob Dylan, and rock music helped him get through the process. During the next few days, with coaching, he sealed the picture with several coats of polyurethane, waited patiently overnight for each coat to dry, and then added a brass hook for hanging his artwork. After connecting to people in the group, Bob began to feel generally more at ease. He still tended to talk only about his favorite subjects, and frequently checked with me on his looks. After a few weeks, gaining more confidence, Bob asked to move to the clerical group to try office work, and we supported his selection of this activity for himself.

Bob responded well to the structure of the new group. He found the routine of photocopying, collating, and stapling to be comforting, giving him the necessary stability to make him feel secure. What he liked the most in the clerical group was using the calculator. He was good at working with numbers and was proud to handle departmental billing records. He had found his niche.

Chapter Thirty-Four

Bob spent 3 months practicing his newly acquired office skills. With coaching, he also worked on his social skills. He was encouraged to talk about topics other than music and his appearance, helping him to interact more positively with others.

Ultimately, Bob was referred for rehabilitation counseling and, after testing high in math skills, was sponsored by the State Office of Vocational Rehabilitation to attend accounting courses at a community college. Meanwhile, Bob entered a supported apartment program where he lived with two other patients under the supervision of a social worker. After Bob graduated, he began working as an accounting assistant.

Bob came back to visit his occupational therapists, proud of his competency and his new successes in life. He was working with his hands in ways he hadn't imagined possible before. Bob had gotten the assistance he needed, gaining self-assurance and changing his life for the better. With help, "Clumsy Bob" had become "Confident Bob." We were proud of him, too. Without his even asking me, with certainty, I could now tell Bob, "You look terrific!"

Chapter Thirty-Five

Find It at the Mall

Paula D. Carey, MS, OTR/L

I met Lillian while she was a resident at the developmental center in which I was working as a new occupational therapist, fresh out of college. Lillian was in her early 50s and had lived at the center for more than 30 years. She had osteogenesis imperfecta, a congenital condition that affects bone development, leaving bones malformed, brittle, and very susceptible to fractures. In addition to this disorder, she was in chronic pain and periodically depressed. She required ongoing assistance with all of her daily activities. In those days, shopping at the mall was certainly not one of Lillian's daily activities.

The day of our first appointment, I walked into Lillian's room and stopped short, appalled at the sight in front of me. Five people surrounded Lillian's bed, trying as a group to lift her onto a stretcher. Lillian was frantic; she had been in bed for the past 18 months because of a serious hip fracture, and she was obviously very fearful of being dropped. "Be careful! Don't hurt me!" she cried out.

I was flabbergasted. There are very specific ways that individuals should be lifted and moved, known as transferring, to avoid hurting either the person or the rehabilitation professionals. But what I saw in front of me was chaos. Each aide was stretching across the bed, sliding Lillian toward a stretcher on the other side. They then were trying, in this extended stance, to lift her onto the stretcher. They had no leverage or balance, and everyone was in danger of being hurt.

"Wait! How can we do this differently and still keep her body aligned?" I asked them, bringing the commotion to a halt. "We've always transferred Lillian this way," said one of the aides.

Well, it looked like the goal of my first session with Lillian had been decided. We talked about ways to transfer Lillian safely. I coached a brain-storming session with Lillian and the aides on what could be done to make Lillian comfortable and safe when she had to be placed on a stretcher. We came up with the idea of a transfer board on which she could be easily slid from bed to stretcher. An adaptive equipment specialist made the board for us. Lillian was thrilled when we used it for the first time, and it worked like a charm. Transfers became less painful and less scary for her and easier for the developmental center staff. That was the first of many steps for Lillian.

As I continued to work with Lillian, we became a real team, not just an occupational therapist and a resident. We each gave and received in this therapeutic relationship, which came to be much more than my "job." Our teamwork, figuring out what her strengths and needs were and what she wanted to accomplish, helped Lillian ultimately to find the courage to venture into the community again.

Lillian told me that she rarely left her room, and it struck me that this contributed to her depression and negative feelings about herself. So one day, I asked Lillian to accompany me on an outing on the developmental center campus. Lillian was thrilled at the idea of getting out, but we had many challenges to overcome. She couldn't stay in an inclined position for more than 15 minutes, but couldn't see much from the flat position. She was dependent on others for her mobility, and because even the slightest bump caused her pain, it was hard for her to trust even those she knew would push her carefully. But Lillian was very motivated. She had fractured her hip just after a new power wheelchair had been purchased for her, and she'd never had the chance to use it. She really wanted to work toward being able to use the wheelchair to get herself around. When I presented her with the idea of an outing, she saw using a stretcher on wheels as the first step toward realizing this goal of eventually returning to power wheelchair use. Deciding that the risks were worth it, we planned carefully to avoid the possible pitfalls of injury and discomfort.

Lillian began venturing out with me. During our trips around campus, she began to talk about her life. She told tales of escapades from her youth, when she moved about easily in a powered wheelchair and was always looking for mischief. These conversations were very therapeutic for Lillian, even more so than the exercises she did to increase the length of time she could sit up.

One day, Lillian told me she wanted to go shopping and out to eat at a restaurant, two of her favorite activities. It was a wonderful short-term goal. Lillian, a nurse, a therapy assistant, and I plotted and planned for weeks to make the trip a reality. Lillian fluctuated between excited anticipation and fear of going out into the community, where she didn't feel safe. "They all stare at me, and they don't understand," she explained. I reassured her, and to help prepare her, we acted out situations she might encounter.

Finally, the day arrived. We headed for the mall in a van equipped with a stretcher on wheels. At first, it seemed that Lillian was right. Many fellow shoppers did stare at her. But as the afternoon progressed, we met many considerate people who took the time to chat with her. Several store clerks welcomed her and praised her for coming to the mall. She loved it! Her adventure left her tired, in pain—and completely giddy with the pleasure of her success!

That was only the beginning. After many months of effort and ongoing occupational therapy services, Lillian began to use and operate her new powered wheelchair on her own. Lillian eventually landed a job at the developmental center and became involved in an educational program to earn a general equivalency diploma. She regularly went to the mall, restaurants, a local amusement center, and church. Lillian began to view herself as what she was—a capable adult.

I had the great fortune to share many of these adventures with Lillian, and they inspired me. Through my journeys with her, I witnessed Lillian's courage and perseverance as she expanded her horizons and once again took part in activities she had abandoned long ago. Lillian enriched my life, helped me develop as a therapist, and changed me irrevocably. She also taught me how you can find a new way of life if you start by shopping for it at the mall.

Let's Do Lunch

Susan Bachner,
MA, OTR/L, FAOTA, CEAC

Helen is one of those people we may read about every now and then in a story on the bottom of page one of a Kentucky newspaper on a slow news day. "Woman Found Neglected in Rural Mountain Cabin" might read the headline above the story. In the text of the article, intrigued readers drawn to the story would find details about Helen, a woman judged to be approximately 40, who was discovered by a social worker in a deserted shack deep in the hills of Appalachia. Arriving to give follow up care to a man who had recently been discharged from an emergency week-long stay in an acute hospital, the social worker literally stumbled upon Helen curled up on the dirt floor near the door of the remote cabin that the man, apparently Helen's brother, called "home."

The Thanksgiving day before she was found would undoubtedly have been Helen's last holiday. She was suffering from exposure, malnutrition, and was acutely ill with the flu when she was discovered. Dressed in rags, she appeared to have lain on the floor for much of the week that her brother was gone, unable to get food for herself or even get to the outdoor toilet. She did not speak, nor did she seem to understand why she had been removed from the cabin and where she was when she awoke the next day in the hospital. She appeared frightened as though she had never seen so many other people or the inside of a hospital room in her entire life.

Helen was an extreme example of a person with what is sometimes described as "Appalachian syndrome," a situation in which dwellers in remote areas of the mountains of Kentucky are in many ways cut off from the civilization that surrounds them in Kentucky's cities and rural farming and horse-raising countryside. Babies in those mountain cabins are delivered at home and have no ongoing medical care, no hospital records, and no contact with doctors or others. Children with disabilities or developmental delays receive no treatment. Mountain dwellers depend on relatives or are isolated without available help and often cannot read or write.

Helen had lived in the mountains with her older brother and their now-deceased parents all her life. As a child, she had developmental delays and various medical problems. As an adult, she was small in stature, quite cognitively limited, couldn't talk, couldn't read or identify pictures, and had no social skills to interact with others or even to use utensils for eating.

When she was admitted to our large residential facility for adults with developmental disabilities, the various staff tried to evaluate her mental, physical, and social status using the customary tests and other evaluation methods familiar to them. It was very difficult to elicit any kind of response from Helen, and that was discouraging to the staff. They had no idea of her capabilities and were at a loss as to how to interact with her or help her. She appeared frightened and disoriented, but was compliant and cooperative, and she tended to follow staff around like a lost puppy dog, as if afraid to be left alone. She was referred to me for an occupational therapy evaluation.

Part of what occupational therapists do is to perform a functional evaluation to find out what the person can do, what she cannot do, and what she wants to do. This is very different in focus and methods from the evaluations done by other disciplines. When the individual is articulate or at least can speak, the verbal communication assists us in the fact-finding and gives direction to avenues yet to be pursued. However, what are we to do when the client's cognition is severely limited and no verbal speech is present? This was the dilemma I faced with Helen.

As the director of occupational therapy at the developmental center, I have the opportunity to get to know clients on a regular basis and to know them as individual personalities with individual wants and needs. Over time, to me they become people with names and distinctive identities rather than souls classified only by their birth defects, physical and chromosomal abnormalities, haywire brain chemistry, and the losses stemming from deprivations of their environment. But achieving this level of familiarity needs a starting point.

Where to begin with learning about Helen was indeed a challenge! The window of opportunity had to be tied into her only observable strength noted to date. Helen, like most others at the facility, was highly motivated to eat. That was enough. Occupational therapists understand the power of doing and the significance of observing the numerous patterns associated with that doing. So I chose to perform the "Let's Do Lunch" evaluation with Helen.

Let's Do Lunch is an evaluation tool that I developed to determine a person's functional status and to provide insights into six different areas that impact a person's performance. Examples of these are a person's physical state, emotional state, neuromuscular condition, and so forth. Even those people with limitations as severe as Helen's are able to participate successfully with the Let's Do Lunch evaluation. What I usually do when I bring someone into my office for an occupational therapy assessment is to suggest that, before we start, first we should go to the facility dining room and have a cup of coffee or eat lunch together. The client doesn't realize that this social invitation is part of my evaluation, and I get to see them doing a natural activity in a natural environment. So Helen simply needed to do what came naturally, something as routine and satisfying as getting lunch in the facility dining room. For me as the occupational therapist, it was an opportunity to gain an understanding of her as a person. Certainly this was our best shot.

At that point, all we knew about Helen was that she was brought to the facility by a social worker after having been discovered living under primitive conditions in her brother's Eastern Kentucky mountain shack. It was imperative that the team know more so that she could be served appropriately. The "givens" were that she was mentally retarded, did not talk, and had a lot of congenital problems. Precious little else was known.

Let's Do Lunch began when we walked into the dining room together. Helen was a little unstable, but it did not seem to be due to any muscle weakness in her legs. She had lots of trouble locating one of the many empty seats. Then with staff help, she did find a chair but refused to sit down on it. Her reluctance was later discovered to be unfamiliarity with furniture; I found out that she also refused to lie on her bed in the cottage. I watched as Helen had difficulty getting into the cafeteria line, finding a tray, and placing food from the serving table on it. While eating—and she was really very hungry— Helen placed the dish within 4 inches of her eyes and only reached for food that was directly in front of her. Anything placed to either side was ignored. When it came to drinking from her glass, she would not put her head back; she seemed to not want to move her eyes. Then, despite her obvious appetite, she left food on her plate. When the remains were pointed out to her, she quickly devoured them! All of these behaviors told me a great deal about Helen's functional abilities. While Helen could not, and will not, be able to speak, she was indeed able to communicate her needs and wants clearly through the structured analysis afforded by the Let's Do Lunch evaluation. I realized that one of her basic needs was that she had serious eyesight problems. From these and other observations that day, I was able to submit a report to the team that included a description of her suspected vision problems. Helen was sent to an eye doctor and bilateral cataract surgery restored her sight. She was now ready for the next step.

Programming was begun to introduce Helen to common amenities; these allowed her to participate more fully in daily living activities. Sitting on chairs and lying on a bed, use of a bathroom, use of utensils for eating, basic grooming activities such as washing her body and taking care of her hair, and working/playing cooperatively with others are some of the basic things that Helen needed to learn. And this was merely the beginning.

After the surgery that restored her vision, Helen began exploring her environment. She was particularly fascinated with water and began to enjoy washing in it, playing with it, pouring it, and drinking it from a glass. She also began to enjoy some social life within her residential community; she seemed genuinely surprised and pleased to discover the presence of other people, and she started practicing appropriate ways of dealing with them. She began going on outings with the group and seemed amazed at the bus, the ride, and the scenery outdoors. She started being interested in looking through magazines and became able to identify some of the pictures. It was as though Helen had discovered a whole new world.

The occupational therapy evaluation Let's Do Lunch, which allowed me to see that Helen could not see, was the start of a whole new life for her. Opening her eyes opened up that whole new world, and Helen is now a participating member of the community at the developmental disabilities center. What a distance she has traveled from the mountains to the city.

Chapter Thirty-Seven

Life, Liberty, and Power Mobility

Linda Lorentzen, OTR/L

Amyotrophic lateral sclerosis is a progressive disease that takes away sometimes a little at a time and sometimes a lot at a time. Over the years I've seen many people deal with ALS; some do it very well, others are so overwhelmed that they forget that they still have each day to live. A lot of valuable living time is wasted. Then there are people like Ruth. Is there quality in a life with a disease for which there is no cure? Ruth's life is a case in point that there most certainly is.

When I first met Ruth, she walked into the occupational therapy clinic in obvious good shape from her years as a grade school physical education teacher. Her ALS had become symptomatic, causing her problems, particularly with right hand weakness. She had already done some homework and found a few adaptive aids on her own. I introduced her to a few others, and that began our journey. That was 3 years ago.

Today she relies on her wheelchair for mobility and is dependent on others for most of her care. But she continues to have her irrepressible spirit. She continues to have a desire to help others. She still actively seeks ways of prolonging whatever function she has.

I must admit that if anyone had told me that Ruth would have adjusted so well to power mobility, there was a time when I would have been skeptical. I remember introducing her to the concept of using a power wheelchair as a means to increase her independence. She looked me straight in the eye and said something like, "Baloney." She wanted to maintain and use her muscles as much as possible. What was hard for her to face was that her muscles just weren't allowing her to live life fully.

Ruth was concerned because she spent much of her day in a reclining lift chair, waiting for people to come and assist her. The hours alone were long and the time between her husband's leaving for work and the time the personal care attendant arrived could be unbearable. Growing up as a hyperactive person, Ruth found having to sit still for so many hours at a time insufferable.

Ruth agreed to be seen in the Seating and Wheeled Mobility Clinic and to try out different mobility options. After careful consideration, Ruth agreed to a power wheelchair complete with a tilt-and-recline system. After we cus-tom-fitted it carefully and it was delivered, she realized that the possibilities were endless. Ruth was ecstatic!

She was immediately able once again to pace back and forth in her living room; she could go to the window to check on the neighbors' activities; she could go to the over-the-bed table for a quick snack and have a drink out of a long straw in a glass; she could go to the speaker phone and dial a number using her mouthstick; and she could reposition herself in her wheelchair through the tilt and recline features. The quality of Ruth's life increased because she could move when she wanted to, not when other people were available to move her. Ruth claims, "I have always felt like I have to move or I'll go nuts, and moving in the wheelchair gives me the same feeling of mobil-ity and control that I used to get by walking."

Ruth describes herself as a caretaker. Her dealings with ALS have not changed this part of her personality. She continually attempts to make oth-ers feel comfortable with her disease and not feel bad for her. She dreads the day that ALS may take her voice, knowing she will have to become profi-cient at using augmentative communication devices and that might make it harder for her to ease other people's worries about her.

Ruth's mother suffered a stroke 6 years ago and has had her mobility severely limited. Ruth's mission has been to find a way she could still go for a walk with her mom. She and her husband did research and stumbled upon a device to help her reach her goal.

When I recently visited Ruth, she invited me to go with her to the garage. A strange-looking contraption was sitting in the middle of the garage floor; it consisted of a two-wheeled metal base complete with a lawn chair and a footrest attached to the base. Her husband proceeded to attach the cart to her power wheelchair with a custom metal hitch. At Ruth's invitation, I climbed onto the lawn chair, and she took off, pulling me down the quiet street in front of her home. Several neighbors outside, obviously used to see-ing her give rides to her mother and others, waved to us.

Chapter Thirty-Seven

Ruth, limited to head, neck, and minimal trunk and hand movement, nodded at her neighbors as we passed. I felt like the homecoming queen, waving, smiling, and chattering as we went.

Now that Ruth has power mobility, her friends think that she is physically better because she can do so many more things. But she's not physically better; in fact, she has lost more muscle power to the disease. She is psychologically better. She's in control of her life because she controls when and where she will move. Now, with her power wheelchair pulling the cart, she continues to give to others.

Is there quality of life with ALS? Looking at Ruth, the only answer can be a resounding, "Yes!"

Chapter Thirty-Eight

A Well-Dressed Woman

Valnere McLean, OTR

All patients are important, but sometimes we meet people who become very special to us in ways that go beyond the rehabilitation setting. My special patient was Jo, who had the distressing habit of continually removing her clothing.

Jo was a 37-year-old blind and deaf woman who had been institutionalized all her life. She was dependent on others for everything and was very difficult to manage. In 1993, she was transferred to a group home, where she received significantly more attention and assistance than she had anywhere else before. She was taught to feed herself and help with her own bathing and dressing.

All of us have strengths and weaknesses, and Jo was no different. Physically, she had normal muscle tone and full range of motion in her joints, although she had some looseness in her shoulders, hips, and knees. She could sit up straight. She had good balance when sitting, but she leaned slightly backwards when standing. She got around the home by sidestepping firmly, moving in circles.

Within her limited repertoire, Jo appeared to learn more about her environment with her feet—she rarely used her hands to explore. She loved to walk. Jo liked contact with other people, and she especially liked people to hold her hand and follow where she took them. She seemed to have an extraordinary sense of smell that allowed her to recognize people. She was in almost constant motion when awake, and she'd been given a chaise lounge in the main living room on which she rested in between her active periods. She loved anything warm, such as sunlight or clothes just out of the dryer. She hated the cold.

Some things that come quite easily to most people seemed to present problems for Jo. She didn't mind having her teeth or hair brushed, but she wasn't willing to do these tasks on her own. She would hold a spoon and bring it to her mouth, but did not scoop up food with it. She responded better to eating when her little finger was linked to her caregiver's finger and her hand was guided through the motions. She didn't like to be strapped into an automobile seat, so she resisted van rides.

There were negative behaviors that were particularly detrimental to Jo's quality of life. She tried to provide her own stimulation for herself by pushing and rubbing her body against objects, walls, and people; by rocking, rotating, and twirling; and by flapping her hands near her eyes and grinding her teeth. Some of her behaviors were self-injurious and thus very dangerous for her body, such as butting her head and slapping and biting herself. She would bite, hit, or pinch when angry or frustrated and had unpredictable emotional outbursts that were difficult to calm. And, causing embarrassment and frustration to those around her, she habitually removed her clothing.

Her psychologist thought she might be "sensorily defensive," a condition in which one or more of a person's senses are easily overstimulated to the point of great discomfort and distress. This would explain many of Jo's seemingly unusual preferences and odd behaviors. In Jo's case, her sense of touch was extremely sensitive; along with other strange sensations, clothing felt like spiders on her skin. Often, when people are sensorily defensive, they try to avoid the cause of their discomfort. It was thought, therefore, that Jo removed her clothing to stop the unpleasant crawling sensations.

I decided to plan a "sensory diet" for Jo, a special schedule of activities that would calm her and would, I hoped, make her feel comfortable for a few hours afterward. Sensory diets are commonly used with people who have Jo's kind of sensory defensiveness. Family members or caregivers can be trained to follow the diets and provide the activities, such as strenuous muscle work, slow rhythmic movements, deep pressure on the skin, joint compression, warmth, wrapping or rolling the body, and jumping. They are commonly used with children to help them avoid future problems, but such activities "diets" are effective with people of all ages. The staff on each shift were alerted to Jo's needs and promised to follow through on the special activities all day long.

Jo responded immediately and remarkably to her sensory diet. But a few weeks into our schedule, I had to leave because of an illness in my own family. Another occupational therapist, working with the dedicated group home staff, took over. I was assured that their work with Jo would continue. Circumstances intervened, and life did not bring me back to the group home. Time passed, and I often thought of my special patient and how she was doing.

One day, I was in the waiting room of a medical center, when I heard a familiar voice behind me. I turned around to a beautiful sight: Jo, calm, fully clothed, looking wonderful, and holding her attendant's hand. The attendant told me that Jo's sensory diet had turned her into a different person. She now fed herself and assisted in her daily bathing and dressing. She enjoyed outings and was involved in social programs for the blind and deaf. And after being helped to pick out her daily outfit with care and attention to the sensations of her body, she was able to remain well-dressed all day long. How could I not feel joy?

Chapter Thirty-Nine

The
Magical Mr. T

Richard J. Russ, MA, OTR/L

Magic is not a subject in the occupational therapy curriculum of any occupational therapy program that I
know of. We are medical professionals who study anatomy, physiology, and psychology. We are taught to help our clients
learn techniques and strategies they can use to improve their
functioning. We help them to better cope with their disabilities
and return to productive and satisfying lives. I've always thought
that what I do is pretty special, but until I met Mr. T, I never considered relying on magic. Now, I think perhaps magic should be a
required occupational therapy course.

In 1997, I was assigned a new client who suffered from severe,
out-of-control diabetes. Because of his condition, Mr. T had two
below-knee amputations, multiple finger amputations although
with some joints remaining on most of his fingers, and he was
blind in one eye. In the hospital, he was fitted with two prostheses for his legs and trained to walk using a walker. Mr. T was sent
home because physically he was able to get around his house
either using his wheelchair or his walker.

Emotionally, however, Mr. T was a wreck; he was very
depressed and expressed many feelings of distress over being only
"half a man." I tried to remind him that he had a very supportive
family that loved him and needed him, but he could not get past

the idea of losing so many body parts and his inability to do much for himself.

As an occupational therapist, I instruct my clients in helpful techniques to adapt to their surroundings. But more importantly, I also listen to them. I get to know what their interests are and use those in our therapy sessions. So I was eager to learn all about Mr. T as well. I found out that Mr. T was retired, was an amateur magician, and had a strong interest in ham radios. Magic had always fascinated me, so I asked him to show me some tricks. He told me he couldn't do any tricks because he couldn't use his hands. However, while giving him a great deal of emotional support, I coaxed him to try to do a trick for me and told him I would forgive him if he made any mistakes. With great reluctance Mr. T tried to perform a trick, and with some difficulty he completed it with smooth enough sleight-of-hand to make it look credible. I saw the excited look in his eye when he was able to pull off the trick and accomplish something he thought he'd never do again. Without any prompting from me, he performed another trick and completed that one pretty effectively as well.

That treatment session became a great success for Mr. T and proved to be a turning point. His wife told me that this was the first bit of enthusiasm he had showed in many months.

When I returned for my next visit, Mr. T had a 20-minute magic routine prepared for me. Although Mr. T had some difficulty with his act, he said he performed much better than he had expected. This was his first real step in getting back to normal daily activities in his life.

During our next session, he took me into his radio room and showed me how to use the ham radio. His wife confided in me that he had spent a lot of time there before his first amputation, but this was the first time since then that he had stepped back into the room. She was excited to see him regaining interest in his former activities and sensed this would be another important step to escape his overwhelming depression.

Building on our previous successes, in the following weeks Mr. T was willing to attempt activities that previously he wouldn't try. Although still discouraged by his physical condition, Mr. T began to adapt how he did things in order to succeed at tasks that previously seemed impossible. With the support of his family and his newfound confidence in himself, he began to take back control of his life, with no sleight-of-hand necessary. Though Mr. T and his wife have since moved away, I am confident that they continue to make magic together!

Yes,
There Are Angels

Wayne Pusatero
Submitted by
Deborah Morawski, OTR/L

No one likes being in a hospital, especially if the recovery is a long one. Nurses are in short supply, doctors are busy, and meals are nothing to look forward to. Except for watching television or having a visitor, there's not much to take your mind off how you feel physically. Although you'd like to be treated with special care, you're surrounded by other people who are just as sick as you are, so you don't always get the attention you may want. It's easy to feel pretty down.

That was my mood in June 1989, as I lay in a hospital bed, facing a 38-day stay. I had undergone total knee replacement surgery for rheumatoid arthritis, but an infection required me to go back into the hospital for a course of intravenous antibiotics. I was very depressed and had just about given up hope.

During the days that followed, I saw so many health care professionals, my head spun. One was an occupational therapist named Deborah. She was just another hospital employee to me at first.

But when my daily rehabilitation began, I became much more aware of Deborah. Right from the start, she made me feel different. She took an interest in me and in helping me feel like a whole person again. During our therapy sessions, we did the expected things, like exercising, learning to use occupational therapy gadgets to perform everyday tasks, and fitting splints for my arthritic hands. But we also talked about many things, not just medical talk about my condition. It was apparent that Deborah was not just another health care employee doing a job. She showed a true interest in my getting better, but she was also interested in me as a person. I began to look forward to her visits each day as I put myself back together. When I was ready to go home, I was sad—I felt like I was losing my only friend.

In February 1990, I started the year off back in the hospital, this time looking at a 30-day stay. Another infection in the knee replacement site again required antibiotic therapy that could only be done in the hospital setting. I knew it would be a pleasant stay when I discovered that Deborah would once again be my occupational therapist. One day, our conversation turned to my skills and abilities. I said that I had experience in computer work, and Deborah asked me if I would be willing to create some forms for her. Of course I said yes!

She turned my life around that day. Each day for the next 3 weeks, Deborah would arrive at my room promptly at 11 a.m. with a wheelchair. She'd whisk me to the rehabilitation center, where I spent 2 hours in front of a computer, creating her forms, typing, and handling other administrative duties that we jokingly called "stuff." For the first time in a long time, I felt useful and, most importantly, needed.

In November 1990, I was back at the hospital. This time, uncontrollable bleeding, followed by anemia, followed by removal of my spleen, caused me to develop severe weakness and minimal endurance. I could hardly walk at all and needed intensive treatment in the rehabilitation center. But despite my setback, I was not depressed because I knew what to expect, and guess who my occupational therapist was? Right! This time around, I was too weak to do "stuff," but Deborah was still there for me. She was very instrumental in gaining admission for me to the rehabilitation center, where I began another uphill battle with my medical condition. When I was well enough to be discharged, Deborah gave me some great news. If I wanted to, I could come back to the rehabilitation center as a volunteer, doing forms, typing, and "stuff."

That's just what I did. I worked as a volunteer from April 1991 until August 1992. Then another milestone in my recovery occurred: On August 12, 1992, I was hired by the rehabilitation center as an employee! One of the best things about my job is that I get to see Deborah every workday. I truly have a wonderful friend in her. Each June 12th, the anniversary of our first meeting, we celebrate. We also exchange birthday and Christmas cards, and we meet for lunch about once a month.

My life improved dramatically thanks to the help of my occupational therapist. Deborah helped me overcome not only physical problems but also personal ones. Instead of focusing only on the arthritis that was plaguing me, she took the time to find out what I wanted to be able to do with my life despite my illness, and she helped me find purpose and happiness.

I've learned that occupational therapists can do more than help you move your arms or legs. They look for the whole person and what that person needs, whether it is physical, mental, or emotional. In my book, they're the angels of the health care profession.

Chapter Forty-One

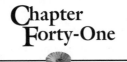

Traveling Light

Richard J. Russ, MA, OTR/L

Life on the street is tough, and you have to travel light. You have to be able to take care of yourself. But how do you do that when you've lost most of your fingers and toes? That was the challenge presented to me by Claude during a severe cold stretch in the middle of a harsh New York winter.

Claude was a young, homeless man. He was admitted to our orthopedic unit after spending several days and nights outside, exposed to the frigid elements. There are outreach workers on the streets in especially cold weather, looking for people like Claude, and Claude had been offered the chance to go to a homeless shelter, but had refused. The price of that refusal was steep. Claude now had a bad case of frostbite, and it was necessary to amputate most of his fingers and toes.

Claude was fitted with special shoes and orthotic devices for the insides of the shoes to accommodate his toeless feet. With some minor physical therapy, he was able to walk on his own almost as well as he had before the surgery. Still, Claude was quite distraught. Being able to walk was not good enough for life on the street. You had to be able to use your hands. But Claude had very few joints remaining on each hand. As a result, he could not hold any utensils to feed himself, brush his hair or his teeth, or put on his clothes. And in no way could he do the many things he needed to do for his protection and ultimate survival in the street world.

The first thing I did was to measure Claude for a simple device he could place on the palm of his hand called a universal cuff. A universal cuff is a narrow piece of fabric with Velcro at each end that is strapped around the palm of the hand and fastened over the back of the hand. It has a pocket at the palm in which a variety of utensils can be placed: silverware, a comb, a toothbrush, writing utensils, and whatever else you need. Claude was a fast learner and was easily taught how to put the cuff on by himself and place the utensils inside the pocket also on his own. I showed him how to use what was left of his hands as well as several new uses for his teeth.

Claude quickly gained competence as well as confidence in his new-found functional abilities, which in turn spurred him to explore additional paths to independence. As I watched his progress, I knew that there were many other pieces of adaptive equipment that could further improve Claude's functional independence and I discussed these with him. But Claude actually liked his life on the street, and that was where he intended to return. As Claude taught me, street life meant traveling light. A lot of baggage, even if it was adaptive equipment, was not suited for that lifestyle. So instead, Claude concentrated on doing everything he needed to with his simple universal cuff. I must say he even taught me a few tricks using the cuff that I had never seen or heard of before.

True to his word, Claude signed himself out of the unit against medical advice and returned to his life on the street. He never said goodbye, or even thank you; that just wasn't Claude. But I was confident that with his attitude and the universal cuff, he was going to make it, traveling light, even out there.

Chapter Forty-Two

Do It My Way

Anne Gaier, OTR/L, CHT

I never expected that the most difficult patient of my early occupational therapy career would become a lifelong friend. In 1974, I had 1 year of rehabilitation experience and thought I had all the answers regarding physical disabilities. I could devise just about any adaptation a patient at our Santa Barbara, California, facility could need.

One day, my supervisor handed me a folder and said, "You have a new patient ready to be scheduled." The patient was diagnosed with Guillain-Barré syndrome, an infectious neurological disorder that causes paralysis of the entire body (or sometimes just the arms and legs) and leaves the person with extreme muscle weakness or total inability to move. The good news about this mysterious disease of unknown origin is that when it has run its course, people generally recover fully, although it takes a long time. My new patient was starting on the road to recovery, having just been transferred from an intensive care unit in Ventura.

"Simple enough," I thought to myself. I'd done this same routine dozens of times before. But my mistake was in thinking that all patients with Guillain-Barré syndrome were the same.

Mr. Dale Bushey was about to change that. A retired World War II army officer, well-traveled and worldwise, Dale was his own man. He was a husband, father, artist, and stocks-and-bonds watcher. He was also a powerful presence in a room.

I conducted an initial evaluation and issued my report. I believed that Dale was ready to begin the monumental task of relearning some activities of daily living, once again gaining control of his life.

On the first day of therapy, I marched into Dale's room, feeling myself completely in charge. After greeting him with a smile and a firm "hello," I launched into an explanation of dressing training. I ended my speech with my first question to Dale: "Do you want to start with upper body dressing first?"

During my talk, his face had slowly turned bright red, and now he huffed at me: "That's what you think! If I can't do it the way I used to, I'm not doing it!"

My mouth fell open. Too late, I tried to chat with him, then gently explain the importance of learning self-care techniques, but to no avail. He wouldn't budge. I had blown my opportunity to connect with him, and each new attempt was met by an emphatic "No." That day, I left with my tail between my legs.

Throughout Dale's stay, we sparred frequently; he usually won. Finally, with the help of my supervisor and Dale's rehabilitation physician, we negotiated a "treatment truce." Following the new ground rules we'd laid out together, we began to work as a team. Dale steadily and gradually progressed in all of his therapies. He was eventually discharged to his loving family, who helped him continue his outpatient occupational and physical therapy programs at home.

I didn't realize it at the time, but Dale had just taught me a valuable lesson in strength, character, and empathy for my current and future patients.

Several years passed, and I rarely saw Dale. Although I can't recall the exact moment, at some point, we renewed our acquaintance and cultivated a friendship. Gradually, I came to know Dale outside of the rehabilitation setting. We would spend our time together chatting about people we both knew. Before the Guillain-Barré syndrome had set in, Dale had loved to carve delicate bone-and-wood sculptures. He'd lost the necessary hand dexterity, so he instead took up painting. I loved seeing his oil paintings, and he shared his techniques and the stories behind the scenes he painted. He enjoyed giving me the latest news about his children and grandchildren. I thrilled in seeing the seasonal changes in his beautiful garden.

We shared in times of crisis as well. When his home was destroyed in the 1990 Santa Barbara fire, Dale talked to me about the devastating losses of a lifetime, of treasures that would be only memories from that point on. He and his wife confided their dreams in me as they planned and rebuilt a new home. A year later, when I moved to Seattle, we vowed to stay in touch, and we have.

As my patient, this strong-willed man who had always been in control and in charge of his life, his soldiers, his family, his body, had taught me to look beyond myself as a therapist and to see my patients as complete people. Thanks to Dale, I began to try to understand why they did what they did. As my friend, he taught me how to garden and convinced me to begin investing and saving for my retirement (which in those days seemed eons away).

Most importantly, Dale gave me the gift of a lifelong friendship, and as time passes, it becomes all the more special.

Please note: Patient's real name used with permission.

Chapter Forty-Three

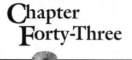

Reflections on Rehabilitation

Peggy Prince Wittman,
EdD, OTR/L, FAOTA

The year was 1963. President Kennedy was shot, mini skirts were just beginning to be popular, the Top 10 songs on the charts were Beatles tunes, and scoliosis, curvature of the spine, was still conservatively treated by spinal fusion, rods, and body casts. At 14, after 2 years in a body brace that had not done enough to keep my spinal curvature in check, I lay in a hospital bed in a university teaching hospital 600 miles from the small town in which I lived. My teenage life had come to a sudden halt and I found myself encased in plaster from neck to knee in a pediatric unit with dying cancer patients and heart surgery patients.

In the midst of this depressing scene, one day a miracle worker arrived. Telling me cheerfully that I needed to gain strength in my arms in order to successfully live flat on my back in bed for the next 6 months, she expertly tied the head of a yarn octopus to the head of my hospital bed and instructed me to braid the arms and legs! I had always loved doing crafts, and suddenly I was doing something I enjoyed again. Nancy returned the next day, excited to find the octopus completed, and bringing with her the first piece of adapted equipment I had ever seen—a pair of prism glasses. Prism glasses fit on the face like regular glasses but have angled glass panels that reflect the images, so that my boring upward view of the ceiling became a forward view, as if I were sitting and looking straight ahead of me. Using these, I regained some of my world; I could see in front of me again, I could watch TV, and most importantly, I could read to keep up with my schoolwork, almost like a normal teenager.

Later, after surgery, again bored by long days with little to do except read and play games with my mother and the student nurses who stopped by a couple of times a week, the miracle worker arrived again. This time Nancy whisked me away on a rolling flat gurney through the hospital maze to a downstairs room where I worked with tiles and proudly made a trivet to take home with me. From that day on, I was hooked on occupational therapy and spent many happy hours there, helping those 6 months of hospitalization to pass.

Nancy, the miracle worker, was, of course, an occupational therapist, and from that long-ago experience I was blessed to discover a career I'd never heard of before; a career that I have found meaningful, challenging, and worthwhile for nearly 30 years.

But even with my career, my days of being a patient were not over. Five and a half years ago, I was suddenly diagnosed with major arterial blockages, and 4 days after my initial outpatient cardiology appointment, I again became a hospital patient. This time my doctor was a cardiac surgeon, not an orthopedic specialist, and my hospital stay was 5 days instead of 6 months. Instead of lying in bed, I quickly became a cardiac rehabilitation client, and my life was changed again in irreversible ways.

This time I knew, intellectually at least, about the curing powers of reflection, writing in a journal, and participating in meaningful activity. Thus, while still in the hospital, I began writing as a way of expressing myself, of holding on to my sanity at times, and of dealing with the many changes happening again in my body, mind, and soul. The following is the last thing I wrote to describe my rehabilitation experience.

"I think that the real power of heart disease is its total disregard for the 'isms' of this world. There is no gender, race, or age discrimination here. I enter the rehabilitation room slowly—I am still not in physical shape to move quickly. I look around at the very mixed group of people (mostly men, but not exclusively, all ages, black, white, Hispanic, Asian) who are to become my next support system, with grave doubts. My 80-year-old mother who has driven me to the rehabilitation center is by far the most spritely of this crew!

"The nurse so hopefully asks why we're here; I give the 'right' answer, while others are more honest—'They told me to come.' I confess I return only because I feel I must—this is, after all, everything I have believed in during my whole professional career. This is rehabilitation—cardiac rehabilitation to be exact—what I teach my students to do with their lives, what I have written about, and what I have countless times told my clients would help them.

Chapter Forty-Three

"The whir of the stationary bikes and the thud of the treadmills become familiar sounds. And those who ride them become my friends. These are the will-to-be survivors, the motivated, the right-to-lifers of my new cardiac world. I become one of them as we struggle to learn to not eat gizzards at all, much less things fried in lard; to adjust to powerful new drugs; to integrate exercising into new lives; to learn about blood sugars and blood pressure and blood clots; to give and take concern for each other. I learn what motivates my new friends. I thought first it must be fear, but I know now that it is courage; Irving's courage to plan ahead to days when he can hunt again, Ed's to once more make his famous hooked rugs for friends and family members, George's to help with his family-run business, Mary's to see her grandchildren, and mine to finish helping raise my daughter, to return to my teaching career, and to finish all the other life tasks that were too nearly cut short.

"The days melt into weeks. I am stronger now; I spend less time in bed when I am home and am able to join friends for lunch. I can begin to think about going back to work; I can again concentrate for short times. This support group stuff really has worked. This rehabilitation process has indeed been helpful. And what else have I learned being here as a 'patient'? That I will miss the staff; that I am impressed with my new-found colleagues. They are, without a doubt, some of the most caring, committed, personable, kind, and knowledgable health care workers I have met on this journey through the wonders and nightmares of modern medicine.

"And I relearn what I have always preached as an occupational therapist. Miles on a treadmill without purpose are useless. The bike odometer alone is meaningless. But when they are linked to my need to stand to teach a class, to remember words so I can lecture, to walk across my daughter's soccer fields, to do those everyday things that make my life uniquely and specially mine, they become powerful tools in this business of getting well. I will always cherish the new-found friends I have made here; I do not know how I could have regained my many losses without their help and support. My 'graduation diploma' will go with me to my office wall to join other professional accomplishments, one newly acquired friend I will continue to see, and this rehabilitation group experience will indeed continue to shape my life as a person and as a professional."

Five years later, these experiences remain with me, influencing my practice of occupational therapy, my teaching, and most importantly, my way of living my life. I consider myself a grown-up version of that teenager in the hospital nearly 40 years ago who was able to get through the long months of hospitalization by being kept productively occupied by Nancy and the occupational therapy staff. I remain impressed by the curing powers of reflecting, writing, and engaging in meaningful activity.

Chapter Forty-Four

The Closet: A "Clothes" Encounter

Gwen Weinstock, MA, OTR/L

You don't usually find miracles in an ordinary closet. As closets go, this one is typical—a big, cluttered mess! Its home is in a locked, inpatient psychiatric unit in a large Manhattan psychiatric hospital in which I worked as an occupational therapy student intern. People needing treatment for immediate mental health crises spend several weeks living in this unit until their symptoms can be controlled with medication, psychotherapy, and occupational therapy. Then they return to their homes or, if necessary, to a longer term treatment facility.

Some of the patients in the unit are admitted on an emergency basis with only the outfit they are wearing, literally the shirts on their backs. To provide something for those clients to wear while they are at the unit, staff members are in the habit of donating clothes. Ironically, their generosity had an unintended consequence. All the donated clothes are stored in that closet next to two occupational therapy activity rooms, stuffed into it as they are brought in, without any attempt at sorting or organizing them. Bags of mismatched shoes, socks, shirts, pants, skirts, and other assorted garments lie on top of one another in a huge sculpture waiting to tumble out and attack anyone who opens the door.

So, when a patient needs an item from the closet it is a challenging and tedious process for the therapist. First, you have to open the closet door carefully so that none of the clothing hits you in the face as it tumbles out onto you. Then you need to go through the bags hoping you can find something that is appropriately male or female, close to the right size, and a bit to the patient's liking. Forget matching outfits or selecting favorite colors or flattering styles. Then all the bags have to be returned to the closet and positioned just right so that the door will close again. The closet, however, was not intentionally messy; the mess just "grew" because the space was filled to overflowing with the haphazard accumulation of bags placed one on top of the other by caring, but busy people.

One afternoon, Harry, a 30-year-old man with schizo-affective disorder, a condition in which people have mood swings and trouble forming relationships, approached me. He had been in the hospital for over a month. Harry was sweet and soft-spoken, and after being in treatment now frequently started conversations with other patients and with staff. A very tall and thin African-American man, he always kept himself and his room very neat and organized. Harry was usually the first to help clean up after group activities, and he had carefully completed many arts and crafts projects that showed how well he was now able to plan, organize, and carry out a complicated activity. However, he had recently mentioned to me that he did not feel fulfilled because he no longer had any personally meaningful tasks in which to participate.

That day, he asked if he could select a fresh pair of pants and a shirt from the closet. Together we walked to the closet. I braced myself for impact while carefully unlocking the closet door. After a minor eruption, the jumbled bags and strewn items settled around us on the floor. We began to search for Harry's outfit. Needless to say, a large-sized shirt and a slim pair of pants were not laying squarely on top of the heap. So we began to dig. I opened one bag. It was filled with women's clothing. That bag was set aside. Harry removed a second bag. The clothes inside were too small. The bag was placed on the floor. We looked through another bag and another bag, and before we knew it, there were bags scattered all over the floor. I saw an opportunity. Thinking that it might be a good purposeful and personally meaningful activity for him, I nonchalantly asked Harry if we could organize a shelf in the closet together. He agreed enthusiastically! So we removed the remaining bags from one of the shelves and put them on chairs and on the floor. We began to look through several bags and boxes to identify the contents.

Another patient passed by. Maria was a large, sweet, shy 29-year-old Hispanic woman with brown eyes, black hair, and a very warm smile, who was diagnosed with depression. This made it hard for her to feel good about herself or to feel hopeful about her own abilities. In training to be an opera singer, her growing depression made it impossible for her to continue in her chosen career, so she was admitted to the hospital. Her growing insight into her depression made her fearful of the life issues she would have to deal with after being discharged from the hospital. Maria ventured toward the closet and asked what we were doing. We invited her to help us organize a shelf. She enthusiastically joined in and began to sort through the women's blouses.

Albert, a usually hostile patient diagnosed with schizophrenia, a thought disorder that often involves disorientation and inability to concentrate or work cooperatively with others, surveyed the scene. Albert was a short man in his 60s with long, white hair and an ever-present shadow of white stubble. He had a long history of alcohol abuse. Albert didn't talk to very many people on the unit, and when he did, his words were often unintelligible. However, the closet organization crew apparently met with his approval, because after observing for several minutes, he asked if he could help too. We welcomed him and directed him toward a box of shoes. Albert sat himself down on a chair and slowly started to match together pairs of shoes.

Several other patients joined in, including Juanita, a 25-year-old woman with schizophrenia who had a penchant for lycra pants and stiletto heels, and Mabel, a large woman in her 50s with schizophrenia who was a regular at our morning grooming group. More boxes were removed from the shelves, and we began to attack the whole closet. Two other occupational therapy student interns saw what was happening and came over to help. They marveled at the concentration and cooperation taking place among these patients who were usually very slow to become involved in group activities. With gentle direction, all the patients were busy at work. One person matched up socks, another folded dresses, and a third sorted through undergarments. Clothes were separated into piles and folded neatly. Doctors and nurses passed by the busy group and shook their heads in amazement. Patients who usually had difficulty interacting with others, following directions, and performing organized tasks were all working together. Some patients were looking through bags, others were sorting, and we noticed several others putting aside items of clothing they liked.

An hour and a half later, the eight of us stood proudly in front of a beautifully organized closet. Flushed with pride in our achievement, we displayed our hard work to the nurses, doctors, and some of the residents. We had accomplished it, every person had contributed, and together we had made a difference. Working together to accomplish this task encompassed what occupational therapy is all about. Occupational therapists take everyday activities that people are having difficulty performing, for whatever reason, physical, emotional, or some other, and help them to do those things again. The feelings those patients expressed—rewarded, purposeful, and proud—made organizing an ordinary messy closet by an unlikely group that afternoon into something quite miraculous.

Chapter Forty-Five

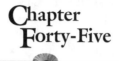

Close to the Edge
Edith Newhall

The two-story atrium at the famous Rusk Institute for Rehabilitation Medicine in New York City is filled with light and has a view of the courtyard. It is ordinarily a relaxing place to be on a busy day. But for several months in 1989, the space was filled with strange apparatus, hoists, forklifts, and other paraphernalia suggestive of a major renovation or a construction project. Only the presence of several large canvases and a determined man with brushes and paints being lifted by the machinery to reach various parts of the canvas revealed the space's busy, not relaxed, true purpose during these months: a studio for the very well-known New York artist, Chuck Close, a patient at the rehabilitation hospital.

Although paralyzed by a sudden illness, Close desperately wanted to continue his painting. His occupational therapist, Phyllis Palsgrove, provided him with adaptive equipment so his body could paint. He supplied the canvases and the lifting equipment from his downtown studio. She persuaded the hospital administration to take unprecedented action and allow the atrium to become the space for him to paint.

The following article by Edith Newhall, excerpted by permission from *New York Magazine* (4/15/91), tells Chuck Close's remarkable story, an example of what can happen when a great artist, a world-renowned New York hospital, and a resourceful and determined occupational therapist work together to make rehabilitation activities a part of real-life:

Two years after he was paralyzed, Chuck Close can paint the way he always did.

On an unexpectedly balmy day in January, sunlight is streaming through the windows of Chuck Close's large studio on Spring Street. As usual, the radio is playing and the phone doesn't stop ringing. The artist sits on the forklift he has always used, putting the finishing touches on a 9-foot-high portrait of the painter April Gornik. Two recently completed canvases lean against the walls: the enlarged faces they depict—painter Eric Fischl and photographer-painter William Wegman—are instantly recognizable to anyone who keeps up with the art world.

Nothing much has changed, really. Except the artist. As he lowers the forklift, he takes an orthotic device off his hand, pulling its Velcro snaps apart with his teeth. When he raises himself out of the forklift, he transfers his body to a wheelchair.

To those who know him, Chuck Close's steady, almost willful, recovery has been nothing short of miraculous. Only 2 years ago, the collapse of a spinal artery suddenly paralyzed him. In the early stages of his paralysis, not even his doctors could have predicted he'd come this far. But for Close, 50, who grew up dyslexic and later developed a style of painting so complex that it sometimes took him 14 months to finish a work, being quadriplegic was simply one more obstacle to surmount, one more problem to solve. "I'm a fighter, and I've always been a fighter," he says matter-of-factly. "These are just limitations that no one would have picked."

Close has already tackled one of the biggest problems: he can paint almost exactly the way he always had. The paintings look remarkably unchanged. Only a few months after he was paralyzed, he started painting again; his new works have been sold—for well into six figures apiece—to New York's Museum of Modern Art and the Modern Art Museum of Fort Worth. This month, he will have two new paintings in the Whitney Biennial and will receive the 1991 Skowhegan Medal for Painting. In October, he'll exhibit a new painting at the Pace Gallery, as he has done about every 2 years since 1977.

Going to lunch in SoHo is not a simple matter for Close. He must maneuver his wheelchair into and out of the elevator, then through the lobby door. But he does it almost daily. Lunch with friends is a routine, like painting ("9 to 5—the whistle blows and I go home"), and Close is a man who cherishes his routines.

Seeing him seated at a table at Savoy, a small restaurant near his studio, I find it hard to believe that Close has experienced limitations of any sort. At

Chapter Forty-Five

6' 3", with a full beard and arms like a wrestler's, the artist is an imposing presence, rather like a friendly bear. Though his large, powerful-looking hands now have no grasp—Close eats by using an orthotic device (a sleeve on his hand into which a fork or spoon is slid and held at an angle)—he orders exactly what he wants and shows no self-consciousness whatever when he spills or drops something. He drinks his wine the way someone might pray, pressing his palms together upright to hold the glass.

Though he has a learning disability that makes it difficult for him to recognize people even after he's met them several times, Close has been painting portraits since 1968. Tight, meticulously rendered portraits painted over grids have given way to looser, almost expressionistic handling of paint. Over the past 4 years, Close has been working on a coarser grid, applying his marks in patterns that transform the face into a field of flickering colors. Viewed from a distance of less than 3 feet, the paintings are almost abstract.

The most significant change for Close has been his attitude toward his paintings. The die-hard formalist who used to come up with "distancing devices" to separate himself from his subjects had finally acknowledged the psychological and emotional aspects of his work. "They were always important to me," he says, "but I tried to approach painting very straightforwardly and not be so terribly involved with who the subjects were. But when I was lying in bed in the hospital, I'd see these faces looming over me and these were family, friends, artists—all the people that I paint. Looking up and seeing the faces of everybody who counted gave a new kind of urgency to recording these images."

December 7, 1988, started out like any other day for Close, except for the chest pains, and he'd had such pains on and off for years. After he leaned against the breakfast table for a while, the pains disappeared, as they always had, so he decided not to worry. He'd been to doctors and had tests (in Japan, he been hospitalized for these symptoms, but the tests were inconclusive).

Feeling better, almost elated, Close left his Upper West Side apartment and spent his entire day walking: down to a 57th Street studio of National Public Radio—he was to be a guest on Weekend Edition—then down to his studio in SoHo, and ending up all the way back uptown at Gracie Mansion, where he was presenting an award to an art teacher. But as he was sitting on the dais, the pains returned more severely than before. As soon as he'd presented the award, he walked off the stage. The police, already warned that Close was not well, escorted him across the street to Doctors Hospital.

At first, Close was treated for what the doctors thought was a heart problem. He was hooked up to an EKG and given nitroglycerin. But by the time his wife, Leslie, arrived, Close had begun to have spasms, and within 2 hours he was paralyzed from the neck down. Leslie Close had him transferred to Tisch Hospital at New York University Medical Center.

Several days and many tests later, Close's doctors were able to make a diagnosis: he had suffered a collapsed spinal artery, which cut off the blood within the spinal column, killing nerves and causing the paralysis.

Close spent the next 6 weeks at Tisch Hospital. His lungs had to be suctioned every few hours to keep them clear. He was given steroids, which made him hallucinate; he gained 30 pounds in a few days (when he went off the drugs, he lost those 30 pounds in 1 day). Throughout his ordeal, he lay wondering how he would paint again. "I remember thinking, How much movement will I have to have if I stick the brush between my teeth? I thought, I'll get the paint on the canvas even if I have to spit it on."

As the weeks passed, Close, whose paralysis was incomplete and asymmetric, began to regain movement. He was transferred to the Howard A. Rusk Institute, NYU Medical Center's rehabilitation medicine unit. There, Close began working with Phyllis Palsgrove, an occupational therapist who sensed early on that her patient was determined to get back to painting. "I'll never forget the day I made him do his laundry. I thought that he was going to kill me," she recalls.

After he'd grumblingly done that laundry, Palsgrove decided not to urge her patient to relearn domestic skills; that used up a considerable amount of his energy. The best therapy, she knew, was to help him achieve the goal he'd already set. "We began to show him that there were ways to do almost anything," says Palsgrove. "We started with writing. I gave him a device that allowed him to hold a pencil; he found out he had more control than he thought he did. And for Chuck, it was relatively easy—after all, his skill had been in his hands. He started thinking that maybe there was a way he could paint. I started asking him things: How did he hold his brushes? Where did he keep his paint? All the time, I was thinking, How are we going to make adaptations for this?"

Palsgrove devised a holder for Close's brushes, and Close designed an easel, which was built by a technician in the occupational therapy department, that allowed him to paint from his wheelchair. Then Palsgrove found a space on the ground floor at Rusk, facing a tree-filled courtyard, where Close could paint in relative privacy. She persuaded the administration to let Close have it. Leslie Close and Michael Volonakis, Close's assistant, brought in the artist's paints, lights, canvas, and other equipment. "We tried to recreate the same kind of atmosphere he'd had in his studio," says Palsgrove. "The lighting, having the photograph beside him, the lighting on the canvas."

Leslie Close remembers the day she saw her husband's first completed painting, a portrait of the painter Alex Katz. Though she had seen the work in progress during daily visits, she had also worried that it might not live up to Chuck's expectations. "It was a profoundly sad, expressive painting. Alex has a sad expression on his face. Although it's incredibly competent technically, I can't look at that painting without crying. The whole experience of his illness and his recovery is in that portrait," she says.

Palsgrove felt triumphant. "He was willing to try anything we could work out. That's probably the answer to it all—he was willing to go along with whatever crazy thing we came up with."

Although Close has had the kind of success few artists enjoy, he has remained very much the person he used to be. He and Leslie are both family-minded, their friends say, devoted to their children, Maggie, 7, and Georgia, 17, who will be going away to college in the fall.

Leslie Close received a master's in history of landscape from New York University in 1980 and was director of Wave Hill's American Landscape History program until 2 years ago. She left her job shortly before Close became paralyzed in order to write a book. Now that her life has begun to resume its normal schedule, she says, she plans to teach landscape history.

Close, on the other hand, has been busy resurrecting his old life. But he's had to make adjustments. He has two assistants, both young artists, who drive him to his studio every morning and take him home at night. Usually, one of them spends the day working for him in his studio. Close can manage a few steps without crutches now, he doesn't expect to regain much more movement, but there has been no definite prognosis. "I need less assistance than I used to, but there still has to be somebody close by me, and I do need help relatively often with my equipment—for instance, to move the hoist over or up and down," he says.

Close had encountered the greatest frustration not inside but outside the studio. "When we are out at our house in Bridgehampton and I'm sitting on the deck watching other people do what I used to do, that can be upsetting," he says. "I used to be very active, and it's very hard to watch someone else doing something that I used to get so much pleasure out of." But he has come to terms with his limitations. "This is something I have 100% of the time, and I don't get away from it. It's a new life now, and it's something I'm learning to deal with. It has divided my life into 'before this happened' and 'after this happened.'"

Close still worries about the effects his paralysis has had on his family. "I might be able to explain it best this way: I sit in a wheelchair... but I often sat down anyhow. I look out at the world, which is virtually unchanged—what I look at is the world I've always looked at—whereas my family and friends look at me and they see someone very changed. They see somebody who's not the way he used to be. I know for my family it's a fresh pain every time they see me in the wheelchair. I'll roll by a mirror and I'm shocked to see myself in that chair."

And it is still difficult for Leslie Close, a candid, intelligent woman who thinks carefully before she speaks. "Chuck is heroic. This has been the most devastating thing I have ever experienced," she says. "Every time I see Chuck in his wheelchair, I feel like crying." But when I ask her if she can think of anything positive that has come out of this, she hesitates only briefly: "I never knew how strong I was—we were. We survived it... life goes on. But it's not over yet."

Reprinted by permission of *New York* magazine, April 15, 1991.

As for Phyllis Palsgrove, every time she hears about a new Chuck Close exhibit opening at yet another gallery or museum, she's very glad that for him it's not over. And she can look back with pride at her resourcefulness and occupational therapy's role in keeping the world supplied with Chuck Close's art.

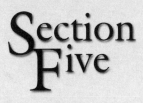

Section Five

Senior Citizens

Enjoying the Rewards of a Race Well Run

Enjoying the Rewards of a Race Well Run

Enjoy the stories of nine older adults coping with illnesses, normal infirmities of aging, retirement, loneliness, changes in living arrangements, and other situations, who are helped by therapists to enable them to conquer these challenges with renewed vigor and hope and to create for themselves a satisfying future.

Potato Pancakes

Vera Cohen, BS, OTR/L and Ellen L. Kolodner, MSS, OTR/L, FAOTA

Mrs. S reminded me of everyone's favorite grandmother. A tiny woman with gray hair in a neat bun, her last gift in her own home to her large and boisterous family was a full-course traditional Passover Seder. She cooked this special holiday meal as lovingly as she had cooked all the family holiday meals for them for her entire lifetime, even though now that she was 83, her daughter was urging her to slow down. A few days later, her life changed forever.

Mrs. S had come to the United States from her native Russia as a young girl; though she lived in this country for many years, she never learned to read or write English. As the years passed, she became the mother of two and then grandmother of four children and took great pride in her abilities as a homemaker and cook. The children were the apples of her eye, and Mrs. S's entire life was devoted to her family. As the family matriarch, she became the center of all family celebrations after her husband died. Her elaborate holiday meals became family legends.

Only days after preparing and serving that large family Passover Seder, Mrs. S's life changed dramatically one morning when illness overtook her and stripped her of all that she had taken pride in. She collapsed at home and was admitted to an acute care hospital with kidney, lung, and other medical problems. When Mrs. S's medical condition improved somewhat, she was transferred to a rehabilitation center attached to an assisted living facility with the plan of returning to her home. "Remember, I'm only going there for a few weeks," she kept telling everyone in her family, "because soon it will be time for our Mother's Day dinner, and I have to start cooking ahead."

Mrs. S was confused and weak, and she could not keep her balance, which made it hard for her to take care of herself, to do simple homemaking kinds of tasks, and to walk safely. So, we began occupational therapy with activities to improve her memory of people, places, time, and general information. Her program of occupational therapy also included weights and upper body activities to improve her strength in her arms for morning care tasks such as brushing her teeth, washing her face, and combing her hair. Mrs. S spent her mornings in occupational therapy doing a variety of activities such as folding laundry, washing dishes, and tossing and catching a ball, to increase the length of time she could do things and to help improve her balance while standing. Other occupational therapy treatment activities included practicing bathing herself, dressing, and safely using a wheeled walker. Ever mindful of her goal to go home, Mrs. S practiced hard and did fairly well with her occupational therapy tasks. "I know I'll have to be able to get in and out of the tub myself, and this tub rail and tub seat will be just the thing to help me," she told her daughter, "and I'd better be able to get to the bathroom myself, too."

Although Mrs. S did well with her therapy, there were still so many things she couldn't do safely by herself that the treatment team and her daughter decided that she would be better off as a resident of the rehabilitation facility's long-term care and assisted-living center. Not entirely convinced, and still hoping to return to her own home, Mrs. S moved into the assisted living section of the facility and was placed on a restorative and maintenance of skills occupational therapy program.

Within 2 weeks it was clear to all of us that she was not doing well. Mrs. S became sullen and began complaining of severe back pain. She just could not find a comfortable place for herself in this new setting. She told everyone who would listen, "I don't like it here," and asked repeatedly "When can I go home?"

Over the next few months, Mrs. S was admitted to the acute care hospital three more times for ever-worsening medical conditions. The second rehabilitation cycle was similar to the first one. The same kind of positive outcomes in occupational therapy were followed by a similar time period in the assisted-living center during which Mrs. S became depressed and then suffered declining health. She still was holding on to the hope of returning to her home, but she understood the reality of her weakening condition. She pleaded with her daughter to keep her furniture and belongings in her apartment "until we're sure I can't go back."

During the third cycle of occupational therapy, it became clear to us that Mrs. S was going to have to adjust to living in the facility rather than at her former home. To do this she would need to find a role and place for herself within the institutionalized setting. Her previous, very precious roles as family matriarch and keeper of religious traditions (i.e. the holidays) were lost to her. Being aware of the importance of these roles to Mrs. S, we felt that we could capitalize on her wondrous talents in cooking to help her replace the lost roles with a newly created role at the facility.

We began by encouraging Mrs. S to teach the occupational therapists and some of the other residents to bake traditional Russian Jewish breads including challah bread, and to cook Russian dishes such as kasha and bow ties and her wonderful potato pancakes known as latkes. These were shared with the staff, other residents, and Mrs. S's family.

Not only were these functional, meaning-based treatment sessions effective in improving Mrs. S's emotional state, but they helped improve her physical condition as well. Moreover, the entire staff looked forward to Mrs. S's cooking. She received many compliments and requests for the recipes and was proud of her accomplishments. She particularly enjoyed having her family join her one week for Friday night prayers with candle lighting and her freshly baked challah. She beamed when she participated in cooking activities, especially when the feast included her legendary potato latkes. Again she could feel like the keeper of her family's religious traditions. Everyone was pleased at how Mrs. S's physical and mental treatment goals of caring for herself, reduction in physical ailments, and emotional adjustment to the residential setting were achieved through participating in these familiar cooking tasks. Cooking and sharing the food was extremely meaningful to her and obviously was therapeutic at the same time.

Mrs. S became a permanent resident of the assisted living facility. Even after restorative occupational therapy treatments were no linger needed and she was discharged from therapy, Mrs. S continued to visit the OT staff to cook. She grew more social with the other residents and staff and loved to contribute her famous potato latkes to parties and special occasions. Mrs. S had finally found a place for herself in her new home.

A year later, after her "official" discharge from occupational therapy, Mrs. S passed away. I visited Mrs. S's daughter's home for the Jewish mourning custom of "sitting shiva" to pay respects. As we ate potato latkes made from her mother's recipe, I gave her daughter some photographs of Mrs. S cooking in occupational therapy. All the pictures showed Mrs. S smiling broadly. Her daughter was very thankful and credited occupational therapy with restoring her mother's well-being and giving her a greatly improved quality of life during her last year at the Center. "With your help she really did find her place in her new home."

We all miss Mrs. S and her potato latkes.

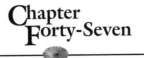

More Scared Than Mean

Constance Martinez-de la Vega, OTR/L

"Leave me alone," she said angrily. I looked at the woman who was lying in bed and realized it was going to be a difficult evaluation. She had been admitted just that morning, and already Sara was getting a reputation of being difficult, cranky, and resistant. Mrs. Sara Church was admitted to the skilled nursing facility, after a short-term hospitalization, with a diagnosis of congestive heart failure and chronic obstructive pulmonary disease. Prior to her hospitalization, Mrs. Church lived independently in a deluxe assisted living residence next to the nursing facility.

I introduced myself to Mrs. Church and her daughter Lara. "My mother is tired; come back tomorrow," Lara told me. Any hope I had of doing an evaluation that day was quickly dashed as Lara stood protectively by her mother's bedside. Mrs. Church did appear very tired and weak. She also looked more scared than mean. I told her I could see that she was very tired and that I would return tomorrow. She managed a small smile of appreciation and waved goodbye.

Lara came to my office later that day. "I just wanted to thank you," she said. Lara explained that her mother had been evaluated by two other kinds of therapists, interviewed by a social worker, and examined by nurses, but not one person listened to her. "You were the only one who listened," Lara said.

Chapter Forty-Seven

The next morning, I tried again. Mrs. Church greeted me with a welcoming "Good morning." "Good morning, you look a little more rested. Are you ready for the evaluation?" I said. "I like you," Mrs. Church said. "You know, you were the only one who listened to me yesterday, and I really appreciate that.

"I really hate it here, and I want to go home," Mrs. Church said in a whisper, as she rapidly drew in her breath and replaced the oxygen mask over her face. "Take your time, Mrs. Church," I told her, "breathe slowly and rest between sentences." "Call me Sara," she said. I explained the role of occupational therapy to her. "You can help me get back home," she said in a rushed voice. Her eyes sparkled at the thought of returning to her apartment.

Sara was determined to get better. We had started her therapy sessions in the morning, so she would have more energy. Some days Sara was so tired she could not move out of bed and would beg me to come back later. I taught Sara energy conservation techniques so that she would not fatigue so easily throughout the day. Sara was sweet, funny, and full of old stories. She often joked that she gave the nurses a hard time because they talked at her and not to her. Sara was not always in the mood for therapy, but I always managed to get her to work with me.

Sara missed her friends. She became very depressed her second week in the nursing home. She really wanted to return to her apartment. Lara was concerned about her mother's health and her depression. Although Sara was making progress toward her occupational therapy goals, the atmosphere of the nursing home really seemed to have a negative impact on her mood. Three weeks into her therapy sessions, Sara was able to put away her oxygen. She was incorporating her energy conservation techniques successfully into her daily activities, but she was still quite weak and depressed. I suggested to Lara that we encourage Sara to exercise more often. I thought we could motivate her to exercise by taking walks to the dining room at the apartment side of the facility in which Sara had her apartment. She could visit her friends and eat the foods she liked by choosing her own menu. We incorporated the walks into our therapy sessions. It took a full week before Sara could make it to the dining room without the assistance of her wheelchair. All her friends at her dining table applauded when she walked in with only her cane to assist her. Sara was so happy and proud, there were tears in her eyes, and Lara was there to share the celebration meal with Sara and her friends. Once Sara was seated, she looked up at me and asked if I would join them. I declined, but before I left, she told her friends, "I am going back to my apartment soon, and this sweet girl is going to help me do it."

The next step of therapy was to make sure Sara could perform her activities of daily living in her apartment safely. Our sessions progressed rapidly, and Sara's mood lifted. Lara commented on how well her mother was doing.

Sara enjoyed being back in her apartment, even if it was briefly for therapy sessions, and loved dining with her friends. Sara performed her exercises faithfully. She used her favorite cane to perform her upper extremity exercises. "I'll do these exercises everyday so I can get stronger and return to my apartment." Our sessions were the highlight of my day. Sara worked hard to get back home. After 8 weeks of therapy, Sara was ready to return to her apartment.

Our last session together was fun and happy. Lara helped her pack for the move back to her apartment. Sara's blue eyes sparkled, and she gave me a big hug before she left. She made me promise to visit and keep in touch. I said I would. She promised to do her exercises faithfully and use all the techniques I taught her so she would never have to return to the nursing home. I visited Sara a few times that year. She was always glad to see me and bragged that she performed her exercises daily.

I relocated to another state in the winter of 1997 and continued to correspond with Sara and Lara. Sara always wrote how much she missed me and how happy she was to be home. She enjoyed visits with her daughter and grandchildren and dining with her friends. When I had not heard from Sara for a number of months, I wrote to Lara. Lara wrote back with sad news. Her mother had passed away in the summer of 1997. Lara reported her mother died peacefully in her apartment. Her mother, Lara said, never stopped bragging about her therapist who helped her return home and how much she enjoyed her therapy sessions. Lara said her mother never stopped doing her exercises, and that her last year of life was spent doing the things she loved most, telling stories, visiting friends, and enjoying her time in her own apartment.

You Could End
Up Anywhere—
Even Meeting
a Woman

Chapter Forty-Eight

Deborah Mandel, MA, OTR

It's easy to tell stories about Roland. At age 74, women and intimacy still baffled him. Roland was one of the participants in the University of Southern California Well Elderly Study, which documented the effects of occupational therapy programs with senior citizens who lived independently in their own apartments. The occupational therapy took place in group and individual sessions. The research team believed that the treatment in the two formats would be synergistic, each would feed the other. Roland's story is a good example.

As a supervisor, I was fed a continuous stream of Roland stories by the treating therapist, Laura. In group sessions, Laura met Roland, who was charming, but also disruptive. "Roland shows up late to group. He barrels through the door, interrupting whatever is going on, talking at the top of his voice about some intimacy problem with his girlfriend." Or "Roland sometimes seems to drift off from the group topic and gets up and wanders around."

In individual sessions, Laura came to know Roland as an artist who, in her words, was intensely searching for clues on how to connect with the world and build successful relationships. Or as Roland himself would express it less euphemistically, he wanted to spend his individual session "getting advice about why women are the way they are." Laura also learned that Roland had been mostly deaf since he was little. Until the age of 74, he had used second-hand hearing aids that either did not work well or were inappropriate. This explained a lot: his sometimes difficult to understand speech, his inattention to group discussions, his loud voice, his interrupting. As Laura worked with Roland, she came to see the many ways that a lack of hearing had affected him and shaped who he was.

One day when Roland bemoaned the fact that his car didn't work, Laura suggested that he take a public bus to the store where he bought art supplies. Laura was surprised by the response from this apparently adventuresome 74-year-old man. "No. No. No. I do not take the bus. Nope, can't do that." With some prodding for the reason, Roland exclaimed, "How do you know when to get off? You could end up anywhere." By now he was visibly agitated. Laura suggested that he only needed to ask the bus driver. "Nope. Nope, can't do that." Why not? Roland looked at her like she was from another planet. "Can't ask questions. You ask questions and they think you're stupid. I learned that when I was little."

Laura tucked this information away until Roland's group was planning their next outing into the community. They decided to visit a museum. Each group member took on some responsibility for the trip. Laura managed to persuade Roland to be in charge of planning the transportation. Together they looked over maps and discussed whether to take the public bus or a local service bus. Roland chose the local bus because the map and schedule were easier to understand. Although he kept blurting out doubts, Laura reassured him that she would be there for support.

On the day of the outing, everybody was waiting at the bus stop. When the bus pulled up, Roland kept deferring to the others to get on ahead of him. Finally, he was the last one. He climbed on, and in his slightly too loud voice spoke to the somewhat burly bus driver, "We're going to the natural history museum, okay?" The bus driver nodded his head. As he took his seat, his chest just slightly puffed out, Laura could see that Roland had turned a corner.

Some months later Roland told Laura, "I gotta thank you, you know. You've really helped me. I can talk to people now." She was confused because Roland talked all the time. What did he mean? "I mean that I can talk to the big guys. I walk right up and talk to that big guy, you know, the head of this place."

I've had a chance to visit with Roland several times since the study ended. He has brand new hearing aids and he's taking ballroom dancing lessons. He goes to the dance at his senior center on Wednesdays and takes a bus to another dance uptown on Saturdays. He's not afraid he'll end up just anywhere. You end up at the dance hall. After all, dancing is a good way to meet women.

Chapter
Forty-Nine

For St. Patrick's Day, Grow a Potato

Mimi Wolak, MA, OTR

I value my Irish heritage, and sometimes it really comes in handy! Although I grew up in a city, as an occupational therapist, I found out one St. Patrick's Day how useful it could be to learn how to grow a potato. The year was 1976. An extended care nursing home facility in rural Nebraska had lost its accreditation due to poor management. One of things it needed to do to regain its accreditation was to hire an occupational therapist, and that was me, a city girl.

One of my first decisions was to start a remotivation activity group on the unit where the most confused residents lived. These kinds of groups, where people can talk about familiar life experiences, are often very helpful in focusing confused elderly people on day-to-day matters and can provide them with the satisfaction of remembering and reliving important life events. Drawing on my own experiences going all the way back to summer camp, I tried just about everything from sing-a-longs to discussions of antique cars. But nothing I came up with created even a spark, let alone any motivation.

Time went by, and when I looked at the calendar, it was St. Patrick's Day. Drawing on my knowledge about Ireland's farming tradition, I thought that it would be fun and meaningful to mark the occasion by planting some flower seeds; certainly this group of farming folk would appreciate flowers! But as we proceeded, it appeared from their lack of enthusiasm that this gardening activity was going to be yet another collosal failure.

Desperate to change the situtation, I remembered that there had been a great potato famine there, which caused a large wave of Irish immigration to the United States. My attempt to discuss the potato famine with the group, however, looked like it was also doomed to fail. That is, until Mable, who always sat mute with her head down, suddenly looked up and asked me if I would like to know how to plant and grow a potato. She then proceeded to explain in great detail how the planting was done. As Mable did so, several other residents chimed in with their own techniques for potato planting and growing success.

By the time the session ended, not only was the group energized and excited, but I knew more about potatoes than a city girl could ever expect to know. I also learned something else extremely important. Book learning and your experience will only take you so far as an occupational therapist. I as a city person had defined connection to the earth as gardening and flowers. I wasn't sensitive enough to realize that these residents shared a history of connecting to the earth by farming and planting what they defined as useful crops, like potatos. This showed me that rather than just talking to or at our patients, we can learn a whole lot more from considering their unique histories and the wonderful and sometimes unusual stories they have to share, if only we are willing to take the time to listen.

Chapter Fifty

A Real New Yorker

Donna Conley, OTR/L

I am an occupational therapist at the Veterans' Administration Day Treatment Center. Our day treatment center is located adjacent to the mental health clinic waiting room. As I passed by one day, I noticed a distraught-looking man with his head down and his eyes filled with tears. He was obviously in the throes of depression. I tried to begin a conversation, but at first he barely spoke, looking away, almost appearing not to hear me. When I mentioned his noticeable New York accent, however, he began to brighten. As we talked briefly about New York, Gino seemed to come alive. He shared stories of the city and of his adventures there. Coincidentally, I was going to visit New York that weekend, and I asked Gino if he had any recommendations for Italian restaurants. He gave me the name of one of his favorite places just as his psychiatrist called him for an interview that would lead to another hospitalization.

I later learned that Gino had a 40-year history of manic depression that often led him to uncontrollable bouts of wildly grandiose highs and suicidal lows. His behavior during these times had led him to legal difficulties and multiple hospitalizations. In fact, it was while he was waiting for hospitalization during one of his suicidal periods that we had that first meeting.

Once he returned from his hospitalization, Gino requested a referral to the day treatment center and became one of our most dedicated "members." During the next several months, I learned Gino's amazing background. During his bouts with depression, he was thrown out of his home when he couldn't afford his rent and became a homeless teenager on the mean streets of New York. When he got older, he founded and later lost several businesses; at different times he owned a restaurant and was the boss of a construction firm. He had suffered through the horrors of state-run mental institutions in the days before medication, where treatment consisted of ice baths to calm the patients and cruelty to amuse the staff. During his long struggle, he landed in prison and lost his civil rights. This was the worst indignity that Gino suffered, he said. He spoke often of his feeling that the label "ex-con" forever marked him as less of a human being, and that he could never be considered a useful member of society again.

As his depression subsided, Gino became extremely active, constantly on the go and involving himself in multiple projects. To focus his energy and assist Gino with reclaiming a sense of purpose, I urged him to begin volunteering. Neither of us could have imagined how this goal would change Gino's life and benefit so many others. He accepted the challenge wholeheartedly. Within a few months, he had gone from collecting day-old bread and delivering it to the poorest people in town to running a full-service program for the poor. His program offered food and clothing to children who lived on the streets, as he had once done. He did whatever he could to make others feel cared about and comforted, including helping people find short-term housing, assisting them with utility bills, and finding job opportunities.

I had to take a leave of absence to recover from surgery. The postoperative discomfort and being at my parents' home had depleted my usual patience. When the phone rang one day, my mother answered it, and moments later called to me, "Some strange man is on the line for you." I immediately recognized the voice at the other end of the phone as Gino's.

My first thought was, "I'm the patient now; I don't have anything to give this man." And then I wondered to myself, "How did Gino manage to find me? Not even at my home number, but at my parents' house?" I had enjoyed working with him for several years, and I was very proud of the efforts he had made to live a productive life despite his mental illness. But on that day, he was still my patient, and it was still not my practice to have patients calling my home. I was unprepared for the message he would deliver.

That day, Gino told me that he had been invited to meet then-President Ronald Reagan. He would be flown to Washington all expenses paid and be honored in a ceremony. My initial thought was that Gino had relapsed and was in the midst of an alarming high and an extraordinarily grandiose delusion. "Poor Gino," I thought to myself. He could almost overhear my thoughts and began to laugh. "No, really! I'm really going to meet the president!"

Chapter Fifty

He reminded me that he had won the local volunteer award for which I had nominated him. That led to his nomination for a national award. That nomination had been made shortly after I left the clinic for my sick leave, and I hadn't been informed yet of Gino's progress. The morning of this call, Gino had been notified that he won, and he would not rest until he shared the news with me. Listening to him, I began to think of all of the city, county, and state awards he had won, and it began to dawn on me that Gino's story was indeed true!

Gino told me often that it was our initial meeting that made him begin to think of himself as a valuable person again. As he put it, "That someone would sit down with a crazy old man and ask his opinion, that made me think I was still worth something." He continued, "And then you told me when you got back from New York that you actually went to the restaurant I recommended, that was amazing!"

Later, Gino proudly shared with me the pictures of himself sitting at the President's table, shaking Ronald Reagan's hand. Seeing him wear his red, white, and blue Presidential Medal, I felt the satisfaction that through occupational therapy, Gino had the chance to add meaning to his life. Gino might not recognize and actually wouldn't use the terms "holistic care," "meaningful roles," or "therapeutic use of self." Instead Gino would put it, he had been "therapized." However you say it, though, his success at both selecting a restaurant and selecting meaningful life activities was more than any of us could have imagined possible.

Chapter Fifty-One

Going AWOL: You Can Go Home Again

Mimi Wolak, MA, OTR

When I entered his room for the first time, Don was sitting on the edge of his bed and his wife was sitting in a chair next to him; they were both sobbing inconsolably. My first thought was that perhaps someone in the family had died. That was not the case, but I was not far off target. It was Don himself they thought was going to die, because according to local folklore, once you had to come to the "Annex," as the extended care nursing home facility in rural Nebraska was called, you were never going to go home; you came there to die. Don Mason was an elderly man whose leg had been amputated due to atherosclerosis, a disease of the arteries that results in decreased blood flow through them, and he was at the facility for post-surgery rehabilitation. When I heard about his fears, as far as I was concerned, my job as an occupational therapist was to convince Don and his wife that he could indeed go home again.

When I questioned Don's wife as to what she needed Don to be able to do for himself in order to care for him at home, her answer was very simple and very practical. If Don could only get in and out of the shower and on and off the toilet, she would be able to take care of him in the comfort and warmth of their home. Don was debilitated and probably going to lose the other leg. But at the time, he was still capable of learning to transfer on his own. I promised Don and his wife that I would teach him how. We worked for the next 3 weeks in the occupational therapy room on proper weight bearing techniques and on strengthening his arms so that he could use them for walking with crutches and for support for the needed transfers. Don was extremely motivated and proved to be a quick learner.

For his 83rd birthday, Don got a special gift—a weekend pass to go home. He confided to me on the Friday before his birthday that he intended to go AWOL; at the end of the weekend, he did not intend to come back, he was going to stay at home. Don was as good as his word. It wasn't quite as simple as perhaps Don thought it would be. It took the help of a home care nursing staff and a devoted and loving wife. But Don did succeed, and in doing so, made a wonderful gift to both the staff and the other residents of the Annex. He taught us all that given the right tools for success, residents did not have to come to the Annex to die; they could come to the Annex to learn the skills they needed so that they could go home again.

Chapter Fifty-Two

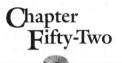

Chicken and Black-Eyed Peas

Vera Cohen, BS, OTR/L and Ellen L. Kolodner, MSS,OTR/L, FAOTA

Hospital food may be nutritious, but as any of us who have ever spent even a day or two in the hospital knows, it is rarely appetizing. Just imagine, then, how it must have appeared to Mr. R, facing a lengthy stay in our rehabilitation facility, deeply depressed, and daily presented with a menu that bore little, if any, resemblance to the ethnic foods to which he was accustomed. Short of starving himself, Mr. R had to learn to take matters into his own hands.

Mr. R had good reason to be depressed. After suffering with diabetes for many years, his kidneys failed, requiring him to undergo dialysis 3 days a week. When circulation in his left leg was severely impaired, he was admitted to an acute care hospital where the leg had to be amputated. That is what brought him to our rehabilitation center.

Mr. R was a retired policeman. He had always been a man of few words, but he had led a very active life, always ready to help others in need. But none of that, other than his refusal to engage in conversation, was apparent when he first began occupational therapy. Mr. R appeared lethargic and confused. He rarely talked, and he was depressed. Worst of all, he had practically stopped eating, only taking a meal on the occasions when his wife arrived with food from home. His weight loss and his lethargy, confusion,

189

and depression seemed to increase as his caloric intake dropped. Something had to be done, and done soon.

The need for Mr. R to practice balance with his new prosthesis turned out to be the key to solving the problem. Mr. R was asked to think of something he would really like to eat and then cook for himself. In the process, he would have to spend time balancing on his prosthesis. The thought of being able to prepare something that would appeal to his taste buds gave Mr. R a new sense of motivation.

He decided on chicken and black-eyed peas, something that had never been on the center's menu. Mr. R sat patiently while he measured out the rice and prepared the chicken and black-eyed peas. Then, balancing on his new prosthesis and using his walker, he made his way over to the oven. After several trips back to the oven to check on the chicken, Mr. R made one more trip to fill his plate and returned to the dining table, with his dish heaped full. The meal was a great success in more ways than one. Not only did Mr. R refill his plate with several helpings, but for the first time in weeks, he was smiling and sociable. The task of cooking something of his own choosing for himself made Mr. R feel like a whole, useful person. Cooking was a therapeutic activity not only because it addressed his need to learn to use his prosthesis; it took into account his whole being, including his cultural and ethnic roots, in a very meaningful way.

Since that first culinary success, Mr. R has made remarkable progress in his rehabilitation and is expected to rejoin his wife soon in their home. When he does, I suspect that they both will eat very well.

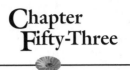

Chapter
Fifty-Three

Operation
Vaudeville

Laurie E. Nelson, MA, OTR

They did not wear uniforms, no one saluted, and they could not order anyone court-martialed. But any general or admiral would have admired and been proud of Ruth's and her neighbors' logistical planning and their ability to organize, motivate, and mobilize their troops, all of whom were veterans—even if their objective was only to cross a road in the dark of night from the East building to the North building in their Los Angeles retirement community to attend a vaudeville show.

I met Ruth when I was working as an occupational therapist for the University of Southern California Well Elderly Study with four groups of older adults living in retirement homes in the Los Angeles area. The study was documenting the impact of occupational therapy programs with senior citizens living independently in their own apartments. The occupational therapy preventive program of health and wellness activities provided the support, education, and experiences that the elders appeared to be craving in order to take more control of their own lives.

Ruth was a member of that community. When I first got to know Ruth, her organizational and logistical skills were still hidden qualities. During our individual meetings in her apartment, Ruth graciously laid out tea and cake for me. It was during those visits that I learned about the occupations—the activities and engage-ments—that had shaped the life of this 80-year-old woman. Growing up, she had enjoyed swimming, lifesaving, body surfing, and dancing. Ruth had wanted to be a nurse, but her mother had enrolled her in business courses instead. That led her into jobs involving accounting and bookkeeping. She had married and raised three sons.

Now, she lived her life at a different pace. She had high blood pressure and slept with oxygen each night. She was able to walk only where there was level ground. Her neck was severely twisted to the right, especially during times of greater stress. Ruth attended a weekly Shakespeare Club meeting in her building, but her participation in community activities had dwindled. Although she owned a car, driving was no longer an option. Ruth told me that most of her close friends had died, and she didn't know her other neigh-bors. Since she liked companionship for social outings, this meant she rarely left her home to enjoy activities of interest.

Through our weekly occupational therapy sessions—conversations while enjoying Ruth's delicious variety of cakes, freshly baked for each meeting—I learned about Ruth, and Ruth learned about the meaning of occupations in her life. She began to take greater control over designing her lifestyle as we discussed topics such as how one's occupations relate to nutrition, physical and mental health, safety, relationships, and transportation.

Ruth became a hostess when we formed a group of community residents, setting up the coffee and snacks and creating a warm and inviting atmosphere for the others. She was consistently present and involved with the laughter and discussions. Behind the scenes, she volunteered to distribute reminders every week to group members living in her building. Each individual brought a unique quality that shaped the group, and Ruth helped make sure that everyone got to the meetings. She created a presence of fun and caring dur-ing the meetings, as well as supplying those delectable cakes. But Ruth was still more of a follower than an instigator or leader.

Ruth rarely missed our outings into the community. These became times of adventure, new exploration, and social connectedness for Ruth and her new-found friends. With enthusiasm, Ruth took her knowledge of occupa-tions on the road. While I watched with pleasure, she tried new types of transportation and was not daunted by unexpected circumstances, for exam-ple when our group had to take a taxi home when caught in the rain after dinner at a new restaurant. Ruth had certainly gained new confidence, knowledge, and skills.

As we neared the end of our program, an important next step for Ruth and the group was to complete an outing without me, their occupational therapy group leader, present. I informed them that I would not be going with them on their next trip.

When presented with this possibility, Ruth was hesitant but up for the challenge. Plans had to be thorough and precise in order for the group members to feel comfortable enough to even attempt the activity. As usual, we made it a group activity to decide on the event. The group chose to attend a vaudeville musical performance to be held at their retirement home later that week. At first I was relieved that they had chosen such a simple outing. I thought to myself, "This will surely be a positive experience for all of them." However, I soon realized that the outing would be anything but simple. That's when Operation Vaudeville was launched.

The musical presentation the group chose was scheduled to take place in the North building. Ruth's apartment, along with many others, was across the street in the East building. This created a major safety obstacle because the event was to be held at night, when Ruth and the others had never dared leave their building alone.

Having worked at this retirement home for several months, I knew that we had already broken new ground by asking seniors to attend activities across the street in the daytime. The North building was always locked, and if the regular attendant at the door was unavailable, Ruth and her friends could easily be stuck outside for a long period of time.

So this outing required intensive planning and teamwork on the part of the seniors in order to accomplish what some may consider a simple task. They developed a strategy. Ruth, Mary, and Laura, from the East building, would gather in their lobby at a designated time. Together, they would cross the street in anticipation of finding Doris, a North building resident, waiting at the door to let them in 15 minutes prior to show time. If for some unexpected reason Doris was not there, they would initiate their backup plan. They could ring Diana, another North building resident, on the intercom. She would be stationed in her apartment ready to receive the signal to come down and let them in. Diana was instructed to wait for their signal until 5 minutes to show time before heading downstairs herself.

Meanwhile, seniors in the North building would commence action, addressing a different kind of challenge. Designated seniors would call those group members with memory impairments. By calling them no more than 30 minutes before the show, they could prompt these members to head downstairs to join the rest of the group.

They went over the strategy and rehearsed their parts until they were certain that the plan was foolproof, then waited for the big night.

It was a success! Ruth explained that even an unanticipated snag they ran into did not throw them. It was an unexpected one-dollar donation collected for the musical performance. This became an embarrassing situation for some, but luckily enough cash could be pooled from among the other group members to cover the costs for everyone. Although they were unprepared for the donation, the rest of the plan worked smoothly and safely. They did add one creative factor, however. The group from the East building brought along their flashlights as they crossed the street.

As we discussed the experience afterwards, Ruth was amazed and proud of her accomplishment. She and her friends had participated in an evening outing without their group leader. It was an empowering moment as they realized that they were able to network and plan and go to an event as an independent group. Ruth recognized the value of community, and how much more freedom she had when she and her peers worked together.

At the end of the discussion, Ruth laughed and compared me (a 28-year-old occupational therapist) with her mother. I wasn't sure how to take that, until Ruth noticed my puzzled expression and clarified her compliment: "When I was a youngster, it was my mother who taught me independence. Now that I'm a senior citizen, you've taken her place and taught me independence again."

Chapter Fifty-Four

A Man and His Dog: The Story of Barney and Bob

Patricia H. Findlay, OT

After the death of his wife, Bob carried on, spending his winters in Florida and summers in a small unheated cottage in northwestern Ontario. He shared this retirement lifestyle with Barney, a small terrier. Barney had been adopted by Bob and his wife a year or two before her death and had accompanied them in all their travels.

Finally the time came when the yearly trip back and forth to Florida was too much, and Bob had to find winter accommodations closer to home. Although Bob was eligible for all levels of supportive accommodation for senior citizens in the city of Winnipeg, Barney wasn't welcome any place. Unwilling to separate, Bob found a private room and board setting in which Barney was also a welcome guest.

They spend their winter days sitting on the couch dozing, watching television, or supervising the activity at the bird feeders just outside the patio doors close by. Barney leads a quiet life, rarely moving, only jumping off the couch to get supper or to go out the patio doors. He then crosses the cedar deck and jumps into the garden to eliminate, barking at the birds on the way to let them know who's boss. Last January, the landlord noticed that Barney was no longer going as far as the garden but was eliminating on the deck itself. The landlord raised concerns about damage to the deck. Bob was also concerned because Barney would no longer jump up onto the couch when told to do so.

Bob was very upset. He saw his choices as either getting rid of Barney, his beloved companion and reminder of the life he had formerly enjoyed with his wife, or moving to less pleasant and far more expensive housing. Aware of the distress the situation was causing, the landlord's wife, an occupational therapist, applied an occupational therapy approach to the problem.

While both Bob and Barney must be considered "frail" elderly, for the most part they manage well. Their health is closely monitored, and they are treated by their respective doctors with appropriate medications. They are fiercely independent and strongly motivated to manage on their own. Bob has cardiac and balance problems, complicated by inactivity, as well as some minor memory lapses. Barney has severe arthritis and a Parkinsonian tremor, mainly in his hind legs. Both have a hearing impairment.

The occupational therapist observed Barney for a few days and came to realize that, while he could jump down off the deck into the yard, about 12 inches, he couldn't consistently jump back up again. This was much worse when the temperature got down below 0°F. It was obvious that the arthritic pain and stiffness were interfering with his function. Once the problem was identified as physical frailty rather than sheer cussedness, the landlord was quite willing to do whatever was necessary to help Barney. Soon he built a ramp out of the locally available material (i.e., snow) between the garden and the deck. With training from the landlord and lots of encouragement from Bob, Barney was soon using the ramp quite effectively. However, on a really cold day he still needed a lot of verbal persuasion.

The task of jumping onto the couch was broken down into two steps by putting a small stool next to the sofa. This worked for a while, but eventually even jumping that distance became difficult for Barney and another solution had to be found. At first Bob stood near the sofa and tried to bend over and pick Barney up. This usually resulted in Bob's losing his balance and falling backward onto the couch. It was more difficult to persuade Bob to change how he did things than it had been to retrain Barney, but eventually he learned to sit down on the stool and then pick Barney up.

Bob and Barney have been able to maintain the lifestyle they want by being willing to change the way they do things and to make minor modifications to their environment. They can now spend their time doing what's important to them—supervising the birds. The birds still pay no attention at all.

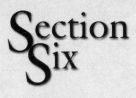

Not Always a Safe Haven

Accidents at Home, Work, and Play

Accidents at Home, Work, and Play

Read about ten unusual, unpredictable accidents and injuries such as falls, sports injuries, and other major traumas sustained at home, work, or play by people going about their daily activities who are fine one minute and seriously impaired the next. Their descriptions of recovery from such debilitating accidents, with the help of therapists, show others how concentration and creativity help people put their lives back together after sudden devastating events.

Chapter Fifty-Five

Doctor, Will I Be Able to Play the Piano?

Denise McCormick

It was not the way I had anticipated beginning the summer. With 2 days of school left, I was frantically trying to organize myself for a move to teach at another school at a different grade level. I was alone in the classroom in the early evening at the end of May, where I had come for just a quick stop to do a little more packing. I climbed up on the radiator. It took less than a second for the climb to change the course of my life for the next year. I put out my hand to steady myself on a board above me that served as a shelf, and it suddenly collapsed. I fell from my perch and almost immediately felt excruciating pain in my wrist.

It took a lot of gritting my teeth and strength for me to pick up my now useless hand and walk to the other side of the building to call my daughters and husband. Our local hospital could not surgically set my wrist, so my husband drove me to Burlington, Iowa, which was a half hour away. The wrist had to be pinned in two places. At 1:30 a.m. we returned home. I was upset with myself and how the accident had immediately turned an ordinary evening into pure chaos.

The next 2 months were slow and agonizing for someone as active as me. I wondered if life would ever return to normal, as I was now suddenly dependent on others for the simplest ordinary tasks. But the worst was not being able to play the piano. I had enjoyed playing for church, weddings, and funerals, but all of that was now definitely out of the question. Secretly, I worried about my ability to ever play again. The cast had covered most of my hand, and the day the cast was removed, my hand was totally useless. The doctor had not told me anything that I could do while the cast was on that might have helped to prevent the total deterioration of my hand. Then, when the cast was removed, he actually asked me if I wanted to rehabilitate my hand myself or did I need therapy. There was certainly no question in my mind that I needed help.

Luckily, when I called Henry County Health Center, they referred me to Joe Whalen, the occupational therapist. I waited through 4 days of nervous anticipation and total frustration before I walked into the occupational therapy room. I had been crying the entire morning because up to this time I had received little information about what lay ahead. I immediately relaxed, however, because Joe seemed to sense my utter despair and quickly started talking about what we would be doing to regain the use of my arm and hand. Of course it had been my right, dominant hand, and with school less than a month away, I was more than a little anxious to recover.

Joe explained that while it had been my wrist bones that I broke, the muscles surrounding and guarding the area had been badly injured as well, and right now they were what prevented me from being able to use my hand. My hand was twice as big as usual from the swelling, and there was scarring where the pins had been in my arm and hand. Words cannot possibly describe the pain I felt when trying to move or work with the hand. Nevertheless, I was eager to begin to get it back to normal, and we got started with occupational therapy right away.

To warm up my arm before therapy sessions, Joe would have me put my arm in a machine called Fluidiotherapy, in which ground corn was heated and swirled around. You put your hand into an opening on the side of the machine, and the warm cornmeal gently swirls around it, warming, supporting, and massaging your wrist and fingers, making movements much easier. To make it more interesting, as well as to improve finger and wrist dexterity, small objects are placed inside for you to find. As you feel them moving around, sight unseen, you pick them up and manipulate them in your fingers to identify them, and thereby move your wrist and fingers within the supportive and comfortable environment. It felt great!

I grew to enjoy my sessions in the Fluidiotherapy, but one of my greatest inspirations was another patient of Joe's. His name is Dennis, and he had been in a car accident. In the accident, he had a broken neck and a very high level injury to his spinal cord. My first day with Joe, Dennis walked in on his own toward the middle of our consultation. I knew what he had been through and realized that he was literally considered a walking miracle. I knew from that moment on that I was in good hands with Joe as my therapist.

During therapy, I learned that there are many parallels that can be made between occupational therapy and teaching. Each individual must be considered for his or her own uniqueness, and for success to occur, those individuals must be validated and supported continuously. My 7 months of occupational therapy included friendship, caring, understanding, and lots of hard work of stretching, massaging, splinting, and doing various activities geared toward moving my wrist and fingers. Of paramount importance also is the creativity of the person in charge to make routine tasks exciting and meaningful. I never ceased to be amazed at the problem-solving strategies employed by Joe when a roadblock would occur for me or for another person. If I had not gone for occupational therapy treatment, I shudder to think what shape I would be in today, both emotionally and physically. The lessons I learned in occupational therapy will carry over into everything I do.

I am eternally grateful that now I am swimming a half mile 5 days a week, lifting weights, and enjoying my life with enthusiasm and vigor. Best of all, I am again back at the keyboard playing the music I love for people I really care for. The one thing I do not do with my hand is use it to grab overhead shelves, because my days of foolishly climbing on radiators and other unstable surfaces are over.

Chapter
Fifty-Six

The Return of
My Ring Finger

Jill E. Van Dyke, OTR

One single accident changed my life forever. Accidents don't usually have positive consequences, at least none that are obvious at the beginning, but mine certainly had great results in the end. If not for my accident, I never would have met my husband; I never would have had my wonderful daughter, Julia; and I never would have learned about occupational therapy or become the kind of occupational therapist with first-hand knowledge about my patients' experiences.

On June 21, 1983, I finished my last final exam of my first year at a community college in Jackson, Michigan. I rushed home to get my Wendy's restaurant uniform out of the dryer. As I ran down the basement stairs, I tried to flip on the light switch, which was situated on the ceiling. Out of habit, as I had done for years, I jumped down the last two steps. The light switchplate had broken long ago, and a metal piece was bent outward. It had never been a problem before, but this time, my ring caught on the metal, and with the full weight of my body bearing down on it, my ring finger was torn completely from my left hand.

My mother, a nurse, knew exactly what to do. She grabbed my severed finger, put it on ice, and sped off with me to the local hospital. There, they stabilized me and put me in an ambulance to the emergency room at University of Michigan Hospital in Ann Arbor. Once there, I was met by two plastic surgeons, Drs. Stevenson and Friedman. They operated on my finger for 6½ hours and successfully reattached it. It was a very welcome sight to see my finger turning pink again with circulation. My family and I were elated.

I would soon discover, however, that the hardest part of my ordeal was yet to come. I spent a full week in the hospital recovering. I remember the frustration of not being able to do much for myself early in the healing process. I will never forget one meal in particular that was served to me, or rather, that was dropped off on my bedside table. How could I forget that big slab of lean ham as the main course? No one seemed to notice or care that I had extensive bandages on my left hand and an I.V. line on my right hand. I could not open any packages or cut my meat. I thought I was going to go hungry, until someone finally answered my call and arrived to help me.

When I first got home from the hospital, I hoped to get back to a normal life, but this wasn't immediately possible. I wanted nothing more than to take a shower. But with all the bandages, I couldn't do it alone. My mother and my sister had to help me bathe. I had never felt so humiliated and helpless in my life. Of course, things got much easier for me as time passed and I regained use of my hand, but it was a long process.

Once home, I was referred to outpatient occupational therapy for rehabilitation. I spent the next 3 months relearning how to use my hand and getting past the almost unbearable pain of extremely hypersensitive nerves following the reattachment.

During rehabilitation, a beige hand splint was fashioned for me. I was worried that people might think I had a fake hand. Because I always was concerned about my appearance, I pretended it was like a plaster cast, and I asked my friends to sign it for me! This made me feel much better because it stopped any confusion about a fake hand.

As an added benefit of my rehabilitation, I met people who would change the course of my life forever. For example, Hildy Martin, an excellent hand therapist, taught me all about occupational therapy. The activities she had me do to help me regain strength and range of motion helped me regain dexterity in my hand. After talking with her and seeing what she had been able to do with my hand, I decided to become an occupational therapist. The September after my accident, I applied to the occupational therapy program at Western Michigan University, and I started occupational therapy school the next year.

As a result of attending occupational therapy school, my life took a whole new turn. As one of my fieldwork assignments, I returned to the University of Michigan hospital and even had the chance to review my old records. One day as I was going down an escalator, I ran into Dr. Stevenson, who remembered my case, and we had the chance to talk about it, this time as medical professionals, rather than doctor and patient. As an intern at a summer camp for children and adults with physical impairments, I met a handsome recreational therapist who was doing his fieldwork internship there that summer as well. Knowing well the value of interdisciplinary cooperation, we soon established several programs together for our campers/patients. After relating to each other as medical professionals all that summer, for the past several years now our new relationship is that of husband and wife and parents of a daughter.

My experiences as a patient all contributed to the kind of therapist that I have become. I never leave a patient's room without making sure that my patients have their call lights accessible; I help them open packages when appropriate; and I always respect my patients' dignity, being careful during their occupational therapy training in dressing or intimate activities of daily living, that curtains are pulled and bathroom doors are shut. For some patients, I acquire different-colored splint material and straps in order to give them the choice that I never had during my rehabilitation. What's more, I can empathize with their feelings of hypersensitivity, pain, and frustration during the long road to healing.

It took 10 years before I ever wore a ring again, and even now I choose to wear my wedding ring on my right hand. While I have scar tissue and a slight deformity in my finger, I have regained complete function of my hand thanks to the occupational therapists who treated me. On June 21 every year, I celebrate—yes, celebrate—the anniversary of my hand injury. I think about how it changed my life and how having had that first-hand experience led me to a career in occupational therapy.

Chapter Fifty-Seven

Socks or No Socks? That Is the Question

Margret I. Kingrey, MA, OTR

D r. P came walking down the hall with his cane. He was an elderly, slightly portly gentleman who had refused occupational therapy the day after he was admitted to the skilled nursing unit 3 weeks before. He had broken his hip in a fall at home and had been admitted for rehabilitation following surgery.

"I only want to walk and go home," he had stated when I first screened him for occupational therapy. "I was one of the first doctors in this valley. That was in 1934. I've been practicing medicine ever since. I ought to know what I need."

Apparently unaccustomed to being a patient, he was pleasant, but firm in his denial of his need for my services. He was confident that he knew what occupational therapy was since we were working with his wife who lived at the nursing home because he could no longer take care of her at home. She had dementia and he acknowledged that we were doing a good job of helping her eat and socialize, but, as far as he was concerned, occupational therapy wasn't for him.

Two weeks after his arrival, however, Dr. P's physical therapist stopped me in the staff lounge to ask if I would reevaluate him. He was now moving around on his own, but was having difficulty putting on his pants and socks. He always wore slip-on shoes, so they were no problem to get on.

"Sure, I'd be glad to. However, last time he refused occupational therapy. I'll try again when he's down in the PT gym next time. When is he being discharged?" "We are planning on discharge in another week, as soon as we think he's safe," the physical therapist told me. "He does have some family and neighbors in the area, but you know those slip-on shoes don't fit that well without socks and we don't want him falling again." She hurried off to work with a patient, leaving me to ponder my approach to someone who didn't realize he needed my help.

Later that afternoon, I armed myself with a stocking aid, a dressing stick, and a smile, then walked into the physical therapy gym. Dr. P was working on some mat exercises. "Hi, Dr. P, your physical therapist says you're having trouble putting on your socks. I thought I might be able to show you something that would help you do it by yourself." "No, thank you," Dr. P responded a bit irritably. "My socks and I are getting on just fine."

"OK," I said, "Glad to hear it." I picked up my gadgets. "Let me know if you want to see how to use this stuff later. Just tell Nora, the physical therapist, or the nurse and they'll call me."

"Sure, sure," he huffed as I left.

Two days after the encounter in the gym, I spotted Dr. P walking down the hall. He did not have his cane with him, and poking out of his shirt pocket like a dress handkerchief was the top of a pair of black socks. I glanced at his bare feet inside his shoes as I smiled and commented, "How about that, you're getting around without your cane. That's great! I notice though that your socks are in your pocket, do you need help getting them on?"

"Oh, I'll find a nursing assistant to help me after awhile," he grinned sheepishly. "That's fine, but where are you going to find a nursing assistant when you go home?" I quipped. "You know I have a very handy gadget for helping with socks when there are no nursing assistants around. I'll see you in the gym this afternoon."

That afternoon I again approached Dr. P while he was on the mat. He offered no objection as I demonstrated how to put the sock onto the stocking aid and put it on his foot, simulating pulling it up. "Now you try it."

Dr. P took a sock out of his breast pocket, put it on the stocking aid, slipped his foot into the space, and pulled. "I'll be damned!" he commented in surprise. "Guess I better have one of those." The physical therapist grinned, "See, now you can do it by yourself."

Dr. P decided that the occupational therapist was a pretty good person to know. After his sock success, he requested more occupational therapy and I worked with him on other activities such as cooking, small household chores, and driving. When he was discharged to his home, he was independent in all of his daily self-care skills, drove his car, and did some light meal preparation.

Several months later, I saw Dr. P at the grocery store near our neighborhood. "Say there OT, how are you? You know I still use that sock thing every day. I'm sure glad you were around since there are no nursing assistants at my house," he chuckled.

We chatted for a bit and then went our separate ways. I was pleased with myself. I taught one of the pioneer physicians in this valley how to put on his socks. What a great profession I have!

Chapter Fifty-Eight

Believe in Me

Jan Keith, COTA/L, AP

I opened the City section of the *Eau Claire Leader-Telegram* and immediately spotted her picture among the obituaries. Was this just coincidence, or a message from God, reminding me of the impact this woman, unbeknownst to her, had on my life? It was August 1996 and my husband and I had returned for a visit to Eau Claire, Wisconsin, after moving to Wyoming 13 months before. This unexpected glimpse of her picture brought back vivid memories of a time 2 years earlier. Little had I realized then that this tiny, frail, yet spunky woman would have a profound impact on my life, both personally and professionally. Neither did I foresee how a casual comment she made would forever bring tears to my eyes whenever I recalled "our" story.

I could tell from the start that Millie was going to be a "problem" patient, not that she was all that different from many of the other patients I worked with as a certified occupational therapy assistant at a 218-bed skilled nursing home in west central Wisconsin. While many of the geriatric patients I treated were highly motivated and cooperative about receiving occupational therapy services, others, like Millie, participated with reservation and subtle (or not so subtle) resistance.

In June 1994, Millie fell at her home with resulting vertebral compression fractures. After her discharge from the acute hospital, at 83, Millie was admitted to our nursing home for rehabilitation. She needed additional nursing and rehabilitation services in our facility to complete her recovery and allow her to return home safely to live on her own again.

As part of her recovery process, Millie's doctor ordered occupational therapy to help her achieve independence in daily life skills, and this is where I came into the picture. In our geriatric setting, daily life skills training generally meant assisting patients to regain their ability to do basic self-care tasks (feeding, dressing, grooming, toileting, and moving using canes or wheelchairs if necessary) as well as the higher skills needed to live on their own in the community, including transportation, meal preparation, money management, and homemaking activities.

Millie's first occupational therapy evaluation showed that she was in a generally weakened state, with poor endurance. Her vertebral compression fractures caused her considerable pain with any movement and particularly with bending, making walking and putting on clothing below the waist especially difficult. My goals in therapy were to help Millie regain strength and stamina through an individually tailored exercise program, to teach her adaptive techniques that would make dressing easier and less painful for her, and to help her learn to move safely and effectively with her walker while doing her household tasks.

This was all fairly routine to me; however, it quickly became apparent that Millie was not going to be a routine patient. While she arrived punctually in the occupational therapy clinic each day, looking prim and proper with her tightly permed, meticulously combed gray hair and wearing her carefully coordinated maroon polyester pant suits, once there she did not retain the image of a docile compliant octogenarian. "This is for the birds," she would say daily as we started her exercise program. "I don't need this stuff. I don't see how this is going to do me a bit of good."

I tried different approaches and different exercises, but Millie's response was always the same. While she was adorably pleasant and chatty with the silver-haired friends who came to visit her, she remained gruff and uncooperative with me and her occupational therapy program.

Despite her frequently voiced opposition, Millie worked on her exercise program and would, at times, practice a new dressing technique. To help increase her strength and stamina, I put small plastic weight cuffs on her arms while she performed the activity of stacking upside-down plastic cones one on top of another to build a tower and while she hung clothespins on higher and higher rungs of a ladder hooked onto a table top. To make her fingers stronger, she found small pegs hidden in thick pieces of therapy putty and did shoulder exercises using a weighted wooden dowel as a barbell to strengthen her shoulders. She made pegboard designs while standing at the counter to increase the time she could spend standing up and tried maneuvering with her walker in small, tight spaces. She practiced using a long shoehorn to put on her shoes without bending and learned safe ways to move without hurting her back. Millie did all these activities and more, faithfully, though reluctantly and not without her constant, "Oh, for heaven's sake! Why do I have to do this anyway?"

I began to dread Millie's occupational therapy appointments and felt a growing discouragement in being unable to motivate her or help her realize the value of occupational therapy. But we stuck with it, she and I, and as the weeks went by, Millie grew stronger despite her verbal resistance. I watched as she became able to move about more confidently with her walker and dress herself faster and with less assistance. After 4½ weeks of occupational therapy, it was decided by those of us involved with her care that Millie was ready for discharge from our facility and could return home to her own apartment.

When the day of Millie's discharge arrived, I was secretly relieved. Although I was pleased that she had achieved her therapy goals, I felt that all I had succeeded in doing was irritating her. Actually, I wasn't even sure if I had had anything to do with her recovery at all.

My personal tradition at the time of facility discharge has always been to say a private good-bye to the patients I've worked with and wish them well in their adventures beyond the nursing home. Most of these "good-byes" follow a fairly common scenario and my farewell to Millie that warm, July afternoon started out typically.

"Hi, Millie," I said, walking through the doorway of her room. "I know you'll be leaving in just a little while and I just wanted to stop in to tell you good-bye. I hope things go well for you at home and that we won't see you here again unless it's as a visitor."

"Thank you so much for all you've done for me," Millie replied sincerely, sitting on her bed, surrounded by boxes and bags of her belongings.

"But Millie," I reminded her, "remember that you were the one who did all the hard work."

"I know," Millie said as she smiled up at me, "but you believed in me."

"...but you believed in me... but you believed in me... but you believed..." Millie's words echoed through my mind that afternoon and for a long time afterward. What a revelation for me! Until that moment, I had felt that I hadn't been able to reach Millie as a therapist. But with her telling comment came the realization that what she had needed most was someone to believe in her... someone who believed that she would recover and return home. Someone who was willing to work with her day after day to realize that goal in spite of her sour attitude and her unfriendly demeanor. My effectiveness as an occupational therapist, at least in Millie's case, had come not through the performance of a highly technical therapy procedure or the use of an innovative treatment technique, but instead through the simple conveyance of confidence and belief in another person.

I never saw or heard from Millie again after that summer afternoon, but her comment changed me by increasing my awareness of the awesome power that we as occupational therapists have to positively affect other people's lives. That comment became a gift that has made me a much more effective therapist. I continue to try to apply "Millie's Principle" to my therapy work by demonstrating to my patients my strong belief in them and in their capabilities. Millie taught me that by believing in the potential in others, and sharing that belief with them, I can give them the amazing power of believing in themselves. That belief and self-confidence are gifts I can return to others, a gift that could help them in accomplishing great things, or as in Millie's case, even when the task at hand is simply surviving your stay in a nursing home and going home again to live on your own.

Grandmother Ora Goes Home

Donna Holt, BS

Grandmother Ora was fixing a simple meal in the kitchen of her one-bedroom apartment when she tripped on her kitchen rug and fell. Somehow, despite her intense pain, she managed to drag herself across the floor to her living room area where a phone sat on an end table. Desperately grabbing the phone cord, Ora tugged until the phone fell to the floor, and she was able to summon the paramedics.

When the paramedics delivered Grandmother Ora to Edwin Shaw Hospital, a rehabilitation facility, the initial admission just showed a woman in her 70s with an arm fracture and a bruised hip. But further investigation revealed that Ora was a very unusual patient. My grandmother had lost her right leg to bone cancer at age 7. At that time, extensive surgery had also been performed to remove cancer from one arm. As a result, her left elbow was permanently bent at an approximately 80 degree angle of flexion.

Ora had started walking with crutches at age seven and continued until she turned 16, at which time she had her first artificial leg prosthesis made. After that, she walked everywhere, and never used a wheelchair. Later, while living in Calgary, Alberta, Canada, she spent almost 3 months in the hospital while a new prosthesis was made for her. Today, technology is much more advanced in the area of prosthetics; they are lightweight, constructed from plastics, and are extremely functional. But the one my grandmother was using the day of her fall was the same one she had gotten way back then in Canada. After she returned to Ohio in 1973, numerous adjustments had been made to it due to wear and tear from daily usage, but the prosthesis itself did not change. It weighed a very hefty 16 pounds and was held to Ora's body by shoulder straps. She was able to dress herself, used a girdle to hold her hosiery, wore a stump sock to protect her body where it fitted into the artificial leg, and put handkerchiefs under the shoulder straps to protect her skin. But over the years, the shoulder strap supports and the weight of that leg had left permanent indentations on her body.

With all that, Ora was a fiercely independent woman. She married and raised a child despite murmurings from relatives who said she would never be able to have a family because of her physical condition. My mother and I am certainly glad they were wrong! Not only did Ora raise her own child (my mother), when she was in her 60s, my grandmother worked as a caretaker for a family with five young children!

At Edwin Shaw Hospital, Ora knew exactly what she wanted. She wanted only to go back to her apartment and take care of herself just as she had done before the fall. She wanted to cook her special soup, which she delivered personally to friends in the apartment building; to play cards and bingo with the other seniors; and to go on field trips with them in a bus. It was a simple, straightforward set of goals, but also an ambitious agenda for someone Ora's age and in her condition.

During her hospitalization, Ora was assessed by an occupational therapist. After an initial period of healing for her arm fracture, Ora began to work toward the goals she had set for herself with the therapist. If she was going to live independently again in her apartment, she needed to increase her arm and hand strength. Arm and hand strength were crucial to dressing and undressing, preparing meals, being able to do her housekeeping chores, and for engaging in her favorite leisure activities. Ora did qualify for some outside home health aide assistance, and the family was willing to help out as well. But as far a Ora was concerned, she wanted to maintain as much of her independence as possible and was intent on doing as much as she could for herself.

Not all of my grandmother's needs were physical in nature. Psychologically, the whole ordeal of feeling dependent on the hospital staff as well as being away from her own apartment and her friends was extremely difficult for Ora. This aspect of Ora's rehabilitation was not overlooked by her occupational therapist, who was holistic (i.e., interested in the whole person) in her approach and cared as much about Ora's psyche as she did about her arm. The twin sets of need came together in purposeful activities that served to increase my grandmother's arm strength, while at the same time keeping her occupied in activities that were meaningful to her. Ora attended bingo, cooking classes, and ceramics and jewelry craft classes at Edwin Shaw. One of my most cherished possessions today is a ceramic dog painted to resemble the colors of my own pet dog that Ora painted for me while she was at the hospital. I treasure it now as a special memory of my grandmother.

Knowing Ora, it was no surprise that she met her goal and was able to return to her own apartment. She needed a little help, particularly with bathing, but soon her neighbors once again received her special soup, lost to her at bingo and cards, and enjoyed her company on outings. That terrible fall my grandmother had taken could have been devastating. She could have ended up having to live in a nursing home and needing to be taken care of for the rest of her life. But thanks to her determination, and the willingness of the occupational therapists at Edwin Shaw Hospital to help her achieve her goal, Grandmother Ora was able to go home.

Chapter
Sixty

Stand Up
and Be Counted

Vera Cohen, BS, OTR/L and
Ellen L. Kolodner, MSS, OTR/L,
FAOTA

M r. M has a tallit, a prayer shawl worn by Jewish wor-
shippers in synagogue. Mr. M also has a very devoted
son who is very observant and attends synagogue on the
Sabbath and on various holidays. When I met him, Mr. M wanted to go to synagogue with his son and pray next to him wearing
his prayer shawl.

But Mr. M, an otherwise very independent 82-year-old
Russian Jewish immigrant, had fallen down the steps of his two-
story home where he continued to live alone after the death of
his wife. He fractured his left leg and injured his right wrist and
was placed in a full leg cast and right wrist brace for support.
These injuries, together with his arthritis, meant Mr. M needed a
lot of assistance with upper body care such as bathing and dressing and was totally dependent on others for lower body self-care.
He needed assistance walking, since he was not allowed to put
full weight on his left leg. Mr. M was accustomed to being independent and had difficulty accepting confinement to a wheelchair and being dependent on certified nursing assistants for his
self-care.

Due to Mr. M's arthritis, occupational therapy focused on
strengthening his upper body and right wrist with light weights,

since he would need to support himself until his left lower leg cast was removed and increased weight bearing was allowed. Self-care using long-handled equipment was also introduced for increased independence.

By the time the cast was removed, Mr. M had improved in self-care. We now wanted to capitalize on Mr. M's religious background to make his treatment meaningful. We knew that during a synagogue service, there were lengthy periods when prayers were said standing. In occupational therapy, therefore, we worked on Mr. M's standing balance and ability to stand through various activities. We had Mr. M stand with a walker and assistance and practiced putting on and taking off his prayer shawl. Mr. M seemed skeptical initially about his ability to complete these tasks, but his confidence improved after standing long enough to complete the ritual and to recite appropriate prayers. Mr. M was very pleased with his accomplishments and exclaimed, "Just wait till my son sees me."

Mr. M continued to progress in therapy. After 2 months, he achieved all of his goals and was independent with self-care, was ambulatory with a walker, and was able to prepare small meals. However, he was unable to climb steps, as demonstrated to the therapist during a home checkout of Mr. M's house. Therefore, Mr. M's son made arrangements for a first floor set-up with a bed and commode and help with grocery shopping and laundry. With his regained independence, Mr. M is looking forward to standing next to his son in synagogue draped in his prayer shawl. Through therapy, he knows that he will once again be able to participate in Jewish life.

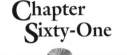

The Power
of Encouragement

Barbara Schroeder, COTA

I live in rural Wisconsin and have been a country girl all my life, happy with the isolated, simple, quiet life. I worked for 25 years at a factory in which I operated various sewing machines, performing repetitive, manipulative, and sometimes heavy work involving both of my arms and hands. One night, I woke up because my hands were tingling painfully. I began to experience pain, numbness, and tingling in my arms. I lost strength in both my hands and felt pressure on the nerves at my elbows. Looking back, I had probably been experiencing symptoms for many years but thought nothing of it. Finally, I admitted there was something wrong and went to a physician.

I was diagnosed with a condition known as carpal tunnel syndrome (CTS), common in people who use their hands regularly in repetitive actions, such as typing, gardening, playing a musical instrument, or, as in my case, sewing on a machine. My physician told me surgery would be required to correct the problem, but that I could return to work within a few weeks.

Unfortunately, things did not turn out that way. I believed that any orthopedic surgeon who had performed routine carpal tunnel surgery could take care of me. But I had a much more complicated case of CTS and should have sought a hand specialist. My surgeon did not prescribe occupational therapy for me after the surgical procedure, and I suffered from complications that kept me out of work for 10 weeks. When, after 7 weeks, it became clear that rehabilitation was necessary before I could return to work, my workers' compensation representative was finally able to get approval for occupational therapy.

I had never heard of occupational therapy before, but Sharon, my occupational therapist, was a kind, compassionate, knowledgeable person. She suspected from the beginning that life would never be the same for me; I could probably never return full-time to my factory job. She began to gently guide and advise me along the way. She gave me information and challenged me in amounts I could digest, then stood back and watched me grow and develop, giving me extra doses of encouragement just when I needed it.

My treatment included increasing my range of motion, strengthening my muscles, and reducing the scar tissue and sensitivity in my hand. It also included psychological counseling, although I didn't realize it. The physical aspect of treatment was expected and helpful, but in the long run, the most critical and useful part of my therapy was helping me find a new purpose in life. For me to remain a productive part of society, I had to give up what had been comfortable, enjoyable, and secure. Sharon gently forced me to look at things objectively and honestly. She guided me one small step at a time in making necessary changes. Without her encouragement and her belief that I could become successful at something new, I would not be what I am today: a certified occupational therapy assistant (or COTA, as we are known in the profession).

When I first expressed interest in becoming a COTA, Sharon answered my questions and arranged for me to observe COTAs in action. That helped me realize I could enjoy something else as much as I enjoyed sewing. However, one huge obstacle loomed in front of me, I would have to attend college. At 43, I felt too old and too far removed from any formal education to believe I could succeed in college.

However, I contacted the local technical college, met with an academic counselor, and underwent academic, psychological, and interest testing. Although my self-confidence was at zero, my test results indicated I had the ability to succeed in any of the programs offered. But because of my physical limitations and restrictions, the only associate degree program I could have taken would have resulted in a testing lab job. I shared my disappointment with Sharon. "I really think you are a 'people' person," she responded. "Why don't you look into schools that offer COTA programs?"

But new obstacles loomed. My husband did not want things to change. He didn't want a wife in college, especially a college in a big city 52 miles away, where the nearest COTA program was located. It wasn't that he was trying to hold me back; he was just a guy with old-fashioned ideas, much like the rest of our friends in town.

Once again, Sharon helped break a seemingly impossible task into small, easily accomplished pieces. I temporarily resumed my sewing job and enrolled in two general education evening classes at the local college. Succeeding in those classes gave me self-confidence and won my husband over. He agreed to support me in my new quest.

Two months after I finished my classes, I underwent surgery on my other hand, this time by a hand specialist. The restrictions he placed on me after surgery brought my sewing career to an end for good. I began taking the general education classes required for the distant COTA program at my local college. My success again helped my husband see me in a new light, and I applied and was accepted into the COTA program after one semester. Although Sharon was no longer treating my hands, she was always willing to offer advice and encouragement when I called.

Making a major career change at any time in life is difficult, especially when it isn't planned. I could not have done it without the encouragement and support I found in my occupational therapist. A wonderful change came about in my life. Now, as a member of that same profession, I know that the biggest part of my job is offering encouragement to my patients when they think they are facing an insurmountable challenge, helping them achieve their goals so they can be happy in life, too. And I'm pleased to report that my husband is proud of the job I do too.

Chapter
Sixty-Two

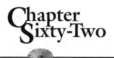

A Friend
in Need is a
Friend in Deed

Mary-Kay Webster, BS

Anita and I met in 1980 while pursuing our bachelor's degrees at Virginia Commonwealth University in Richmond, Virginia. "Pursued" is probably an overstatement. I vaguely knew that Anita was majoring in something called occupational therapy. But our relationship did not depend on discussing our majors, future plans, or career goals. We lived in the "now" of a lively music scene on a moderately progressive campus with many wonderful music venues. We rarely let our studies interfere with our extracurricular search for as much live music as Richmond had to offer.

In fact, my only memory of Anita's course work involved a combination of one of her class craft projects and our favorite band, Roomful of Blues. The morning of the project deadline, Anita unveiled her masterpiece. Using a piece of leather, she had etched the figure of a fringe-skirted wrangler with ruby red lips and heavily lashed eyes, turned longingly toward a full moon above. The wrangler's black cowgirl boots wrapped the lower fence rail of her perch, and her lasso hung in suspended animation arching moonward. It was a skilled, artful, pictorial of one of our favorite Roomful tunes, the provocative "Fine an' Healthy Thing." Its relationship to occupational therapy eluded me at the time. It was only later, as a patient, that I came to recognize that Anita's project embodied many traits shared by most of the occupational therapists I have encountered—skill of fabrication combined with creativity, innovation, ingenuity, and a strong sense of individuality.

Not too many years later, I was anything but a "Fine an' Healthy Thing." As a result of a diving accident, I suffered a major spinal cord injury, leaving me a person with quadriplegia, impairment of all four limbs. It was then that I was grateful that, notwithstanding all the good times we had chased, Anita had indeed pursued her occupational therapy degree and become a skilled practitioner. One of my earliest memories after the accident is of Anita at my bedside, one hand supporting my left forearm, her other hand supporting my seemingly lifeless hand while she encouraged me to flex my wrist.

From her very first reaction, trying to increase and develop my muscle strength, Anita's primary objective, both as an occupational therapist responding to a physical disability and as a friend, was to maximize the level of independence I could realize, considering the limitations I would be facing. In the initial stages of my rehabilitation, the occupational therapy focus was on strengthening muscles that were obviously still functioning, while continuing to monitor and stimulate those that potentially had flickers of return. But Anita did not approach it just as a task in exercise. Her contribution was to tailor some of those exercises in ways particularly meaningful to me. For example, remembering our college craze for music, Anita brought in a child-size xylophone that made exercising shoulder and arm muscles much more pleasurable and offered an outlet for the inevitable frustration of my new situation.

Later, as my level of disability became more predictable, Anita was able to share different ways of looking at issues that could only come from someone experienced with rehabilitating people with physical disabilities. Maintaining my appearance was important to my morale. Sometimes, the simplest solution provided the answer. Personal grooming, particularly brushing my hair, was much easier using a round brush rather than having to struggle with the additional burden of keeping the bristle side of a one-sided brush angled toward my hair. Earrings without posts were easier to get on and off. I also wanted to maintain contact with family and friends. Anita showed me that conventional telephones with the old-style hand-held ear and mouth piece were easier to hold with my limited grip. When it was time to return to work and resume my career at an accounting firm, Anita was right there beside me, analyzing my work site for the most ergonomically sound ways to do my job. Over time, Anita continued to help me develop the skills to find the simplest answer to whatever obstacle came my way.

Chapter Sixty-Two

Sometimes, simple was not available, and the alternative was a more sophisticated option called "assistive technology." Again, Anita's guidance proved invaluable. Assistive technology covers a wide range of products like wheelchairs, especially power wheelchairs, environmental controls such as remotes and touch lamps, adaptive driving equipment, and kitchen aids such as cutting boards with sides that keep food from rolling away, just to name a few. Like most people in my position, I was overwhelmed by the decisions that had to be made as to how much assistive technology to introduce into my life, what technology to look at, and what technology was the best fit for me. I will be forever grateful that this became Anita's specialty within occupational therapy. Her sage counsel and efforts to keep the kind, level, and amount of technology a consumer-controlled decision continues to make my life easier.

I will never be a "Fine an' Healthy Thing" again, if that means being able to use all four of my limbs the way I could before my accident. But my life and level of independence are immeasurably greater than they would have been without occupational therapy and a friend like Anita. It was a rather extreme way to discover what Anita had been doing back in college when we weren't listening to music, but I am grateful that the profession of occupational therapy was available at Virginia Commonwealth and that Anita picked that as her major. I am particularly lucky to have someone as creative, intelligent, and capable as my best friend Anita committed to its practice.

Chapter
Sixty-Three

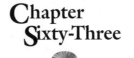

Someday Soup
Kimberly Eberhardt, MS, OTR/L

On a summer day in 1996, Chuck Hince injured his spinal cord in a surfing accident on Martha's Vineyard and arrived on the rehabilitation floor of Boston Medical Center paralyzed from the neck down. Chuck had no arm movement and his spinal cord seemed to be cut entirely, making his injury appear to be complete. The outlook was discouraging. However, Chuck wasn't seeing things that way.

In fact, he was making long-term goals for himself before I could even write them on his first occupational therapy evaluation. "If they say there's a chance that something will come back if I work at it, I'll do it." Chuck vowed that he would never stop working at getting some movement back someday. "I took the initial devastation of, 'Gosh, I may never move again' and said 'Okay, watch, just watch.'" This was Chuck's interpretation of his situation.

It was almost as if Chuck's muscles were listening that day. Soon after, the left biceps muscle could be felt straining to move. Chuck was regaining the use of his dominant left arm. Chuck's routine by then included a daily lunch workout during his OT treatment session with me. "The most frustrating thing about being a quadriplegic is learning everything over again after you already knew how to do it all," Chuck explained. But he wasn't

225

Chapter Sixty-Three

discouraged. "Someday, we'll tackle soup, Kim," he told me. "Yes, someday soup! " The phrase became our motto.

During our lunch treatment sessions in occupational therapy, we made the most of the available muscles Chuck had by using a deltoid aid exercise device. I put this piece of equipment, which consists of a supportive sling on a shoulder height stand, next to Chuck's left arm. His arm and shoulder were supported in the sling so that he could move them without having to hold the arm and shoulder up in the air, fighting gravity, at the same time. Using the device, he practiced doing many of the things he wanted to try to relearn, including feeding himself various kinds of foods. This was the first activity that established a sense of accomplishment and normalcy in his life since his injury.

Assisting Chuck in gaining independence in such a meaningful, purposeful occupation, eating by himself, I found his enthusiasm contagious. Many other patients on the unit, both those with injuries of greater and lesser severity, were also encouraged. Comments from others such as "Chuck is my hero," and "If Chuck could do it, I can too," made me appreciate the inner strength of this outwardly strong individual and his remarkable ability to motivate others by his example. It also brought home in a very concrete way both to him and to me the powerful impact occupational therapy had in helping him begin to realize his potential to regain the power to do things.

Not long after this major achievement, Chuck concentrated in the occupational therapy sessions on learning to move his power wheelchair with his left arm and was soon able to accomplish this goal as well. Then he began working in occupational therapy on gaining right arm movement, and by practicing tasks daily, he did it! During his 3 month stay, Chuck continually surprised us all with the remarkable gains he made despite the daily obstacles he faced.

"Not being able to scratch my own face and trying to get a nurse to do it at two in the morning; hitting the bed rails with my head, arms, and legs due to spasms in bed; spilling food on myself when trying to put the fork in my mouth—these are just some of the things I deal with on a daily basis... There is so much people don't know about spinal cord injury. But, this is what I have and I've got to deal with it!"

The producers of the news program 48 Hours were so impressed with the eternal optimism and admirable efforts of this motivated young man that they interviewed him and filmed a special on this part of his life. Christopher Reeve and his wife, Dana, had arranged to meet the 27-year-old who had touched the hearts of persons with disabilities around the world. On May 15, 1997, Chuck's triumphant story was told on national television. The country not only watched, but applauded as Dan Rather called him "a superman of strength, courage, and candor"; Chuck and Christopher Reeve were then highlighted on the program's finale, which achieved one of the highest ratings of the season. Chuck's story touched the hearts of many that night. The show ended with a comment on his positive attitude and with Chuck's promise that, "You haven't seen nothing yet."

I'm proud to say that this is an understatement. Chuck continued his occupational therapy program. Recently, I had the opportunity to visit him. Chuck is now able to eat by himself without using the deltoid aid and is even able to pick up finger food. He is regaining the use of his forearm and wrist. His next goal is playing the piano. "If I can only play the piano again," Chuck told me, "I'd be the best I could ever be."

As a pianist myself, making music at the keyboard is something I hold close to my heart. This is truly one activity that symbolizes the powerful meaning of what we as occupational therapists strive to do on a daily basis. We try to help a person be as independent as possible in those things that are important to that person. If there is a flicker of a movement, just a slight palpation of a muscle, we'll use it. This is why I do what I do. I find it so rewarding when people are able to focus on enhancing their abilities, instead of dwelling on their disabilities.

As an occupational therapist, I have always valued the significance of tapping into a person's own inner motivation in an effort to achieve independence. I believe that Chuck's perseverance will take him wherever he wants to go. Chuck was a wonderful person to work with because he already had this innate driving force and capitalized on it to achieve the many commendable goals he set for himself. Yes, remember the name, Chuck Hince. I have a feeling we will be hearing from him again. Chuck is going to do great things. That's just the kind of person he is!

Chapter
Sixty-Four

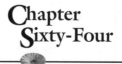

Commuter Nightmare
Bhavisha H. Patel

What was remarkable about Bhavisha Patel was not merely her dramatic plunge from the platform at Philadelphia's 30th Street Station directly in front of a newly arrived Amtrak train. Nor was it that while recovering from her injuries she had the courage to get right back on the train to resume her daily commute again. What really attracted everyone's attention was the torturous looking device attached to her leg and thigh to keep them in the proper position to heal. Here is her amazing story in her own words.

My "flying leap" occurred on June 18, 1996, at 6:50 a.m., I was getting ready to board the Amtrak train for New York City at Philadelphia's 30th Street Station. This had been my daily routine since March of that year, because I am a lawyer who practices in Manhattan and lives in Philadelphia. I wasn't even wearing high-heeled shoes that day, but had on my comfortable "commuter flats" with my professional blazer jacket and skirt.

When the train pulled into the station, I started walking along the platform, positioning myself to get on board. The crowd of people on the platform surged around me, each person with the same intention of boarding the train. Suddenly, I felt myself sailing off the platform. Time slowed down. Everything was happening in slow motion. I was flying in the air; the coffee I was carrying flew out of my hands, and I saw it hit the edge of the platform. Before I knew it, I was on the tracks, in front of the train, 6 feet below the platform, in excruciating pain and unable to move. I knew I had broken my right leg because the thigh bone was quite visible, sticking through my skin. Luckily, a good Samaritan managed to jump onto the tracks beside me; he then lifted me off the tracks, carried me to the edge of the platform, and was able to place me back up on the platform.

I was rushed to nearby Hahnemann University Hospital by ambulance, where I was diagnosed with a compound fracture of the right femur. Early that afternoon, a 12-inch metal plate held in place by 12 screws was inserted into my leg to bring the shattered thighbone together. A full leg cast was put on my leg. The next day, when the anesthesia wore off, I knew that I was living in a new and different world. I could not walk, not even to get out of bed to go to the bathroom. I faced a long rehabilitation, with no guarantee of full recovery at the end.

The third day of my hospital stay, I received occupational therapy for the first time. The initial session was simple. We worked only on getting out of bed. During the second and third occupational therapy sessions, I was taught how to sit in a wheelchair and how to sit on and get off the toilet seat. Everything was basic. I had to relearn the simplest movements—getting out of bed, sitting down on a chair, walking with crutches, and using the bathroom.

I returned home from the hospital with a cast that ran from the top of my thigh to my toes. Despite the lessons at the hospital, I was still bed bound, unable to get out of bed without assistance. I could not go to the bathroom without help. I could not get myself out of the bed and into the wheelchair without help. I could not walk into the kitchen to get myself something to eat without help. I relied on my friends and a home health aide worker for my needs.

In the beginning, my friend assisted me out of bed and to the bathroom and back to bed in the morning. Once he left for work, I was bound to the bed, until the home health aide worker came. She too would help me out of bed, into the bathroom, and back to bed again. There, I would wait again, until my friend returned from work at about 7 p.m. For most of the day I was alone and helpless.

My home situation changed dramatically when occupational therapy, which had started in the hospital, resumed. A week after my discharge, Sharon Finer walked into my life. She brought with her a number of tools and strategies that were designed to help me function independently at home and face the prospect of returning to work.

My first lesson was how to use a "leash." It was a simple device with which I could hook my broken leg and with its help get out of bed. Next, I learned how to transfer myself from the bed to a wheelchair, sit on the wheelchair comfortably, and how to get on and off the toilet seat. I had been given a bed-side commode to bring home from the hospital, but I was too shy to use it. Sharon understood my hesitance.

Unfortunately, like most homes, mine had no special handicapped facili-ties. Sharon suggested dismantling the commode and placing its frame with its side handle bars and built-up seat around and over the regular toilet in my bathroom to allow me to get on and off the seat. It was wonderful. I was able to have some semblance of independence again in something that really mat-tered to me. I could go to the bathroom without having to wait in embar-rassed agony for someone to come home. I was no longer bed bound. I was able to sit up in a wheelchair for part of the day. Sharon also made modifica-tions that allowed me to shower again. She brought me a shower bag and a bath chair and had a hand-held shower installed. All by myself I was able to feel clean again!

Sharon's help did not stop here. At the beginning of each visit, we set a series of goals to be accomplished. The goals incorporated my own concerns and needs. I was especially anxious to get out of the house and return to work. We worked on going up and down the stairs and in and out of the doors of my apartment building while ensuring my safety. She taught me how to walk on the uneven sidewalks of my neighborhood and negotiate curbs. Soon, I was ready to return to 30th Street Station. Sharon recognized how traumatized I had been by the fall. It was important that I get myself ready to return to work, even though it meant revisiting the scene of my disaster.

Sharon ensured that I could safely transport myself to and from the train. She taught me how to get in and out of cabs, and together we revisited the location of my accident. My return to 30th Street Station was important, since I knew I had to face my fears and bury the pain in the past. When that first trip to 30th Street Station and the platform where I had fallen was over, I could get back on the train.

Unfortunately, this was not the end. In early fall, tests revealed that my femur was not healing. I underwent a second surgery, this time including a bone graft. A year and a half later, the metal plates and screws were removed.

Then in January 1998, disaster struck again. The thighbone in my right leg came apart due to incomplete healing. I was sent back to the hospital, diagnosed with a nonunion fracture, and underwent another surgery. This time a Llizarov device was placed on my leg. This brace was the closest thing to a medieval torture device I had ever seen. Resembling four 12-inch-in diameter wagon wheels complete with spokes, stacked one on top of anoth-er with 2-inch spaces between, it was used as an external fixator to support and hold broken bones in place while they heal. It had seven wires on each rim. The wires ran from metal casing outside of the leg, through the skin and bone, and out the other end. It was an effective but absolutely ugly-looking device, and in addition it was heavy and painful to wear. It required constant cleaning at the sites where the spokes entered and exited my leg to prevent infection. The device also prevented me from wearing slacks (except for the very loosest sweatpants), and my skirts had to be extra full and long to go over it and to cover it. When I sat, my leg had to be straight out in front of me because my knee could not bend, and I was in danger of unwanted exposure if my skirt got caught on it even a little bit.

Once again, Sharon was there for me. I was discharged from the hospital but I was not a candidate for a rehabilitation facility because technically I was "independent." However, I was given an occupational therapist; happily for me, it was Sharon again. I undoubtedly needed Sharon, even though just a year before we had worked together on similar techniques for getting mobile and independent. The first few weeks after the second break was a new low for me. I was not sure of the prognosis and started to live in the fear of not ever healing. Just as bad was my daily battle with the cumbersome Llizarov device at which I could not even bear to look. And I still had to face getting back on the train and going back to work.

Thanks to Sharon, I had time to recover from my trauma and deal with the emotional downs. Sharon had experience dealing with Llizarov patients. She recognized that along with the device came significant new demands that had to be met. At the same time, I was relearning the routine tasks that would lead me back to a somewhat normal daily existence. As always, Sharon's exercises and training addressed basic, simple needs. In fact, I had to relearn everything that Sharon had taught me a year before. Without. Sharon's help, I would not have had a clue how to rebuild the fundamental, most important parts of my life.

She brought with her experience, intelligence, and creativity. It is important to emphasize that part of Sharon's genius as an occupational therapist was the fact that she recognized that my most important needs were also the most fundamental. In order to start healing physically and emotionally, I had to start to live my life again, taking small steps and returning to self-sufficiency. From the outside looking in, it might appear that Sharon simply applied "common sense" to the problem of moving an injured body out of bed and into motion. However, in the difficulties I faced, I know that Sharon was a healer who gave me the opportunity to deal with my ordeal of healing my femur by freeing me of my greatest worry, the loss of my independence.

Today I am pleased to report that the broken leg ordeal is behind me. The Llizarov device was removed after 5½ long months, but it did its job and my leg is now well healed. Thanks to Sharon, I was able to resume my daily commuting with the device, and at the time was well known to the "regular" commuters and all the conductors as the lady who had that horrible "thing" on her leg and took up two seats. For now, I am happier to be known as the lawyer who commutes to New York from Philadelphia. I am back on my feet again, I watch my step very carefully when I am on the train platform, and the only commuter nightmares I have are late trains and snowy winter days when the trains get stopped because the track switches freeze.

Section Seven

On the Road

Automobile Accidents

Automobile Accidents

Meet eight people seriously injured in automobile accidents that left them with brain injuries, spinal cord injuries, and other severe physical traumas, whose lives are saved but who need ways to make their lives meaningful again. The persistence and determination they apply to successfully redesigning their lives, with the help of therapists, will inspire everyone who has ever sat behind the wheel or on the passenger side of a car and worried about the driver speeding toward them.

Chapter Sixty-Five

Twin Therapy

Deborah Goldberg, MA, OTR/L

Frankie, 7, Kristen, 6, and the 4-year-old twins, Jason and Justin, were all that parents Kathy and Frank Mayer could ever hope for—active, healthy, friendly, and happy children—miracle kids, they often called them. But since August 6, 1996, Jason has proven time and time again what a true miracle he really is, for on that day tragedy struck and his fierce and successful fight for his own survival began.

On that bright sunny summer day, the family was outside their Deptford, New Jersey, home packing their car for their annual seashore vacation. 4-year-old Jason was riding his Big Wheel tricycle on the front lawn when he suddenly lost control of it and began rolling rapidly down the sloping driveway. At precisely that moment, a truck was approaching on this normally quiet residential street. It happened so quickly. As Frank and terrified twin brother Justin watched in helpless horror from inside the fenced yard and Katherine screamed frantically from the front porch, Jason and the Big Wheel slid under the moving pick-up truck, whose driver did not realize he had run over the preschooler. In minutes that seemed like hours, Jason was dragged 55 feet before Frank managed to jump the fence, run down the street, catch up with the truck, and finally get the driver to stop.

Chapter Sixty-Five

Katherine was sure at that moment that Jason was dead, snatched away from the family in that split second between enjoying the sunshine as he played in front of the house and his plunge into the street. But miraculously, Jason didn't die.

But Jason's medical and physical condition were extremely critical. Jason's skull was fractured and layers of skin and flesh from his chest, arms, and hands were torn away from his small body. Moments seemed like eons as the whole family waited helplessly until the ambulances arrived, and Jason was finally taken to a local New Jersey hospital. There, surgeons wanted to amputate his entire right arm. Luckily for Jason, the surgical team could not be assembled in time, so he was airlifted to Children's Hospital of Philadelphia, a very specialized hospital facility for pediatric surgery and children's diseases. There, the team of surgeons performed a myriad of operations including transferring skin, muscles, tendons, and nerves from his back and leg to save his arm and to reconstruct the rest of his deformed body to the best of their ability. They also relieved a blood clot that had formed in his brain. The only thing amputated was his right pinkie finger, but the rest of his hand and arm were saved entirely. Jason miraculously survived these intensive procedures and escaped death.

Following 3½ weeks of acute care, Jason's medical condition was finally stable enough to allow him to be transferred to Children's Seashore House, a pediatric rehabilitation hospital affiliated with Children's Hospital of Philadelphia, where I work. At Children's Seashore House, Jason participated in intensive rehabilitation programs that included extensive occupational therapy.

As Jason's occupational therapist, my goal was to provide a nurturing environment that would encourage Jason to regain age-appropriate skills and provide education, training, and emotional support for the family. Exercises to maintain and increase his movements and the ability to move his joints to the fullest were critical at this stage.

However, before any therapy could begin, I had to make sure that Jason could trust me. Understandably, Jason was extremely fearful of strangers, especially those who poked, prodded, hurt, or stared at him. Therefore, individual occupational therapy sessions with Jason evolved into whole family sessions. Not only did the immediate family participate, but grandmothers, grandfathers, aunts, uncles, and cousins joined in the activities. Especially vital to these sessions was Jason's twin, Justin. Justin became an integral part of therapy. He attended all occupational therapy sessions and was included in every activity. I was hoping that if Jason realized that this environment was safe enough for his closest brother to play and learn, then he would feel safe as well. I also counted on his natural closeness to his twin to keep him playing with Justin as he had before the accident.

Initially, nothing I offered appealed to Jason. He would tightly wrap his heavily bandaged arms around his mother's leg, never offering even a glance in my direction. The closer I came, the louder he cried. With this challenge, I redirected the sessions away from Jason and focused on demonstrating exercise techniques that Kathy and Frank could do with Jason in his room. I also arranged that Jason's pain medication would always be administered immediately prior to his occupational therapy sessions so that when I did hold him, it would be as comfortable for him as possible.

Meanwhile, time was ticking on. Scar tissue was beginning to form along Jason's right arm, and the potential for muscle tightening and the risk of permanent fusing together of healing tissues, known as contractures, was increasing daily. Exercise and movement were now absolutely essential to prevent future deformities. With Mom and Justin at his side, Jason became less fearful and more interested in the activities and games that I offered to help keep his body parts moving. Justin and Jason particularly enjoyed waving their arms and hands to catch and pop the bubbles that I blew near them. Shaving cream was another favorite medium that allowed Jason the creativity to smear with his fingers and draw anything he imagined while at the same time it was soft and smooth enough to protect him from potential pain.

In the months that followed, Jason and Justin increasingly and actively participated in occupational therapy sessions, with mom Kathy more and more able to simply watch from the sidelines. Justin continued to be a true asset to the therapeutic environment, as he indirectly encouraged Jason to speak, smile, and challenge himself. Activities soon progressed to obstacle courses and scooter board races, where the twins would boisterously push and pull themselves down the hallways while lying on their stomachs on twin scooter boards. Baking cookies, making play dough clay, weaving pot holders, and designing greeting cards were some of the many projects they worked on together that helped Jason regain use of his right arm and hand. The constant reassuring presence of his warm, loving family around him also seemed to help Jason deal with the emotional trauma of his accident and his recovery process.

Activity was also encouraged outside the occupational therapy play room. I repeatedly stressed with Jason's parents that recovery depended on round-the-clock commitment to movement. I provided exercise "homework" in the form of games, and I gave them a list of appropriate holiday toys.

Finally, I was able to form a solid, trusting relationship with Jason, and he and I were able to engage in play and to talk to each other even if Justin did not attend a session or if Mom had to leave for a much-needed coffee break. I was now able to touch and hold Jason with ease. Hand splints and casts were custom fitted to help Jason place his limb in the most functional position while resting. I ordered specially constructed tight-fitting elasticized therapeutic undergarments for Jason to wear as "second skin" to reduce the chance of developing thickening skin scars.

After many months of rehabilitation at the Children's Seashore House, it was finally time for Jason's discharge to his own home. This brought its own excitement as well as a new focus. Starting kindergarten at the local elementary school along with Justin became Jason's next ultimate goal and challenge. With continued outpatient occupational therapy services, we worked on skills he would need for success in the school environment. Jason developed age-appropriate scissors skills and was able to write his name. He was also able to use the bathroom independently and to dress himself fully, including buttons and zippers. Frank and Kathy were happy to report that Jason made new friends in school and had no trouble adjusting to his new environment. His teachers were pleased to see how well he kept up with his peers, despite his physical limitations, which by this time were minor.

When Jason reached the 1-year anniversary of the accident, his close friends and family came to Children's Seashore House to help celebrate his astounding recovery. Jason and Justin decorated the invitations, prepared cupcakes and fruit salad, and made a papier mâché pinata. August 6, 1997 arrived and Jason was smiling from ear to ear.

Today, Jason is making normal progress in school in the same grade as his twin brother and is looking forward to a life of age-appropriate physical, social, intellectual, and emotional development. Despite the accident that almost ended his life, Jason showed me, his family, and most importantly, himself, that he has the inner strength to overcome life's greatest challenges and prove that he is indeed a miracle.

Chapter Sixty-Six

Hi Ho Beanie

Elizabeth J. Healey, OTR

Beanie is not exactly your mental image of an occupational therapy professional. She is only 12 years old, weighs 1,000 pounds, and moves about on four legs. But you'll never convince Quincy that Beanie does not deserve some kind of occupational therapy certification or degree, even if Beanie is a somewhat unconventional medical professional—an Arabian mare with the steadiness of a mule and the heart of a lamb.

Quincy, Beanie, and I met at the first occupational therapy horseback riding program I taught. My first sight of Quincy was when she maneuvered herself out of her car and into her wheelchair. She wheeled across the grass enthusiastically and greeted me with a broad smile and a warm, "Hi, there." She then slowly approached Beanie, reassuring the horse with her soft words. Quincy told me that a car accident 18 years ago left her partially paralyzed, and it had been at least that long since she had been able to ride a horse.

I must admit that as I watched Quincy that first day and saw the volunteers chosen because of their height and strength and their proven reliability, dedication, and good sense struggling to support her on the horse, I realized that Quincy's wheelchair status would be a totally new experience for me and would pose a special challenge; I feared that our plan would end in failure. I wondered how I could delicately tell Quincy of my doubts about her future as a horseback rider.

I accompanied Quincy to the parking lot following that first ride and gently suggested that she might have better success in our new cart-driving program. "Please don't take this away from me," she pleaded, tears welling up in her eyes. "I've known the feel of my car wheels and wheelchair wheels for 18 years now, but the feel of the horse moving under me was so incredible and wonderful. Please let me try!" Her impassioned words remain with me to this day.

Even with the possibility of failure looming, I felt compelled to let her try again. With Beanie's help, Quincy gave it her all. This was the beginning of what only can be described as a miracle. Beanie and Quincy went on to develop a bond of love and trust that superceded any physical limitations.

While Quincy is impaired in her lower extremities, she has superior upper body strength and soon learned to move up a 3-foot-high ramp and transfer herself independently from the wheelchair to the saddle on Beanie's back. One-inch Velcro straps attached to the saddle loosely held her legs in place just above the knees. Safety grips built into the straps could be pulled quickly by a volunteer on either side of the mare if an emergency were to arise.

Quincy rode Beanie for four sessions each week, and by the end of the first 7 weeks, Quincy was able to ride without her "sidewalkers," the volunteers who had initially held her in the saddle. Quincy's abdominal and trunk muscles, which had been virtually untapped or unresponsive to typical clinical stimulation, began functioning in response to Beanie's natural movements. The side-to-side, up-and-down, and forward-and-backward movements elicited muscle responses, which allowed Quincy to sit independently on Beanie's back. This was just the beginning. Quincy progressed with the other class participants, two who walked with canes, two who showed signs of moderate paralysis, and one with a severely deformed and fisted hand. By the end of the following summer, all six adults had advanced in their equestrian skills, including jumping.

The final day of that riding season concluded with a show that brought Beanie and the other horses, all of the riders, and their family members together. My class rode in a drill set to music, and their families, friends, and volunteers observed the miracle in motion. When the routine was over, the riders beamed with pride at their accomplishments. Beanie stood tall, too, head erect as if she knew what she had contributed. For me, the great joy of that day was mingled with some sadness: I now had to graduate this class of champions. These riders no longer needed the program, and many others waited to fill their places and discover their own miracles.

Despite many other classes I have supervised since that year, I still think a lot about Quincy and Beanie. Quincy's stamina and passion for horseback riding and the bond that she made with Beanie made such a difference in her rehabilitation. I have seen many successes over the years, but Quincy's story will always be quite special to me. Although she doesn't know it, Quincy continues to inspire me to inspire others to make their own miracles come true.

Chapter Sixty-Seven

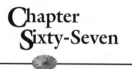

Best Seat in the House

Cindy Martin, COTA/L
Submitted by Valerie B. Whiting,
OTR/L, LMT

Chair caning is an intricate craft that requires nimble fingers and intense concentration on details. There aren't too many who possess the necessary skills these days, which is a problem for those who need repairs to antique chairs. I am always on the lookout for such wonderful old-but-in-need-of-repair chairs at flea markets and crafts festivals, and am therefore also on the lookout for a craftsperson who can restore the caned seats to their former glory. Both of my needs were satisfied recently at a local fall arts and crafts festival.

I have always been an avid enthusiast of such arts and crafts festivals where I enjoy getting lost among the crowds as I wander from booth to booth. Last fall, drawn to her booth by the quality of her work, her use of natural materials, and the functional nature of both her baskets and chairs, I stopped to watch a talented basket weaver/chair caner in action. When I arrived, she was demonstrating chair caning on an antique oak chair by creating a traditional cross cane pattern. Her fingers rhythmically wove the cane from side to side. She made the weaving look so easy! It was clear that not only did she love what she was doing, but she was also highly proficient in her craft. Her wares included a beautiful chair seat that was done in a daisy weave pattern, a more intricate design requiring a more advanced level of skill. She also had many examples of her unusual baskets on display.

It was when I talked to her about her craft and how she acquired her skills, however, that I realized I could chalk up another occupational therapy success story! Here's what she told me.

Approximately 5 years ago, a head-on car crash left her unable to return to her legal secretary position, which made her a single parent without a source of income. The accident had resulted in several crushed vertebrae and some broken bones in her leg and foot. She had learned her craft as a means of therapy to help her refocus her attention and to fill the dark hours after her car crash. She was taught chair caning in occupational therapy, and she used those principles to teach herself basket weaving. After struggling with her first few projects, she finally started to perfect her craft, and, after she mastered the chair caning skills, her friends and family began to inquire about purchasing the chairs she had created. She also started recaning chairs for a few friends and found herself becoming more and more involved with both the process and the entrepreneurial aspects of the activity. She soon turned her passion for the craft into a profitable business venture. What started out as occupational therapy to help her recover from an accident then became a full-time job for her.

In addition to her hands-on craft activities and her appearances at craft shows, she travels around the Southeast lecturing on chair caning and sharing her talent with anyone who is interested. She also teaches, giving private and group lessons in both chair caning and basket weaving. She is very quick to share the story of the tragedy that turned into a personal miracle for her and to explain how the purposeful activity she learned helped to once again make her life worth living. She's most eager to recount how occupational therapy moved her from a job sitting at a desk to a career creating beautiful seats for others to enjoy.

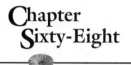

My Ugly Duckling

Michelle Ponsolle-Mays, MS, OTR/L

We all know the story of the Ugly Duckling—a hatchling that judged from the viewpoint of ducks was ugly, but which grew up to be a beautiful swan. I think a lot about that story when I work as an occupational therapist with my right hand.

Nearly 11 years ago, in an auto accident, I sustained a severe, complicated injury to my right, dominant hand. After two initial surgeries, I was prescribed occupational therapy treatment. Because I had no prior knowledge of this profession, I entered the therapeutic alliance a naive individual. However, I had the good fortune to meet Karen, an occupational therapist with specialized credentials in hand therapy, with whom I would work closely over the next 2 years.

As I reflect back on this difficult period, one afternoon in particular stands out in my mind. As at many previous sessions, I was seated across from Karen, prepared to begin my treatment. However, this time was different. I gazed down at my right hand resting on the tabletop and suddenly regarded it in a totally different light than ever before—I became aware that I was permanently disfigured. I had just simply never accepted this as a possibility until that very moment. Overwhelmed by this realization, tears welled in my eyes, and I whispered, "It's so ugly."

Without missing a beat, Karen stopped what she had been doing, placed everything aside, and gently began to talk to me. She explained that my emotions were a normal reaction to my injury. I was experiencing feelings in "stages," not dissimilar to those that individuals with a terminal illness experience. Karen reassured me that this was a normal response and that we could discuss the process during therapy sessions. Acknowledging that I was going through a difficult time, she assured me that I wasn't alone; we would work through it together.

When Karen finished, I was utterly speechless. Karen had given a voice to my despair. She had dared to speak about a side of disability that no one else would. For the first time since the accident, I felt as if someone could truly empathize with my plight. As a result, a therapeutic alliance was formed that would shape both my physical and psychological recovery in the months to come.

From then on, discussing the emotional side of my physical changes and challenges became as much a natural part of my work with Karen as were activities for my hand. As time passed, so did my desire to learn. I wanted to teach others to perform their valued daily activities in the face of adversity. I now knew from personal experience the importance of addressing both emotional and physical needs of people recovering from disability. Believing that I could draw from my personal experience as a means to help others, I began exploring occupational therapy educational programs in the hopes of beginning a new and gratifying career.

In 1996, I graduated from Columbia University in New York City with a master's of science degree in occupational therapy and was elected class speaker for our commencement exercises. After having been employed at The New York Hospital—Cornell Medical Center, Westchester Division, Department of Therapeutic Activities, I am presently a self-employed practitioner. Each day, I try to treat my patients with the same care and concern Karen showed to me. And when I now use my right hand to help someone with an activity, what I see is no longer ugly—it is my personal swan.

Chapter Sixty-Nine

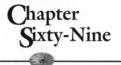

A Beautiful Flower Blossoms Slowly

Julia Waggoner Santini, OTR/L

brie is her own woman, a true individual and I'm sure she was always like that. She even begins her name with a lowercase "b". Unfortunately, I never knew the person brie was before a drunk driver hit her as she walked home from a movie one evening. She sustained massive head trauma, as well as a fractured collarbone and broken long bones in her leg, the tibia and fibula. She spent a few weeks in an intensive care unit before being transferred to the rehabilitation hospital in which I worked.

When I first met her, brie was in a coma. Her gaze was fixed, and she only responded to pain, if at all. Her arms were flexed up tightly under her chin. I was limited in what I could do for her in her comatose state: position her, reduce muscle tone, and try to increase her interaction with the environment through coma stimulation techniques.

Even while she was in a coma, I began to learn more about brie. Her family and friends told me about her free-spirited ways. They filled her room with her favorite things, like her funky clothes, extensive hat collection, an apron from the bakery in which she worked, spices with which she liked to cook, and a much-loved teddy bear. She had eclectic musical tastes, from Squeeze to Björk, to her favorite—Neil Diamond.

248

Gradually, she began to come out of the coma and interact with us a little. I looked forward to seeing what she would respond to each day. One of her greatest pleasures had been rose water baths, so I decided to give brie her first one since the accident. Her nurse and I submerged her in a whirlpool tub and helped her pour a bottle of rose water into the bath. I was certain she enjoyed it, because she smiled for the first time and was able to move her arms and hands more than she ever had before.

One day, as I was wheeling brie through the hospital, we passed a door that led to a courtyard. She pointed excitedly, and even though it was raining, continued to ask through gestures and smiles to go outside. I pushed her wheelchair around and around the courtyard in the rain. It was wonderful to see this young woman, who spent most of her day with her head slumped forward, turning her head and looking blissfully to the sky so raindrops could fall on her face.

Most exciting of all was the day we realized that brie could communicate. She had been using facial expressions and incomprehensible gestures to try to express her needs. The day we tried giving her a communication board, we discovered that she could point to the words "yes" and "no" with a good deal of accuracy using that special board that contained common words and the alphabet. This was wonderful. Up until then, because her ability to follow commands had been limited by her physical impairments, we weren't sure how much she had understood us. All of a sudden, using the board, she could now tell us if she was in pain, wanted to rest, or if she wanted to listen to her music. We felt as if we'd broken down a brick wall that had closed her in, and we were now, for the first time, a part of her world and she could be a part of ours.

After 2 months and much occupational therapy, brie could hold up her head; assist in her grooming, dressing, and bathing; stand with help; and wheel her own chair. She could use her left arm to do some simple tasks like putting CDs into her stereo by herself. She still was pointing only to "yes" or "no" on the letter board, but she had the most effective nonverbal communication I've ever seen. brie's insurance company decided that she had "reached her maximum benefit" from inpatient rehabilitation and had to transfer to a skilled nursing facility. She still had a long road head of her.

I didn't comprehend just how much groundwork we had laid for her recovery until several months later. brie was transferred from the skilled nursing facility, where she was not improving, to a residential brain injury center. At the center, her functional abilities began to improve by leaps and bounds. She could hold long conversations using her letter board, and when I visited her, I got a chance to experience her sense of humor for the first time. She learned how to use a computer and wrote me a letter: "Well, I guess I'm lucky to be alive, and fully functional (well almost!)," she wrote. "I have good memories of you and the place where you worked. You were always the biggest hope for me..."

I keep that letter on my desk; it inspires me and reminds me why I do what I do. Working with brie was like watching a beautiful flower blossom slowly. I was, and still am, in awe of her strength and spirit.

Chapter Seventy

A Message from T.J.

Stephanie M. Milazzo, MA, OTR, CHT

When T.J. Tomblin arrived in the emergency room, what concerned the doctors and nurses most was that he seemed to have fractured just about every bone in his face as a result of being struck head-on while driving a school bus. It wasn't that they didn't notice the severe fracture of his right wrist, it just didn't get their priority attention, at least not until T.J. loudly and insistently made sure they saw things differently. "I am a drummer. I don't perform with my face. I use my hands. Just fix my wrist." The surgical team had to agree to do just that —treat T.J.'s wrist first —before he would allow them to work on his face, a face which ended up requiring extensive reconstructive surgery involving insertion of 16 plates.

I am an occupational therapist who specializes in hand and upper extremity rehabilitation. In April 1994, I received a call from T.J.'s orthopedic surgeon who relayed T.J.'s story to me including the dramatic message during the emergency room saga.

Thomas J. Tomblin was a professional drummer who had his own 18-piece band known as the T.J. Tomlin (without the "b") Orchestra. This orchestra specialized in big band/swing music from the 1940s. In the early 1990s, T.J. was supplementing his income and obtained medical coverage for his family by driving a school bus in the daytime for special education students. In February 1994, T.J. was driving his bus with one student aboard when the bus was hit head-on by a young woman who had suffered a burst blood vessel in her brain. The surgeon went on to tell me that T.J. was a musician who had contributed his talents to several albums by other artists, that being a drummer was the most important thing in his life, and that T.J. was "eccentric"; nonetheless, he asked me to please try my best to return him to the drums.

I met T.J. for the first time later that day. Even 2 months after surgery, his right wrist and hand were swollen more then four times to the size of his left and he could not grip anything including his drumstick. On that very first day, he insisted emphatically that he had to return to playing the drums again as soon as possible "I can not imagine my life if I can not play." I tried to reassure him that there are other things he could do in life besides playing the drums. But T.J. was not to be diverted, "You don't understand, playing the drums is my life. When will I be able to play?" It was at this point in time I realized just how important this was to him. I promised him that I would do my best, but I also warned him I could not do it alone. It was necessary for him to pull his own weight. My favorite therapist speech is: the results are 1/3 the surgery, 1/3 the therapist, and 1/3 the patient's responsibility. Anything less, and the goals cannot be met. T.J. assured me that he would do whatever it took.

Every day during the treatment sessions, T.J. would ask me, "When will I be able to play?" I secretly hoped he would be able to play by December of that year and somewhat hesitantly said, "Maybe December" (keeping my fingers crossed). The next session T.J. came in and changed the date; he said, "Maybe I'll be playing by October." I forced myself to say "maybe," knowing I would not be able to argue with him. This went on incessantly at almost every treatment session.

T.J. worked very hard at his therapy and endured much pain during his treatment sessions. One day he asked me if he could bring in a cassette player with earphones of his recordings to distract him from the pain. I said "Sure, whatever it takes," and it worked. He was able to endure the pain without complaints.

T.J. had a doctor's visit several weeks after he began therapy. He came in after his appointment shouting, "The doctor says I can now tinker with the drums." I was very concerned that the physician might not have appreciated that what he meant by "tinker" was not what "tinker" meant to T.J. I contacted his physician immediately by phone, relaying my concern, but his doctor reassured me that T.J.'s wrist was well healed and would sustain real drum playing. However, T.J.'s problem at that point was that he could not hold the drumstick in his fingers because, although the swelling had reduced significantly, he still could not grip the drumstick sufficiently to play. Occupational therapy came to the rescue! I adapted his drumstick by building up the handle and putting it into a universal cuff to allow him to grip it. I have never seen a happier person than T.J. that day.

Amazingly, 2 months after I first met T.J., in June 1994, he was playing the drums again professionally, a full 6 months earlier than expected. He asked me to attend his second professional appearance, and I did. It was at this event that he announced to his audience: "My occupational therapist is here, and I have to give her a special thank you for giving me my wrist back and my life back." No one has ever given me a greater thank you, or a more public thank you.

T.J.'s therapy was far from over. He continued treatment until January 1995. However, it was back on that day in June 1994 that his personality completely changed. Before he returned to playing his drums, T.J. had been a very determined, but also a very angry man who felt that his life had been taken away from him, even though he was walking and breathing. For him, his music and his life were one and the same. To deal with that anger, his occupational therapy back in those days never stopped at the wrist. We had treated T.J. as a whole person, encouraging him to vent his feelings. That part of my job became much easier, though, after he resumed playing. Restoring his ability to make music, and perhaps all the satisfying, loud, forceful therapy on the drums, allowed his anger to dissipate and his determination to once again dominate his life.

After more than 3 years, T.J. continues to visit me at the clinic every few months to keep me updated. He has since retired from the bus company, has traveled across this country and through Europe with his band, and has produced and recorded his own CD entitled "A Message from T.J." When he visits me and meets the new patients I am treating, he tells them how lucky they are to have me as their occupational therapist; he has become my ultimate cheerleader. Indeed, you could say that he's always out there, beating the drum for me and for occupational therapy!

Chapter Seventy-One

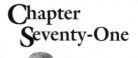

Allison's
Road to Recovery
Allison Brown Mann, OTR/L

Quick thinking, skilled doctors and nurses, tenacious parents, and any number of miracles saved my life. But occupational therapy and a determination to live brought me back to life.

By all accounts, I could have died many times that October evening in 1986. I never saw the car coming at me as I pulled my car out at the intersection, never knew the other car was there until it broad-sided my car on the driver's side. I could have died because the angle of the impact caused my seatbelt not to lock, and as a result, I was thrown forward with deadly force. I could have died when the seatbelt wrapped itself around my neck as it recoiled. I could have died when the force of the crash flung my door open and I was thrown from the car, being strangled by my seatbelt. I could have died when I swallowed my tongue and couldn't breathe.

But I didn't die. Quick thinking by two men who saw the accident saved my life, first by disentangling me from the seatbelt, then by prying my mouth open and freeing my tongue from my throat with nothing more than a spoon hastily fetched from his kitchen. Surgery over the next 24 hours would, as best could be hoped for under the circumstances, put me back together again and start me on the process of healing.

Although I was alive, my ordeal was just beginning. I had suffered massive internal injuries, fractured and broken bones, and multiple head injuries. Later, it would be determined that I had suffered multiple cerebral hemorrhagic contusions of the frontal lobe and subcortical areas due to the force of my brain being tossed against the inside of my skull, injuries that can result in severe brain damage. At the time, however, my mother, Pat, a registered nurse, knew just that the problem was very bad—in the ambulance on the way to the hospital, she and the emergency medical Technicians kept calling my name, but I did not respond.

The first task was to stabilize my condition. Within 2 hours of the accident, I was in surgery, then listed as being in "very critical condition." The next morning, I was back in surgery because of internal bleeding from my liver and internal clotting in my arteries and veins. The doctors and nurses were working diligently with me, giving me the best that the hospital had to offer, but my mother realized that things were really critical and that I needed to be taken to a major trauma center if there was to be any hope of my survival.

Fates that had seemed to favor me the night before now seemed to turn against me. Barricades seemed to appear at every turn. The surgeons who were needed for second opinions were tied up in other surgeries. My mother and father, Doug, didn't know anyone they could call at Georgia Baptist Medical Center, where they wanted me to go, to get me admitted. Fog and rain had grounded the Life Flight helicopter that would have transported me to Georgia Baptist, and the assigned surgeon would not approve my release that night. The neurosurgeon was pessimistic, telling them, "We are losing her. She has been to surgery twice. In spite of all efforts, she is bleeding from everywhere. It will take a miracle to turn things around."

The doctor couldn't have known how prophetic his words would turn out to be. At the same time he was talking to my parents, a prayer vigil had begun at my church. Within an hour, my bleeding had stopped. An hour after that, a trauma specialist at Georgia Baptist had been contacted and agreed to accept me as a patient, and the grounded Life Flight crew had agreed to transport me by ambulance to the trauma center.

There was more good news almost from the moment that I arrived at Georgia Baptist on the evening of October 13, 1986. A CAT scan showed that despite all of my internal bleeding, my brain condition hadn't deteriorated significantly. I was settled into the surgical intensive care unit, where I was comatose for much of the next month. Though I couldn't have known it that first night, I was about to move into recovery mode, with the help of an occupational therapist named Janie.

Chapter Seventy-One

Janie, an acute care occupational therapist at Georgia Baptist, had the enthusiasm of a newly graduated occupational therapist, which she was. One colleague observed that this enthusiasm seemed to radiate from her bright blue eyes and could be seen in her day-in and day-out commitment to her patients.

I met Janie on October 14 and seemed to bond with her immediately. From the first, Janie worked tirelessly, doing things like moving my legs and arms to preserve muscle tone, providing coma stimulation (touch and word exercises that stimulate the coma patient's brain functions), and fashioning splints for my bruised body. Janie also acted as teacher and counselor, offering my parents encouragement and teaching them ways that they could help with my therapy.

Janie continued to see me almost every day, and when I was transferred to acute care almost a month after arriving at Georgia Baptist, Janie was there, continuing my therapy.

It wasn't easy. The ICU stay had included many medical complications. Six separate doctors each monitored a different medical problem, from infections, breathing difficulties, pelvic fractures, bladder problems, and the closed head injury. Particularly worrisome was bleeding complicating the pelvic fracture that led to the need to immobilize my leg in a bent position, which would later take almost 3 years to straighten. For another thing, my voice was extremely soft after having had tubes in my throat for 23 days, so talking was an ordeal. Furthermore, I tired easily and was sometimes uncooperative. At times, I grew frustrated at my own limitations and lashed out at Janie, who always seemed able to absorb the frustrated outbursts and move on. In the end, despite the obstacles, a strong bond developed between Janie and I, and slowly but surely, small milestones of recovery—my first day on a tilt table, giving me a feel for how it felt to stand upright again—began to pile up.

My small successes heartened my parents, but they remained concerned; I was still totally paralyzed on my left side, I had lost many of my academic abilities, and I was unable to do any of the activities of daily living. As I fought through the fog and agitation of coma recovery, my parents began to wonder, "Will we ever see our Allison again?" Janie and the other therapists on my team offered what encouragement they could, but the question lingered. But no one except my parents counted on me and my determination to recover and return to college.

The first signs of big changes are usually small—a tiny bud on a tree branch signals the coming of spring, the barest spit of rain signals the imminence of a downpour. For me, it was a small wiggle of the big toe on my left foot, the first time I had moved the toe in the nearly 2 months since the accident, that heralded my eventual recovery. Just a small wiggle, it was a sign that hard work and grit might lead to something big.

I was transferred to a rehabilitation unit and a new team of occupational therapists, led by Gail. The tasks before us were immense, since it was a long way from a wiggling toe to full recovery. First and foremost, I had to learn how to shower, to dress myself, to brush my hair, put on makeup, and prepare for a new day, then learn to walk, write, and regain my speech. Days were grueling. Every morning before 7:30 a.m., Gail arrived, ready to help me through these tasks. Then it was off to breakfast; then more occupational therapy, physical therapy, and speech therapy; followed by lunch; then more therapy; followed by dinner; and then an evening activity to boost my spirits.

But again, despite my small successes, my parents continued to be haunted by the question, "Will we see our Allison again?" In February 1987, 4 months after the accident, a neuropsychologist tested me and concluded that I would never return to Auburn or any other college. My parents were crushed. Very gently, my mother tried to explain to to me what the doctor had said.

"Mom, what will I do?" I desperately asked, tears filling my eyes. I had never even entertained the thought that I would not go back to college.

"That is just an opinion," my mother replied, trying to comfort me. "You'll go back to school. Just wait and see."

As it turned out, I wasn't quite out of miracles yet. Always a goal-oriented person, I set tough goals for myself each day and week. Soon, Gail had me dressing and grooming myself in occupational therapy. In physical therapy, I practiced leg exercises and walking in the parallel bars. Working with the speech therapist, I began writing for the rehabilitation newspaper in the hospital. Every night, my parents and I practiced visualization, until I could literally "see" myself riding in my wheelchair to the hospital exit on the day of my discharge. And in perhaps the biggest miracle of all, on March 13, 1987, 5 months after an accident should have ended my life, I rode in that wheelchair down a hallway to an elevator, and then into an elevator that took me to the first floor, and then out of the elevator to a door that would take me out of the hospital. At the front door, I paused as if to gather strength. And then, against all odds, the girl who should have been dead slowly lifted herself out of the wheelchair and walked out of the hospital.

I had lived. Now I needed to come back to life.

When my parents first began to discuss how they would care for me after my discharge, they were advised to look at several long-term care facilities for victims of head trauma. None of the facilities seemed right for me, however, and they began to think about a home care program. They were quickly discouraged by the rehabilitation staff and doctors, who recounted the difficulties, catalogued the obstacles, and noted all of the pitfalls of home care. Just finding the therapist and team members in a small town in Georgia would be impossible, they said.

Chapter Seventy-One

Determination in the face of obstacles may be a learned trait or it may be inherited, but whatever its source, my stubborn streak had clearly come from my parents, who, despite the opinions of the "experts," set out to do the impossible.

My parents had been told that finding a neuropsychologist to lead the team would be impossible. No problem. A few inquiries in the local school system led them to Lynda, a school psychologist who had known me as a gifted elementary school student and was now completing her doctorate in neuropsychology. The team had a leader.

My parents had also been told that finding a teacher skilled in the type of learning disability I had would be impossible. No problem. Lynda led them to Michelle, a teacher of children with the same type of learning disabilities. Michelle signed on to the team.

They had been told it would difficult to find a physical therapist and an occupational therapist to come to our home. No problem. Barbara, an acquaintance who was both an occupational therapist and a physical therapist agreed to do both jobs for me.

Volunteers filled in the gaps. Two of my friends who were teachers came by in the mornings to tutor me in English and to drill me in simple math. Another friend came over in the afternoons to do arts and crafts with me to build motor skills and buoy my spirits.

And of course, my family pitched in everywhere at once. My father became the afternoon physical therapist, worked with me in a pool at the local fitness club, and schooled himself in computer programs that would help me with my rehabilitation. My mother worked with me to reinforce the various lessons in math, English, speech, and occupational therapy and to constantly encourage me to continue my progress. My sister, Amy, who had survived the accident with relatively minor injuries, became my confidant and cheerleader.

Finally, the rehabilitation team that the hospital staff had predicted would be impossible to assemble was in place, functional, and ready to roll. Skeptical, the Browns' insurance company sent a neuropsychologist from Philadelphia to review my program. After talking with everyone involved, he told Lynda that he had been prepared to report that it would not work, but that after seeing the plan in action, he was happy to report that he thought it could work.

And what of my commitment to this program? Monday through Friday, I was up at 6:30 a.m. and dressed and at the dining room table ready to begin therapy at 8:00 a.m. Many days, therapy lasted until after 5:00 p.m. (in itself a minor miracle; most head trauma patients lack that level of stamina). By May, 6 weeks after my home therapy had begun, a neuropsychologist who evaluated me in a grueling day-long series of tests reported that I was making "an impressive neuropsychological recovery" and that the pace and extent of my recovery (both how far I had come and how quickly) were "very close to amazing."

Nevertheless, there would be one more set of tests. I had to weather yet another surgical crisis in September 1987, when a calcification that had formed as a result of a blood clot was removed from my left groin. Even though I was in intensive care for 2 days following the extensive surgery, within a week my determination of spirit had me walking up the hall of the hospital. And I resumed my rigorous rehabilitation activities within 3 weeks of the surgery.

Now the girl who should have been dead still had one more obstacle to clear on her path to recovery—returning to Auburn University. In January 1988, I enrolled in two courses at a local junior college where my mother taught nursing. After a ride to school with her, a morning of classes, a ride home, and some lunch, it was back to therapy. At the end of the quarter, another miracle—the girl who was told she might never return to school had earned an "A" in English!

In March 1988, after an 18-month hiatus, I did return to Auburn to complete my freshman year. My roommate from the previous year arranged for me to move into the dormitory with her. The sorority I had pledged the previous year invited me to join again. With the support of the Auburn University administration and faculty advisors, my grades climbed back to where they had been before the accident. Life returned to normal, or as normal as life can be for any college student.

Then I discovered that perhaps the greatest miracle of all was normalcy. For the first time in a long time, I began to think about a future beyond my recovery. I decided to investigate a career as an occupational therapist.

Postscript: During my junior year at Auburn, I transferred to the University of Alabama at Birmingham to study occupational therapy and graduated magna cum laude in 1993. I now works as an occupational therapist at Crestwell Nursing and Rehabilitation Center in Georgia.

In December 1994, I met Art Mann, the son of my parents' friends. Art's parents and my parents had been friends since high school, and Art's dad had been a groomsman at my parents' wedding but we had met only once as toddlers. Art and I were married in January 1996. I had been warned by my doctors that damage to my pituitary gland suffered in the accident would make it difficult for me to conceive. Miraculously, but perhaps not unexpectedly, in early 1997, I became pregnant without any medical intervention, and on November 17, 1997, gave birth to Chandler Austin Mann.

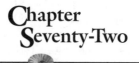

Still
Climbing High

Karen Crane Macdonald,
PhD, OTR/L

I t was September 1992. The truck driver claimed he didn't see
me as he changed lanes, that I was in his blind spot. I was traveling in the slow lane, and I never really saw what happened,
but I certainly felt it.

Six days earlier, I could hardly believe I was presenting a paper
at a national conference on education! This was what I'd been
working for as an occupational therapist for more than 15 years:
speaking at a conference, traveling, meeting people, inching ever
closer to my goal of completing a doctorate in occupational therapy, so I could teach at a university, write, and do research. I
could feel all of the hard work, ambition, and devotion to my
cherished career coming together to put within my reach the
achievement of my long-held goals and dreams.

That all changed in an instant when the truck collided with
my car. On that day, the car-carrier truck in the next lane of the
expressway broad-sided my car not once, but twice, as I was driving to a birthday party to meet my fiancé's family.

Out of nowhere, my head smashed against the left window and
then (even with seatbelt on) I "rebounded" hard all the way to
the right, my whole body thrown like a doll. I was, I guess, reflex-
ively screaming and crying; it felt like a hammer hitting a thumb,
but this was my head! I remember thinking that my car was going

to go out of control off the side of the highway, and grabbing the wheel to steer back into the slow lane. At that moment, on my left in my peripheral vision, I saw a black wall moving toward me. In a split second, he hit me the second time, and I was jerked with maximum force forward and then sharply snapped back, rebounding again. Somehow, I slowed the car and stopped, groggily thinking... "I've been in an accident." I had swirling thoughts and an early memory of the advice in my driver's education course, "If you're ever in an accident, get their license plate." I went to find a pad and pen and discovered that nothing worked right—I could barely move or think—and then the driver of the truck and a witness began shouting "Are you all right?"

Confusion, police, ambulance, stretcher, rain on my face—when did it start raining? Hospital, pain, pain, lost, confusion, why is everyone shouting at me? Where is someone? Pain, my head was exploding and hammering as I writhed in pain.

The accident left me with a massive brain injury, months of painful recovery, and shattered life dreams. Outwardly, however, I guess I looked okay, the way people with closed head injuries sometimes do. I was diagnosed with a concussion and whiplash that Friday night. In a total fog, I went to my orthopedist on Monday, who immediately recognized that something very serious was wrong and sent me to a neurologist. I would subsequently undergo weeks and months and years of neurological testing, physical therapy, speech therapy, occupational therapy, social work guidance, endless other testing, balance and gait therapy, dizziness exercises, and support groups... all for a head injury and whiplash that took only a few moments to change my entire life.

I faithfully and patiently (as possible) tried to tolerate all the treatment, pain, indescribable violent nausea, and reeling dizziness whenever I tried any movement. All the while, because luckily there was no outward sign of disfigurement, people commented, "But you look great!" (Years later, they say, "You sure look so much better.")

During those years, I grasped at promises from anyone treating me—"in 6 months you will see change"—then that was changed to 2 years, then 5 years. I plodded through those years, fully believing that when the magic number appeared, I'd be cured. I've since come to discover that many of the symptoms will always remain. Some can be kept to a minimum by adaptations, but most activities are not possible unless they are kept to a very brief time and are done with assistance or modifications.

That's where my occupational therapy education and the help of several occupational therapists who treated me was really invaluable in keeping me able to pursue my dreams. Changes in my function from the head injury were both physical and cognitive. Strength, endurance, balance, walking, and coordination were major problems for me; memory learning, sequencing, attention, judgment, and processing were also incredible challenges. All routine activities had to be done in a special sequence that eliminated as much turning or leaning as possible, because any leaning caused maximum "seasickness" which rendered me unable to do anything until I stopped and rested. Because I loved my career and my work, I tried working a modified schedule for 3 years and somehow got through each hour, but I finally had to admit defeat, leave my job, and tearfully receive disability payments.

As must be evident from my description thus far, a head injury is incredibly frustrating and challenging to live with. It is equally difficult that it is an "invisible injury" that is unseen and therefore often not understood by others. A short list of my ongoing symptoms and struggles that persist to this day includes: limited strength and endurance; difficulty with walking, balance, coordination, and speaking; and a variety of thinking and reasoning challenges (especially memory, organization, and problem solving). My daily living tasks still must be painstakingly structured, carefully planned and paced, and then broken into tiny concrete steps. I make lists of my lists, just to get through each day. But it works.

I had many difficulties and bad experiences, but there were also good experiences. Because I am an occupational therapist, I was able to figure out some things for myself, and I received significant help from other occupational therapists, including friends, colleagues, and those I saw professionally. I was helped by the early involvement of an orthopedist, neurologist, physical therapist, neuropsychologist, speech pathologist, and social worker during the first several months of pain and massive confusion. However, without my background in occupational therapy, I am convinced that I would not have made the progress that I have made toward managing my daily tasks and continuing toward my dream of completing my doctorate and returning to part-time employment.

After I completed a 6 month medical leave and was attempting to return to work on a part-time basis, my insurance plan covered occupational therapy, but for two sessions only. I knew that I needed occupational therapy treatment desperately to help me to relearn how to do activities of daily living, work, and community management skills. Unfortunately, these two sessions left me very disappointed, because two sessions couldn't possibly address the enormous number of problems I knew I still had. I decided that I would have to call on all my previous occupational therapy skills and try to treat myself!

I used the best of my own knowledge and clinical experience to force my mind and body through purposeful activities during the first year. To increase my ability to sit and balance myself for longer periods of time and to increase my neck and shoulder range of motion, strength, and motor coordination, I set times daily for crocheting, hand quilting, and relearning knitting. For mental reasoning and thinking challenges, it was planning and doing every single self-care task. What a major success it was to do my first load of laundry! I attempted light reading and pored over magazines and picture books on some of my favorite topics such as antiques and decorating to help me tolerate visual stimulation and to help me remember items.

Occupational therapist friends and colleagues who visited offered excellent suggestions for easier to harder activities and assorted "thinking-perceiving-moving" tasks. They suggested helpful card games such as Solitaire, jigsaw puzzles, Scrabble, and ideas that ranged from crawling with my vision blocked to macrame. I tried every exercise and activity I or anyone else could dream up! Progress was slow and evident, but real function was still a distant and foggy goal.

Meanwhile, life went on! During all of this, real life proceeded! This included dating "my beloved," a beautiful wedding, moving to a new home, attempting to continue to work part-time, and somehow staying attached to making progress on my doctorate.

After the indescribable blur of the first year, I started to realize that despite all of my best efforts, faith, prayers, and support, I was still having significant struggles with daily and long-term projects. I started to pay to see an occupational therapist privately, and she changed everything. Over the nearly 5 years that I have seen her, she has changed an enormous number of things in my life from "nearly impossible" to "somehow possible." And the list keeps growing.

With an emphasis on improving my brain functioning and thinking processes, she has worked closely with me as I identify problem areas, and then I follow her lead for problem solving. We brainstorm solutions, she listens to my feedback, and we continually adapt until we hit upon a way of doing things that is realistic and do-able. Because of ongoing difficulty with putting steps in order, planning, and pacing, she started by getting me in the habit of making a daily checklist of "To Do" items. For example, using my strengths of being very visual, we color coded what was to be done and added another color to record what was already completed. Over the years, this system was adapted many times to help me manage at work and to help me progress in school. We made systems for daily, weekly, and annual projects. It is as if I need a structure for "programming" myself for action, and I've learned that no task consists only of a single step. But now that I know how to use the system, I can handle any task, no matter how complex, and that feels like quite an accomplishment!

Despite my best efforts, the cumulative challenges of working in the clinic were too much for me, and I decided to leave my job in the clinical environment, to focus my remaining skills on completing my doctorate. With hindsight now, I can see that I may not ever be able to return to the complex physical and mental demands of the clinic. In the quieter atmosphere of my home office environment, I used my remaining ability to slowly proceed with scholarly work, with the goal of completing my doctorate so I could have a future career of writing and roles in teaching or research.

During the process of my rehabilitation, countless occupational therapists offered support through weekly visits, daily calls, and establishment of a fund that helped to finance my private occupational therapy sessions. Their ongoing helpful tips helped me to adapt, adjust, accept the disability, and to keep living, with meaning.

This experience of dealing with my own disability has helped shape me into a person with patience and a passion for personal and professional growth. It has taught me to care about the adversities of others and has given me the insight to cope with my own. My experience with having and coping with this life-altering physical disability led me to focus my doctoral dissertation research on other women who have faced various life-altering disabilities. I have now interviewed and studied an amazing group of women who have survived and coped with such traumas. My goal was to learn from them and to share with others in the future the kinds of things that help people adapt to such life-changing events. My completed dissertation documents their first-hand experience of living with and recovering from disabilities, written from the unique perspective of one who has been there personally.

In May 1998, with my husband, family, and friends in the audience, I proudly walked down the aisle in my cap and gown at the New York University commencement to receive my doctorate in occupational therapy. The culminating moment of years of dreams, work, and focused activity, it was a very short walk at the end of a very long journey. Cheered on by this triumph, I know that my journey back from disability has not ended my march; on the contrary, my journey toward the challenges of tomorrow's achievements has just begun.

Brain Attack

Stroke and Other Head Injuries

Stroke and Other Head Injuries

These are the stories of eight people whose lives and personalities were altered by injury to the brain. These people needed to relearn who they were and what they could do next. Whether return to former life activities or lifestyle redesign was the outcome, with the help of their therapists, they regained control over who they were and how they would live.

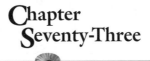

Chapter Seventy-Three

The Father of the Bride

Josephine Cohen, MA, OTR/L

Aaron is the strong, silent type. He is also a very determined and successful person. His large frame and excellent physical strength had made it natural for him to play football and wrestle in high school. After marrying, he had built up a successful lumber and mill business and provided well for his wife, son, and daughter. His son was married and also worked with Aaron in the family business. Life was good, and Aaron was very much used to being in charge of that life. That is, until his stroke shortly after his 61st birthday.

Aaron's stroke was a result of a brainstem lesion that affected his balance and swallowing. Three months after the initial stroke, he suffered a mini-stroke that involved his left leg and left arm, in addition to developing pneumonia. Aaron had full range of motion in his left arm and hand, but he had little or no sensation. If he wanted to use his hand, therefore, he couldn't feel where it was; he had to look where he was placing it. When he didn't, he felt clumsy and out of control, because his hand would bump into furniture or other objects, often causing severe and dangerous bruising.

I learned later just how frustrating all this had been for Aaron and also how hard it had been on his wife. It was not uncommon for her to keep the car windows tightly shut on her late night drives home from the hospital, so that she could scream out loud her hurt and frustration.

I first met Aaron while I was working as an occupational therapist at an outpatient rehabilitation facility, when he was referred to me for hand therapy. By then, 3 years had already gone by since his strokes, and he had received some speech and physical therapy, as well as biofeedback training to help him walk. His arm and shoulder range of motion was very good, but there still was no sensation in his left hand. Most noticeable was that this big, strapping man walked with short, halting steps.

True to his personality, Aaron set himself a rigorous program. With the help of his very supportive wife, Aaron was up and out of his house each morning by 8:30 a.m. He would drive to swimming and physical and occupational therapy sessions. He followed those up with lunch with friends, and then appeared every afternoon at the family business just to "check up on things."

When I left my job at the outpatient facility, I continued to treat Aaron at home, as part of my private practice, as did the physical therapist. As a hand therapist, my focus was not on Aaron's gait and walking. I concentrated on finely coordinated functional hand activities, including typing for strengthening his fingers, checkbook balancing, writing checks, and filling in crossword puzzles for increasing his eye-to-hand coordination and his perceptual skills. Aaron threw himself fully into doing these things, often persisting for long periods each day, long after most people would have given up. I think he considered me a friend with whom a strong bond had formed.

All our goals changed, however, when the physical therapist and I learned that Aaron's daughter was about to be married. Only by chance did I ask him about walking her down the aisle. Aaron's response was not what I expected from this strong-willed, hard-driving man. All he said was, "Her brother is going to walk her down." There was no explanation offered. It was only by talking to Aaron's wife that I learned why he answered that way. Aaron was not sure he could make it successfully down the aisle, and the risk of showing weakness in public and possibly "spoiling" his daughter's magical moment was just not something he could tolerate.

I shared this news with my physical therapy counterpart who assured me that despite his own uncharacteristic misgivings, Aaron was physically up to the task. That was the beginning of our "great conspiracy." The two of us entered into a pact that would not be broken until our mission was accomplished—Aaron was going to walk down that aisle and deliver his daughter to her bridegroom.

For the next 2½ months, we were relentless. We brought up the subject at every therapy session in order to explore his reservations. We both drilled him in walking, concentrating on his gait pattern and on his endurance to go the distance down the aisle. I addressed the issue of what shoes Aaron could wear that would be appropriate for both his gait and the occasion. We insisted on practice, practice, practice. There were times when I was sure that Aaron was going to fire us both, but we were willing to take that chance, hoping that our confidence would rub off on him.

Right up to the day of the wedding, we weren't sure we had succeeded. Aaron just refused to discuss the issue or tell us what he was going to do. A few days after the wedding, I could stand the suspense no longer. I called Aaron to ask how the wedding had gone. In his typical strong, silent type role, all he told me was, "It was very lovely."

My only recourse at that point was to call Aaron's wife. When I told her why I was calling and what Aaron had, or more exactly hadn't, told me, she was genuinely surprised. "Didn't Aaron tell you? He walked our daughter down the aisle, and there was not a dry eye in the room. One woman was openly sobbing."

So why wouldn't Aaron tell me himself and give me the satisfaction of knowing what had happened? Probably because Aaron knew I would call his wife and get the wonderful news of his accomplishment from her. I was so pleased that Aaron had utilized my colleague's and my support and encouragement to maintain his sense of his own strength and self-sufficiency that was the essence of his being. The team effort had been a success. As an occupational therapist, I could respect that need for dignity, and I have maintained a friendship with Aaron and his wife that continues to this day. After all, the father of the bride, his wife, his physical therapist, and I share a memory to cherish forever.

Chapter
Seventy-Four

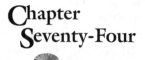

Never Give Up
Linda Carver Morse, OTR

There are some things they don't teach you in occupational therapy school, like dodging a tossed splint or a long-handled reacher, accompanied by a barrage of angry words, all flung by a frustrated patient with stroke. These were skills I had to learn on the job when I first started treating Mr. B.

Mr. B was one of my home health patients. He was a 56-year-old man who had a stroke on the right side of his brain that left him able to walk, but only with a four-pronged quad cane, and with a painful and nonfunctional left arm. It was true that he suffered from a physical paralysis. But his inability to use his arm seemed as much, if not more, due to emotional factors. Mr. B was struggling with the natural and typical anger and depression resulting from the fact of having had a stroke and its impact on his way of life.

Helping Mr. B sort through what he wanted and needed to do in order to continue on with his life was an ongoing process; all the while I found myself having to dodge the flung splint and the tossed reacher being thrown my way and being the target of a hail of angry words. Yet creating a therapeutic relationship in which it was safe for Mr. B to express himself appropriately, while gently channeling and guiding him toward the light of hope and affirmation was crucial before getting down to the nitty gritty of his occupational performance. So I kept at it doggedly, continuing with both kinds of occupational therapy goals, emotional and physical, until Mr. B managed to improve in his physical skills sufficiently to warrant discharge from occupational therapy home services.

I did not fully recognize just how successful I had been with Mr. B until 4 months after his discharge. The theme for the annual New Hampshire Occupational Therapy Association meeting was "Community Experiences with Occupational Therapy." Consumers who had been recipients of occupational therapy services were invited as speakers and instructors. I was surprised to see that Mr. B was to be one of the speakers and privately wondered just what he would say.

When his turn came to speak, I was delighted to hear Mr. B state that occupational therapy had been invaluable to him. He told everyone that he wanted to impart a very important message to us all. That message was, "Never give up on your patients." He somewhat sheepishly admitted that he had been the worst patient; he told how he had cut his splint in half, had thrown his clothes around the room, had thrown things at his therapist, and how he had ranted and raved. Yet through it all, he said, his therapist was as determined as he was and stood by him and enabled him to function. Mr. B concluded that he was now happy to report that he could fully dress himself, prepare his own meals, and work on his computer, all because his therapist never gave up.

I came away from that session recommitted to a very important OT principle. Often after a serious illness or an accident, a person must first sift through the barrage of violent emotions that can plague and dampen the spirit. Unless the treating occupational therapist can put on mud boots and wade through that journey with the patient, the light at the end of the tunnel—truly functional behavior—may never be realized. And no matter how hard it seems and no matter how long it takes, you can never give up.

Chapter
Seventy-Five

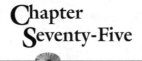

Baby Talk
Jacqueline Davis Templin, OTR/L

New mothers can be insufferable when telling stories about their babies, and I suppose I was no exception. Everyone in my life was subjected to ceaseless tales about Casey, my wonder baby. Some complained that my constant babbling about Casey was putting them to sleep. But one person, Dorothea, actually had a very different reaction.

Dorothea was 78 when she suffered a severe stroke, which left her in a comatose state. Her doctor and family were very surprised, because up to that time, she had been very healthy and active and had taken total care of herself, her husband, and her two dogs. She had a house full of beautiful African violets, sang in the church choir, and visited her two daughters and five grandchildren frequently. She was in the middle of sewing a Halloween costume for her granddaughter when she developed blurred vision, complained of a headache, and then lost consciousness.

After a hospital course during which Dorothea did not "wake up," her family sent her to a skilled nursing facility adjacent to the hospital. Her doctor told the family to find a long-term nursing home placement for the future. In the skilled nursing facility, occupational therapy was ordered for range of motion to keep her joints mobile and for sensory stimulation to try and arouse her on some level. Although she did not speak or follow any commands, she did have a sucking reflex and an adequate swallow and was able to drink small amounts of thick liquids.

Dorothea was one of the first patients on my schedule following my return to work part-time after the birth of my first daughter. This was well before managed care, and I was able to spend a full half-hour with Dorothea three times a week for several weeks. As I passively ranged her thin arms or applied resting splints, I would narrate every detail of my new baby's life. "Hi Dorothea, my name is Jackie. I have a new baby daughter named Casey. She is 5 months old. Guess what she had for breakfast this morning? That's right. A banana. Today she wore a purple jogging suit. Last night we read *Goodnight Moon*."

I moved on to offering Dorothea various scents to arouse her olfactory sense. Scents included snips of African violets brought in by her family; vials of potting soil; familiar cooking ingredients such as vanilla, coffee, or nutmeg; and even noxious odors like vinegar or ammonia. All the while, I would continue with mundane trivia about Casey to my captive audience. Before long, Dorothea had been told every aspect of my baby's existence.

Different tastes were introduced to Dorothea via homemade juice pops, and we included every flavor from sour lemon to sweet cherry. Her response was mechanical sucking and swallowing, but she did seem slightly more alert during these sessions. She seemed to like the ice cold feeling on her mouth.

Dorothea's husband or daughters would usually visit in the early afternoon, and they were eager to learn new techniques that might help her. We even arranged to have the dogs come in one afternoon. Of course, her family also suffered through new-baby stories and were also subject to baby pictures, which I brought in and showed to Dorothea frequently.

Dorothea made very little progress, but we persevered with treatment for 10 weeks with tactile stimulation, positioning, musical tapes, news on the radio, and my 3-times-a-week, detailed accounts of my daughter's life. As plans were being made for a permanent nursing home placement for Dorothea, Christmas came and went. You can be sure Dorothea heard of every gift in Casey's stocking. On New Year's Eve, I entered Dorothea's room and started massaging her fingers. As I told her of our plans for the evening and who was going to babysit, Dorothea opened one eye. She said, "I know your baby's name is Casey. What did she wear today?" I couldn't believe this was happening. I excused myself, ran to the nursing station, and called her husband, who came right over. Dorothea later asked for a sweet popsicle, not one of those sour ones.

Dorothea made an amazing recovery. After a 2-month stay in a rehabilitation center, she returned home to her family, dogs, and plants. On a warm, sunny day, I brought my daughter to meet Dorothea. She reached out, gave her a hug, and told me she had to wake up—so I would stop telling her all of those baby stories!

Chapter Seventy-Six

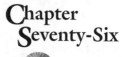

You Are My Sunshine

Julie Chelte, OTR/L

Kelly suffered a severe stroke leaving her with both expressive and receptive aphasia—she could neither speak to express her own ideas nor receive messages to understand what others were saying to her. In addition to leaving her unable to communicate, the stroke paralyzed her right side and caused apraxia, the inability to use objects properly or to plan motor tasks. When I first met the 62 year old, she was lying in bed, appearing pale and weak.

That morning, I attempted to perform my evaluation of her, but Kelly was difficult to rouse. I tried to explain to her that I needed to get her out of bed and into a wheelchair, but she couldn't understand what I was asking her to do. In the end, I had to lift her from the bed and set her in the wheelchair. Kelly couldn't perform any of the other simple tasks, such as combing her hair, either. Kelly moaned and screamed, but I could not tell if she was crying in pain or frustration. Exhausted, she became unresponsive again.

For weeks, her lethargy continued. She seemed to have given up, lacking any noticeable desire to improve her well-being. Her medical team met weekly to discuss her progress or lack thereof, and over time, we became increasingly frustrated when her physical and mental condition did not improve. Kelly's HMO insurance company representative wanted us to send her to a nursing facility and set a 3-week deadline, which was fast approaching.

One morning, however, everything changed for Kelly. Her speech therapist rushed to my office and told me excitedly, "Kelly can sing! She sang a song!"

I could barely believe the news, but I remembered that often people with Kelly's condition are able to sing but not talk. I went to Kelly's room and asked her to sing for me. I had been told that Kelly was singing "You Are My Sunshine," so I tried to get Kelly started. When she began to sing, the words weren't clear, but I could clearly recognize the melody.

"That's wonderful, Kelly! I'm so proud of you!" I told her. Kelly smiled as she reached for my hand and put it to her cheek. While I was sure she didn't understand what I was saying, I knew she could understand the excitement visible on my face.

However, whether or not she fully understood the importance of this breakthrough, Kelly seemed to have found within herself a new determination, which I wanted to cultivate. So Kelly's musical "career" at our facility began. We practiced singing simple songs together daily. Her repertoire expanded, but "You Are My Sunshine" remained a favorite. At the team meeting for Kelly's third and possibly final week, we informed Kelly's doctor about her initially minor but potentially major progress, and the HMO agreed to extend its coverage for another 3 weeks.

In the following week, in addition to singing to warm up, we worked on Kelly's self-care, reteaching her to groom and dress herself. Soon, Kelly was able to follow simple one- and two-step commands. Working hard day after day, sometimes to the tune of "You Are My Sunshine," Kelly finally began to overcome her apraxia and motor planning difficulties. She also began to try to use words to communicate and was having some small success with simple words. She still kept singing.

Muscle strength began to return quickly to Kelly's right leg, and she began to help herself in getting around. In less than 2 weeks, she was walking. That was the good news. The bad news was that along with increased muscle strength in her right leg, her right arm muscles began to develop increased tone. This pulled her into the typical "hemi posture" in her upper body—fingers, wrist, elbow, and shoulder flexed, with the arm held close to the body. In this position, unfortunately, because the muscles that hold her shoulder upright were still weak, the weight of her arm pulled her shoulder downward, and a painful subluxation of her right shoulder began.

However, for some reason we did not completely understand, as her muscles improved, Kelly experienced a setback in her language abilities. Now that she was fully alert and making progress in her physical rehabilitation, she became increasingly frustrated with her speech problems. No matter how hard she tried, she couldn't find the right words. For example, she'd say clearly, "I am you, and you are me," and then shake her head in anger and cry from the frustration of not being able to say what she meant. When asked to repeat words or attempt to speak again, she would give up and stop trying. Her speech pathologist was having difficulty getting her to participate in their 30-minute daily sessions. She even refused to sing. Day by day, Kelly spoke less often and finally she reverted to moaning and expecting people to guess what she needed. The sound of music from Kelly had stopped.

I spent an hour and a half every day with Kelly trying to get her to communicate and every now and then she would sing. But after some time, Kelly began to try to mimic my words. "Juice. Juice," I would coax her, and Kelly would eventually catch on and respond, "youss." I would praise her success, "Good, Kelly, you're getting it." She would grab my hand and pull it to her cheek, her way of showing me she appreciated my efforts.

One morning to my surprise, Kelly asked me in a clear voice, "How are you?"

"What did you say?" I asked her, still amazed by the clarity in her voice.

"You are me, and I am you," she said, then shook her head, realizing that was not what she intended to say.

"I am fine, Kelly, how are you?" I asked hopefully.

"Yes," she said, "My name is Kell...eee."

"What is my name?" I asked her, hoping to stimulate her further.

"You-lee. You-lee. You-lee," she responded with some effort, struggling to pronounce my name for the first time. And then, she sang "You Are My Sunshine."

After 6 weeks at our facility, Kelly was ready to return home with her husband and continue her therapy on an outpatient basis. Kelly was able to perform all of her self-care tasks (dressing, bathing, grooming, using the toilet) and getting around on her own with the support of a walker. Her right arm remained totally motionless and extremely weak, and her speech still needed work, but her husband was still thankful for his wife's progress. "I know Kelly would like to tell you how grateful she is to all of you for showing her that she's still a woman with a life worth living," he told her medical team, "And I'm grateful to you that I have my wife back."

"You are my wife, and I am your husband," Kelly said. Then she shook her head and instead of giving up, tried it again. "You are my husband, and I am your wife," she said smiling at her husband.

As we said our goodbyes, Kelly looked over at me and called out, "Youlee!" And for the last time, she pulled my hand to her cheek. I realized that moments like these are the most rewarding of my career. As they left, I found myself humming "You Are My Sunshine."

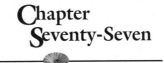

Mr. Zip-Zap
Anne Gaier, OTR/L, CHT

"Zip-zap," he said, standing in front of me in the occupational therapy department. With a grin as wide as a river, my patient pointed to his untied shoes and repeated, "Zip-zap."

It was 1974, and I had been working as a therapist for about a year in a rehabilitation hospital. I especially enjoyed working with older folks and felt I had the best occupational therapy job in the world. I was always ready for a challenge, and at the moment, this man definitely had my attention.

Mr. Yalta had suffered a stroke that resulted in right hemiplegia and aphasia, which left his right arm and leg partially paralyzed and made it almost impossible for him to find the right words or to speak clearly. A tall, quiet man, because of the aphasia he tended to be almost monosyllabic in his communication. It had taken several weeks of hard work before he was able to dress his upper body on his own, and even more time to advance to full-body dressing. He was very proud of his accomplishments in self-care skills, but he knew that to be allowed to go home, he had to be able to dress himself completely.

Now he had surprised me by putting on his socks and shoes by himself. "Zip-zap," he insisted. But what did he want? I noticed that his shoes were untied and made a mental note to bring elas-

279

tic shoelaces to dressing training the next day. After all, if he could already put on his shoes, maybe he could learn to finish the task using elastic laces and a shoehorn. Then he would be independent in dressing, and one step closer to going home.

Undaunted, Mr. Yalta became more persistent: "Zip-zap." Suddenly, it clicked: He wanted Velcro adaptations for his shoes! His roommate's shoes had just been adapted with Velcro, a new material that, because of its ease and versatility, was becoming very popular with rehabilitation therapists and their patients. With Velcro, Mr. Yalta's roommate was able to put his shoes on without help. I smiled and said, "Aha! I will arrange to get 'zip-zap' for your shoes."

Now we—both occupational therapists and the general public—take Velcro for granted. We can easily find purses, wallets, sports clothing, diapers, and more with convenient Velcro. Today, you can buy a pair of athletic shoes with Velcro closures at any local shopping mall. But in the 1970s, Velcro on commercial items didn't exist. Even therapists in a rehabilitation unit had to ask a physician to write an order for Velcro closures for patients' shoes. The shoes then had to be taken to an orthotist for modification, then delivered to the patient at the hospital.

I was able to arrange all this and finally received the shoes with Mr. Yalta's special adaptations. I still remember how pleased he was the first time he got to "zip-zap" his own shoes. Mr. Yalta continued to improve, eventually becoming totally independent. He returned home to his wife and the family bakery. And in the occupational therapy department, we have fondly remembered him as Mr. Zip-Zap.

Please note: The patient's name has been changed to protect his privacy.

Chapter
Seventy-Eight

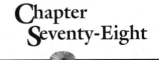

A Spiritual Nature

Peggy Dawson, OTR/L

"That we humans can help each other is one of our unique human capacities. We must share in other people's suffering. To show concern, to give moral support, and to express sympathy are themselves valuable. This is what should be the basis of activities; whether one calls it religion or not, does not matter."

These words, spoken by the Dalai Lama, ring particularly true to me. After being the occupational therapist for many years, I became a patient. I was once a university professor, teaching occupational therapy, until my doctors found a cerebral blood vessel, malformed and slowly leaking. I underwent brain surgery without incident, but postsurgical complications arose. Within hours, I had severe left hemisphere swelling with intracranial pressure. I developed total paralysis of my right side, a condition known as "hemiplegia." I almost died; in fact, I had a near-death experience.

While the initial sensations and images surrounding the near-death experience were over in a matter of minutes, its presence in my life continued to be very strong. Physically, I experienced extreme discomfort, was paralyzed on one side, and now had a brain injury from the swelling, but I also had a feeling of exhilaration. An exciting new opportunity had been revealed. The event had somehow transfigured me, as if I had been taken apart and reassembled in a more expansive way.

After I was stabilized, I was moved to a rehabilitation unit, where I settled into a state of generally "good spirits." Becoming a head-injured, hemiplegic patient afforded me a rare and valuable opportunity to experience the symptoms I had observed and treated in so many others. Hemiplegia is a condition that most occupational therapists think we know a lot about. But actually experiencing it is absolutely crazy. For example, I had always thought there was no reason for patients to cry when they were unsuccessful in dressing themselves. I assumed they broke down, not because they felt a profound grief over their inability to perform a formerly simple task, but because some internal flash of frustration combined with a short-circuited brain caused the crying.

I learned differently one morning when I tried to put on my tennis shoe. I bent in my wheelchair, doing my best to dress. I had a bad headache, and my lifeless right foot might as well have been a hooked trout. In my efforts to get my foot into the uncooperative shoe, I literally chased it around the room. I wheeled from place to place, time after unsuccessful time, until I completely melted into the most well-deserved tears of my life. I had an overwhelming sense of personal ineffectiveness and loss. It was a most terrible phenomenon to consciously will what had so recently been a healthy right side to move and see that it would not respond. I had a fatigue that went clear through my skeleton.

Uncomfortably, I recalled the many times I, as a clinician, had played "cheerleader," encouraging—sometimes almost demanding—that a patient "stay up just a little longer" or do "just one more thing." I'd had no sense of the relentless tiredness he or she must have felt or how physically ill he or she could become trying to comply with that seemingly simple request.

Great trauma can open the doors to great transformations. During this time, despite the difficulties, I often felt an energy that carried joy, even playfulness. As a gag, an occupational therapist friend sent me temporary tattoos for my shaven head. At first, I wasn't in the mood for head decorations. But I came to appreciate those tattoos while I was in the rehabilitation unit. Soon, nearly all of the nurses and many of the patients were wearing them. One, a farmer with above-the-elbow amputation of both arms, wore tattoos on his new prostheses: red hearts that read "Mom." I chose a large red heart with the word "Bad" running across it in block letters on a white banner. That tattoo went on my paretic right leg, of course.

It seems that great meaning in our lives is directly correlated with the ability to complete small, everyday activities. These everyday activities provide the essential bricks in the larger structure of life goals and plans. Day after day, I wanted to make meaning of my life in the same ways I had before surgery. I frequently asked my therapists, "Will I ever write again?" "Will I walk?" "Will I ever be able to teach again?" My therapists' responses showed tremendous patience. They didn't say, "Let's wait and see," nor did they let me waste my time wringing my hands. Instead, they said, "Let's not wait for the hand, the mind, or the legs to come back. Let's just accept what is. Let's just begin right here and build now." They taught me that compassionate patience is not stopping a life, waiting indefinitely to pick up where the patient left off in some now-outdated plan. Instead, we must gently redistribute our hopes and focus on new goals that are concrete, realistic, more immediate, and more attainable.

A friend of mine who is studying the Burmese language told me that many Asian languages use the same word for "head" and "heart," the communication between the mind and the feelings being assumed. This Asian idea was nowhere more exemplified than in the various ministerings that issued from the treatment plans of my occupational therapists. Had my near-death experience not been so recent, I might never have realized the deeply spiritual nature of my chosen profession.

Occupational therapists are kind and understanding; we support our patients by holding their hands, patting their shoulders, smiling at them with encouragement, and guiding them across the rivers and hazards that we know lay within the landscape of specific disabilities. However, we can provide only a rough map of the terrain of illness. Each patient will encounter his or her own particular dangers and difficulties. The biggest problems or challenges may be those not addressed in the clinical setting because the clinic is a very limited world.

My occupational therapists offered me guidance that I especially appreciated: A visit to my "real world," my office. My old, haphazard system of organization now worried me because my memory had since been impaired. I wondered if I would be able to complete a paper that had been accepted for presentation at an upcoming conference. Although one visit to my office didn't give me the answers, it did demonstrate a way to explore these questions.

One of the goals of all religions is to help human beings improve their general condition. Similarly, most if not all forms of spirituality encourage us to appreciate each other and to participate in the wonderment of the moment. My favorite occupational therapist accomplished all of these things and more. She gave me not only techniques for change, but also a new, loving, calm acceptance of who or what I was at that moment. All of my therapists' well-grounded encouragement soon became my own hope.

"Stand up straight," my therapist would command with mock sternness from across the rehab gym.

"You've got to be kidding," I would respond. Our voices, hers prodding, mine good-naturedly complaining, would collide in a jovial exchange. Her delight when I was finally able to stand and completely dress myself, including the elusive right shoe, became my own joy.

Slowly, my body mended. I did not present my conference paper, but my hand began to work. I soon could hold a brush to fix my daughters' hair. Because of difficulties with memory, I could not resume my teaching job, but I regained enough strength in my right side to once again play basketball with my young sons. I regained enough sensation and range of motion to embrace my husband of nearly 30 years. I took a job as an occupational therapy clinician, hopefully one who touches the lives of others.

To these many feats, my therapists today would probably modestly enter the words "good progress" in my chart.

But I know all these moments are holy.

Chapter
Seventy-Nine

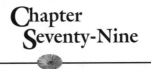

Discovering the Good in Bad Times (In Memory of Emily Marie)

Laura Rutherford Renner, OTR/L

It is true that bad things happen to good people, and we don't understand why. That is certainly how I felt when my schwanoma, a benign brain tumor, was discovered.

I had gotten great satisfaction over several years working as an occupational therapist at Magee Rehabilitation Center in Philadelphia with patients who had suffered strokes, orthopedic and spinal cord injuries, and other disorders. Now, I was looking forward to the next phase in my life—the birth of our first child in just a few weeks. But with the tumor diagnosis, my world was about to be turned upside down, and my most frightening nightmares were coming true. Yet, during those terrible times, wonderful friends and occupational therapist colleagues taught me that even during the worst of times, we can discover that there are good people who do good things that help us deal with pain and loss and recover a positive approach to life.

I was pregnant in late Spring of 1996 when I began to experience difficulty walking, writing, balancing, and staying awake at my job. A tough 8-hour day working with patients now seemed unbearable. At first, I thought these symptoms were the norm for

285

expectant women, but I soon realized that my symptoms were too severe to be written off as just the usual effects of pregnancy. My husband, Richard, and I finally convinced my obstetrician that something was wrong. He ordered a CAT scan that revealed a large brain tumor.

Almost faster than I could absorb what was happening to me, I was flown to Thomas Jefferson University Hospital in Philadelphia, where neurosurgeons confirmed that I had a benign schwanoma. Over the next few days, the obstetric and neurosurgery teams developed a plan to treat both me and my baby. Although Richard and I were still in shock, things appeared to be under control.

But they weren't. The normal prenatal testing I received daily in the hospital started to show problems. I was now 8½ months along, so the doctors decided to deliver the baby by a caesarean section. When they did, it confirmed the suspected anomalies. Our newborn daughter, Emily Marie, had Apert's syndrome, a very rare birth defect characterized by malformations of the skull, as well as other life-threatening complications. Six days after she came into our lives, Emily Marie died. However, I didn't have much time or ability to grieve at that point because I had to ready myself for my own upcoming brain surgery, and I was mentally and emotionally numb from all the medication. But even the surgery did not happen as scheduled. On the morning of my surgery, the C-section incision site was infected, and the operation was postponed 2 more weeks. The ordeal of it all, and the prospect of an additional wait, was devastating for me.

Back home, my husband and I sadly opened the bags of baby gifts that out-of-town relatives had sent for the baby shower that never happened. Unexpectedly, I came across Emily Marie's hospital bag and found her comforter, her little "onesy," and her tiny stuffed bear. The finality of it all suddenly hit me like a ton of bricks. Emily Marie was gone, and I might never have children of my own. I also began to realize how much of my own prior life was possibly going to be denied to me as well, as the enormity of my own symptoms became more apparent.

In my life before the discovery of the brain tumor and before Emily's death, when not busy treating patients, I had been an artist. Now, I could not paint or write, I could not walk by myself, and I had to tilt my head to avoid choking while eating. I was annoyed that I needed help to cook, to get to the bathroom, to dress. I was despondent.

To help me cope despite all the losses, therefore, I had to summon up my occupational therapy experience and focus on my determination to do things for myself. Sometimes, I was too focused and put myself in harm's way by trying something a bit too risky. But I tried not to give up hope.

It was at that low point that I discovered, even in my despair, that so much good surrounded me. I had so many friends. People I barely knew seemed to care about me. My work mates were a huge source of friendship and support. They sent fruit baskets and flower arrangements. After the C-section, they stayed with me in the hospital. These good people piled up against the window and along the wall of my tiny room. When they didn't fit in my room, they sat in the waiting area. I was exhausted and I often fell asleep halfway through their visits, but those visits—and those people—meant so much. During the month that I sat at home waiting for rescheduled surgery, my husband and I were greeted five evenings a week by wonderfully prepared dinners that were hand-made and hand delivered by my fellow occupational therapists. For an entire month, we had no need to prepare an evening meal, and we usually had enough to feed our families and visiting friends as well. My co-workers also combined their resources and presented us with thoughtful gifts. The most memorable and cherished is a delicate silver candle holder inscribed "In Memory of Emily Marie." In the darkest shadows of our loss, the kindness of friends helped light a pathway through our pain.

After my first surgery in October, I improved dramatically. However, I still required occupational and physical therapy through the following month. In a role reversal, I received treatment at Magee's outpatient facility. These had been my colleagues, so I was not surprised to see so many familiar faces. But for the same reason, it was terribly awkward for everyone. After the first day, I did not want to return. The next morning, I sat pouting in the living room waiting for my ride, making hateful faces at my husband for making me go.

My day consisted of occupational therapy, physical therapy, speech therapy, psychological counseling, recreational therapy, and group activities. A friend and former co-worker treated me in my first occupational therapy session. Bob's plan was simple based on occupational therapy theory and practice: assist the patient to resume her activities of work, play, and leisure. His first choice for me was work activities. Bob instructed me to empty the occupational therapy cabinet of all the objects and sort them according to treatment categories. Then he questioned me: what kind of disorder would I be treating with each particular object and activity? It was a major challenge for me because my short-term memory was impaired, perhaps by the anesthesia I'd received (I'd been "under the knife" for 13 hours). This obstacle proved to be only temporary, but initially it had a great impact on my ability to engage in spontaneous word retrieval. The activity Bob chose was successful in reshaping memory connections of the highest order. My co-worker's attitude meant the world to me. Someone with a positive vision of my future believed in my abilities and reestablished my self-confidence that I would eventually be able to resume my occupational therapy career. It was an important step on the road to recovering my positive approach to life.

I took another such step several months later. One of the cards that I received during my recovery was from someone I had known when he was a patient at Magee Rehabilitation Center. Glen's thoughtful words were written, I'm sure, with much difficulty since he was a person with quadriplegia, paralysis of his body below the site of his spinal cord injury, as a result of a diving accident. His reaching out to me with that card stuck in my mind for months afterwards, and I knew it was time to return the kind attention lavished on me by my friends and co-workers. When I was ready to travel by car on my own, I called Glen and set up a time to visit.

It occurred to me after talking with him in his home and swapping horror stories that, although there would always be a scar in my heart where Emily Marie belonged, I still had much for which to be grateful. Glen and I exchanged stories about our experiences in the hospital—the first time seeing your injured self in the mirror, the inability to do the smallest things, like brushing your hair for yourself, and requiring assistance to eat a small morsel of food. For me, these predicaments were thankfully in the past and something I could write about as part of my amazing recovery.

But for Glen, although there will be some limited physical recovery, many of these kinds of obstacles will remain with him for the rest of his life. He had been living on the third floor of his parents' home when he was pulled out of the water after his diving accident on that fateful day, and he has never been up to that third floor again. The thought of his plight makes my head want to spin around 365 degrees. But because of the gains he has been able to make as a result of the occupational therapy treatment he received, it doesn't seem to do that to Glen. He, too, has been helped to deal with pain and loss, and he, too, has recovered a positive approach to life.

Despite his injuries, Glen holds down a part-time job in landscape design and hopes to get his license to operate the van that's parked on the street in front of his house. He often spends weekends in the spring and summer hang gliding with friends in a special recreational program. Grinning, he says that he'd like to see my head shaved to reveal the constellation of tattoos administered to me for my radiation therapy.

Glen's face is handsome and disarming. His good looks were often the topic of conversation among Magee female employees within office cubicles and at shared lunch hours. I wonder if he knows this. For many people, good looks are all they need to carry them far in life, and Glen may have once been in that group. Glen's good looks gave him a jump-start in the right direction, but his own achievements since his accident are what have made his life full of promise. I think Glen would agree with me—our lives and bright futures are what occupational therapy is all about.

Chapter Eighty

Julia Speaks With Her Eyes

Joyce Sabari,
PhD, OTR, BCN, FAOTA

Welcome to my voice of silence.
Life is a precious shell.
Hold it for as long as you can.
Remember, it is only a shell
Which contains the powerful mind.
It says you can do anything
Be anything.
So say what you will say.
Julia Tavalaro

Julia Tavalaro, accomplished poet and author of Look Up For Yes (Penguin, 1998, with Richard Tayson) is unable to speak or move any of her limbs. When multiple strokes left her paralyzed and uncommunicative, she was a 27-year-old housewife and young mother with no literary background.

It was 1967, a time when people with severe disabilities, particularly those who could not communicate, were considered to be "vegetables." After medical intervention failed to restore any of her physical function, Julia was sent to a back ward at a municipal hospital for long-term custodial care. For 6 years, she was bedridden, fed through a tube, and treated as if she were brain-dead. To her family and friends and to the hospital staff, that's what she was and would always be. Astonishingly, what no one knew was that Julia's brain was very much the opposite of dead. For those 6 years, Julia lived a nightmare—alert and aware of everything going on around her, yet unable to move or to communicate her awareness in any way to those who came and went from her room.

I am proud that, from 1973 to 1981, as Julia's occupational therapist at Goldwater Memorial Hospital, I was able to play an important role in giving her back her humanity. Working closely with Arlene Kraat, a speech pathologist, I helped enable Julia to communicate and resume active participation in life. The day that Arlene noticed the merest movement of Julia's eyeball in response to Arlene's words, and called me in to help evaluate whether Julia could possibly be alert and aware, was probably the most joyous day of the preceding 6 years of Julia's life. When we determined that Julia could indicate "yes" and "no" by looking up and looking down, the world reopened to her. It was a moment none of us will ever forget.

After that breakthrough, I did the typical things occupational therapists do. I set up a positioning system that allowed Julia to sit comfortably in a wheelchair. I worked with her to develop the ability to eat foods by mouth. I carefully assessed Julia's potential for any kind of voluntary movement that could be harnessed for use to control a communication system or a power wheelchair. When we determined that she could develop useable head motion, I devised exercises and activities that would help Julia gain motor control. I scoured the growing literature about available technology for people with severe disabilities. Together, Julia, Arlene, and I tried out numerous devices and strategies. Many of the things we tried did not prove feasible for practical use. But we did enable Julia to reliably communicate with a switch-based scan system and to actively read and manipulate the pages of a book. After many failed attempts, Julia finally was able to use her head movements to drive a power wheelchair.

It wasn't until years after I had left the facility that Julia was given the opportunity to use her abilities to develop her talents as a creative writer. Volunteer poets from New York University and an organization called Very Special Arts began to conduct ongoing writing workshops with Goldwater residents. Julia attended these sessions on her own, driving her wheelchair to the classes and using her communication system to tap out poetry—letter by letter.

Julia had a great deal to say and an unusual talent for expressing her profound insights. The workshop leaders, and then others in the writing community, noticed and nurtured Julia's gift. Her works have been published in international poetry journals. She has been featured in articles in *The New York Times*, *The Los Angeles Times*, and numerous syndicated newspapers.

In 1997, after Julia worked for 2 years with Richard Tayson, a gifted poet himself, Kodansha Books published her book, *Look Up For Yes*. In 1998, the book was printed in paperback by Penguin Publishers. This success enabled Julia to leave Goldwater Hospital. She now resides in a private nursing home and enjoys a close relationship with her family.

I am grateful to Julia for including several vivid recollections of our relationship at Goldwater Hospital in *Look Up For Yes*. In particular, I thank her for the following passage:

"During my last occupational therapy session with Joyce in March 1981, she touched my shoulder and said, 'You might want to view my leaving as a door opening for you, Julia. Though it may be scary to go through that door, I think you'll find a higher degree of independence if you take the chance and wheel across. My leaving might give you a clear indication of what you can do for yourself.'"

I am proud that my words and deeds were a source of empowerment for Julia.

Occupational therapy is about mundane activities, like eating, doing simple daily choices, and exerting control over the routine tasks of daily life. When I worked with Julia, I never imagined that someday she would be writing poetry or that she would publish a book. My hope was that, through our work, she could tell others what she wanted for breakfast. My occupational therapy treatments were typical and ordinary, but they I am proud that they gave Julia the ability ultimately to do spectacular things with her eyes and her brain.

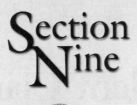

Good People, Bad Things

Violent Crimes, Wars, and Catastrophes

Violent Crimes, Wars, and Catastrophes

Here are nine stories that detail injuries suffered in drive-by shootings, bombings, war ambushes, plane crashes, terrorist attacks, and other catastrophes that happened to people who had no connection to the disastrous events other than being in the wrong place at the wrong time. Recovery from the physical and psychological damages of these disasters amidst the haunting question of "Why me?" took effort and required faith on the part of the victims and their therapists that life could be safe and secure even in the face of unpredictability and chaos. These stories can inspire confidence in all people who worry about the same issues.

Chapter Eighty-One

Their Bullet, My Life

Zoe McGrath, COTA

I was in my second quarter of certified occupational therapy assistant (COTA) school when my part-time employer Ann called. "I have accepted a new client who needs your help. His name is Cruz. While Cruz was a senior in high school he was shot in the head in a drive-by shooting. He is 22 years old and can no longer attend the special education school because he is too old for the school. He now attends our center while his mom is at work. He is paralyzed from the neck down, but has some movement and sensation throughout all of his limbs. He has varying degrees of impairment in their movements, is legally blind, unable to speak, and has severe short-term memory loss. We want you to make a communication board, a very simple one with large pictures, for him to use to tell us when he needs to go to the bathroom, is hungry, and so on," Ann explained. She had called me because while in school I worked when needed for an adult day program called The Center, where I had worked with the nonverbal clients for 3 years prior to going to COTA school.

I went to see Cruz the next day. As I approached him, I saw a large letter board with 5 inch by 5 inch letters in alphabetical order on his lap tray. I wondered, if he can spell, why would large pictures be necessary, but I proceeded. "Hi, Cruz, my name is Zoe.

Chapter Eighty-One

Ann asked me to come and see you." I went on to explain the large picture idea. Pointing to one letter at a time, Cruz responded "Hell no, I don't need pictures, I can spell." I agreed with Cruz, said "Goodbye," told Ann he didn't need the pictures, and went back to school.

The following year I graduated. I returned to The Center to work full-time. My job was to make sure that all 20 adults and five children with cerebral palsy or traumatic brain injuries had a way to get around independently and a way to communicate. I started with the clients with the most simple needs, such as lightweight manual wheelchairs and letter boards. I moved on to teaching sign language to some others and finally to fitting a seating system for a power wheelchair with five different switches to control the chair and adapting a voice output computer for a man with cerebral palsy who was nonverbal. Lastly, there was Cruz with his traumatic brain injury.

"Zoe, everyone else has a power wheelchair and a computer to talk, I want that," Cruz spelled out. I thought for a moment and remembered all the reports that were sent about Cruz. They said he probably wouldn't live more than a few days following the shooting, he wouldn't come out of the coma, he would remain a vegetable, he shouldn't go home with his mother, he could never use a communication device, and he could never use a power wheelchair because his brain damage and short-term memory loss were too severe. I sat looking at his big brown eyes with dashing eyelashes and decided if he had the wherewithal to tell me what he wanted, he deserved the chance to prove it. And did he ever.

Cruz and I spent the next year and a half turning both of our lives upside down—for the better. First, we decided Cruz could use a voice output computer called a Touch Talker. With a budget of $500, we were stalled, but only for a short time. I called people all over the country and found a woman selling one for $1000. I explained Cruz's history and our budget, and she kindly sold it to him for $500. We built the overlay in alphabetical order. With a yellow background, black letters, Velcro scratchy dots, and a little memorizing, Cruz could spell out his thoughts, hit a button, and speak. He was elated. Next we ordered a power wheelchair, funded by the state medical assistance agency in California, which funded Cruz's medical needs. A big orange ball compensated for Cruz's decreased fine motor coordination. With daily training to operate both devices, in a few months, Cruz was cruising around talking to everyone. It had been 6 years since he could move and talk on his own. Cruz didn't care how he was doing it, he was just doing it. As time went on, Cruz's short term memory improved and we realized glasses would help improve his vision.

Then one day Cruz decided he had accomplished more than anyone thought possible and he wanted to do more. "I want to go to schools and talk to kids about what happened to me. I want to tell them to stay away from guns, gangs, and drugs. I want them to learn from me," Cruz said. "OK. Cruz, tell me what you want to say and we will program it into your Touch Talker," I responded enthusiastically. It sounded like a great idea to me. As I waited to write what he said, Cruz came to realize he really didn't fully know what had happened to him the day he was shot. We then contacted his old friends and relatives and pieced together the puzzle. As the pieces began to fit, Cruz's brain continued to heal. He was literally coming to life. A year later, Cruz visited his first youth group. He spoke in Los Angeles, California, to a group of gang members. They cried as Cruz spoke, and they vowed to change. Cruz never felt so alive. "I love this. I can't believe their reaction. I really made a difference." So then we moved on to contacting more schools.

While in the process of developing Cruz's speech, Cruz and I spent every free evening and weekend together. First it was all work. Then Cruz and I started enjoying taking trips to the beach, going to the movies, going out to dinner, and just being together. Then one night while at my house watching movies it happened. We kissed. I don't know how it happened, it just did. I had fallen in love. We had fallen in love.

Clearly, our relationship changed and it was time for me to move on and for Cruz to leave The Center. I moved in with Cruz and his mother, and I changed jobs. Cruz didn't need me anymore at The Center, he now had me at home. By 1996, Cruz and I decided we were ready for our own life together. We now have our own home.

My life is occupational therapy now 24 hours a day. I work in a skilled nursing facility full-time and live and breathe progress in the making at our home as I marvel at each new step Cruz takes. I have found the most wonderful and loving man with all of the fulfillment I could ask for, thanks to occupational therapy! Cruz and I realize we have many hurdles in front of us. But with love, compassion, and occupational therapy we plan to jump those hurdles together and to reach the finish line.

Their Bullet, My Life
a speech by Cruz

Hello, I am Cruz. I am 28 years old. I am an ex-high school football player. As you can see and now hear, I am unable to walk or talk by myself. I wasn't always this way. In fact, up until I was 17, I lived a life probably similar to yours. I grew up in East Los Angeles. I hung around after school and in the summers with my homeboys. I wasn't a perfect kid. I stole little things from the market and once the cops even caught me underage without a license, in my Mom's car, running a stop sign.

The love of my life was and still is football. All I wanted my whole life was to play pro ball, so in school I worked hard to get good grades, worked out, and strengthened myself to play football. I started high school at Garfield High, but in my 10th grade year I was caught smoking pot in the bathroom and was sent to our rival school, Roosevelt High.

I started playing varsity football for the Roosevelt Rough Riders in my 11th grade year. I had fallen in love with Washington. I was their star running back. In one game, I ran 185 yards on 13 carries and made four touchdowns. They called me Chocolate Thunder. I had some really great friends and a couple of girlfriends. Some of my friends were in gangs, and like everyone else I hung out with, they sometimes smoked pot and experimented with other drugs. But, most of all I loved high school and playing ball.

By my 12th grade year, I was being scouted to play college football. UCLA offered me a full scholarship, and I was ready to take it. I hadn't really thought about a major because after UCLA, I had my eyes on the Raiders. I was going to be the next Eric Dickerson. But all of my plans and dreams were shattered on November 4, 1986, at about 6 p.m.

I don't remember that day now, so what I am going to tell you is what my family and friends have told me. November 4th was a school day in 1986. After dinner, a friend came over and wanted me to go for a ride with him on his new moped. We rode around and stopped to hang out and talk with another football buddy at the housing project in which my friend lives. As were hanging out and talking, a car drove by with several men inside who began randomly shooting. At 6 p.m. that night, my two friends were shot in the leg and as I tried to run away I was shot in the head. The bullet entered the left side of my skull, shot through my brain, hit the inside of the right side of my skull, and turned around and shattered. This was the last time I could walk by myself, talk by myself, see perfectly, and plan to live the life I had always hoped for.

They never caught the guys who shot me, though there were rumors later that these guys were shooting at a rival gang or retaliating against a bad drug deal. Even worse is that some people say one of the guys knew me, but didn't realize it was me when he started shooting. I guess I was just in the wrong place at the wrong time. I am an example of what guns can do. I am a son and a brother. I had a girlfriend at the time. This could just as easily happened to your brother, sister, cousin, boyfriend, or even girlfriend. Once a bullet is shot, it doesn't discriminate. Please stop the violence and increase the peace.

For the next 4½ months I lay in a coma, machines feeding me and making me breathe. For the next year and a half I was in a rehabilitation center. Those 2 years are a blur to me now. They were bringing me back from the dead. After those two years, the doctors told my mom that I would never walk, talk, feed myself, or even be able to think. They said to put me in a convalescent hospital and leave me there. They said I would certainly never be able to drive a power wheelchair or use a communication device. My mom didn't believe them and brought me home. I didn't really realize what had happened to me until I was enrolled in a special high school for the disabled and saw everyone else unable to move and talk and I realized I was the same. I don't ever remember being depressed about what happened. I just thought "The hell with the guys that did this to me, and I have to make the best of it."

About 6 years ago, after leaving the high school for the disabled, I was enrolled in an adult day program. They provided me with activities throughout the day while I sat in a manual wheelchair unable to move. I could only communicate using a letter board, and then only when someone else was willing to follow my pointing to the letters. I told them I wanted more. I came to understand that they thought that walking and talking weren't in my future. But I knew my previous doctors and therapists were wrong. I knew I could use a power wheelchair and a computer to talk—I just needed a chance to prove it. With the day program and my mom's help, we started the process. Shortly after that, the day program hired an occupational therapist—Zoe.

Zoe became my escape from silence and immobility. Zoe listened to my dreams. We obtained a voice output computer first. At last I could voice my thoughts, no longer did I have to wait for someone else's eyes to listen to my fingers. Then came my powered wheelchair, and I could again chase the girls and feel the air fly through my hair. I felt I was coming alive again. Zoe and I then set out on the journey of developing this speech. We spent a year after work and on weekends talking about my past with friends, family, and alone. Then we began what many people called "the impossible," getting me up on my own feet, taking my own steps. We started with three people and a walker holding me up. With Zoe cheering me the whole way, I can now walk independently with a walker or while holding Zoe's shoulders. To continue to improve, I work out on weight machines and walk in a swimming pool. I plan to walk on my own someday. And now I am learning to talk; though I have a small vocabulary now, Zoe and I know that together the sky is the limit. Most things come slowly to me, but Zoe and I realize we have the time and giving up is not an option. As my life is coming back together, I am now able to concentrate on goals I set for myself so many years ago. On August 21, 1996, 10 years after losing a scholarship to UCLA because an angry man thought it was okay to shoot aimlessly into a group of kids, I started college. I hope to work with computers someday. I also share my story with people like you as much as possible. Though much was taken from me with that one bullet, in October of 1993, something happened that I thought I had lost forever... I met a woman and fell in love.

Yes, by October of 1993, Zoe and I had fallen in love. We dated like everyone else. We went out to dinner, to the movies, to the beach, and we traveled. In January of 1994, I was diagnosed with diabetes. Zoe moved in with me and my mom to take care of me. With Zoe's belief that I can do anything I put my mind to, and my will to get better, I have learned to care more for myself. In April of 1995, Zoe and I purchased our own van to accommodate my wheelchair. In August of 1995, Zoe and I moved into our own home. Now it is just me and my precious love living our life together. We hope to have children someday. I would love a little "Cruz the Third" running around.

I'll never be the same as before, but we all have to be the best we can and reach as far as we can go. With inner strength, people believing in me, and the Lord's help, I hope to do it all. I just thank the Lord for letting me live. Please remember that one bullet, their bullet, did this to me, but it is my life to live. Though we can't control our own destiny, no one else should be able to take away a life with a gun. I don't want this to happen to any of you. Please stay away from guns, drugs, and gangs. Don't give up. Stop the violence and increase the peace. We're all in this life together.

Chapter
Eighty-Two

Teens Hear It From One of Their Own

Ron Carson, MHS, OTR/L

Antonio is lucky to be alive, although "lucky" did not accurately describe his condition when I first met him in a hospital bed with his mother seated vigilantly nearby. A bullet fired in anger by another teenager had passed dangerously close to Antonio's brainstem and spinal cord.

Antonio comes from a rural South Carolina town, and for some young men, such an environment can be a breeding ground for trouble. Antonio was a victim of his turbulent and dangerous lifestyle of the street. It was, in fact, his lifestyle that led to a bullet fired into the back of his head.

While Antonio was not paralyzed, the near miss had ravaged his central nervous system. He could neither sit upright nor hold up his head without support. He had minimal strength in his legs, no abilities with his left arm, and only some slight movement on his right side. In short, 18-year-old Antonio was basically helpless. He could not get around on his own or care for himself in any way. Nonetheless, he was friendly and open and appeared willing to face the challenges that lay ahead.

And challenges there certainly were. The young man who survived the bullet also survived the many weeks of intensive and painful occupational and physical therapy, including strengthening activities, balance training, daily living training, aquatic

Chapter Eighty-Two

therapy, and psychological intervention. Amazingly, Antonio endured physical challenges beyond normal comprehension and responded with the vigor
and determination of an 18-year-old. After only 7 weeks at the rehabilitation
hospital in which I worked as an occupational therapist, Antonio was ready
for a new start in life. One part of Antonio's recovery process, however, was
delayed until just prior to his discharge at which time, amazingly, he walked
out of the hospital under his own power, requiring only the occasional use of
a cane. When he left, he was also able to feed himself and only required assistance for opening containers and packages.

Because the treatment team feared that as a result of Antonio having
escaped so seeminlgy unscathed by his violent encounter with the bullet, he
was at risk to return to his street life environment, we decided to show
Antonio that other lifestyle choices were open to him. His therapists all concluded that if Antonio could talk as an advisor with other at-risk teenagers
about his experience, both he and they would benefit.

The team wanted Antonio to learn self-respect and self-esteem. By having Antonio overcome his fear of speaking to his peers, we believed he would
gain self-respect and confidence. We hoped that this would help Antonio
better fight the inevitable peer pressure he would face when he returned
home. If Antonio walked away from the rehabilitation hospital with a sense
of both physical and emotional achievement, we believed he had a greater
chance for a full recovery. Without a boost in self-esteem, we felt that
Antonio's hard work at physical recovery might simply provide a mechanism
to return to his previous lifestyle.

We also were convinced that at-risk adolescents could learn a lot from
Antonio, for example, that the glorified Hollywood image of being shot is actually a myth. Through Antonio, these at-risk young adults would see and hear
the real-life trauma and pain inflicted by a bullet. We believed that Antonio's
talk might provide an invaluable service to the community and hopefully prevent some future teenage shooting tragedies.

Antonio had always willingly accepted the physical challenges placed before
him during his rehabilitation, so we anticipated that he would approach our
community education suggestion with the same energy. However, Antonio was
at first unwilling to go through with the presentation. Only after hours of careful prodding did he finally accept the challenge of speaking with his peers at a
local community agency, The Institute, a center for troubled teens.

During the following week, we assisted Antonio with developing an outline for his presentation. Antonio's demeanor indicated to us that he had
reservations about giving the presentation. We gave him several opportunities to back out, but he remained committed to the concept. He told us that
his mother also wanted him to go through with the speech, so he seemed
determined to complete the talk.

302

As the day of the presentation approached, however, there was concern on our part that Antonio might not follow through with the task. He was hesitant to complete the outline, and his enthusiasm diminished. Because of Antonio's previous successes with physical rehabilitation, we secretly believed that he would meet this emotional challenge. On the day of the presentation, Antonio seemed prepared, and he walked to the van without assistance.

Antonio did not speak much during the 30-minute ride. When we arrived, Antonio let out a grunt of disapproval when he saw the students he would be addressing. He nervously began to ask questions about where he would be giving the presentation, who was going to be there, and whether he would be standing or sitting. It was clear that he was apprehensive about giving his talk. In fact, at first Antonio refused to get out of the van to meet the director of the Institute. After some gentle prodding, Antonio reluctantly made his way to the trailer where he was scheduled to speak.

Antonio was about to face his fear of public speaking, so there was tension in the air. As the teenagers began streaming into the trailer, they showed great poise and character. As they passed by Antonio, they introduced themselves and offered him handshakes. These simple gestures helped to calm Antonio's nerves.

Antonio and I were introduced to the audience by our neuropsychiatric counselor. After outlining some of what Antonio would be discussing, he asked Antonio some direct questions. Reluctantly at first but then with more confidence, Antonio answered the questions, beginning a 45-minute conversation between the group of at-risk adolescents and one of their peers. Antonio and the other teens were open with both their questions and their answers. They discussed the events leading up to Antonio's shooting, his rehabilitation, and his future prospects. Antonio was forced to confront the reality that his previous lifestyle had directly led to his physical condition and that he might endure a lifetime of disability because of it.

Perhaps for the first time, the teens heard from one of "their own" about the negative side of life on the streets. Antonio provided a living testament that such an existence is not like the way such life seems on television. The counselors and other staff were careful to convey to the students that Antonio should not be viewed as a hero. We did not want anyone to think that there were rewards to living a street life. There was a strong sense of emotion and intensity as Antonio confronted the group with his experiences. At the conclusion of his talk, Antonio was met with a rousing round of applause.

The Institute's counselors were very effective at putting the event in perspective. They challenged Antonio to return the following month to retell his story. They mentioned that many of their students in the past had promised to reform their lives but many had failed. To succeed, Antonio would need great courage and strength. One counselor gave Antonio his telephone number and promised assistance whenever Antonio needed it.

My pride in Antonio grew that day. He had achieved so many physical gains during his short stay at our facility, and now he had conquered seemingly greater mental and emotional hurdles. He told me earlier that the presentation was important to him because he had never told his entire story, and he needed to get it off his chest. As I now looked at Antonio, I imagined a young man who had won his battle against adversity, giving himself a second chance on life. Of course, only time will tell if Antonio can meet the challenges he faces. I am confident that his rehabilitation team has given him the physical and mental tools to accomplish whatever goals he sets for himself.

As Antonio prepared to leave us, I felt both joy and sadness. Like a father whose son leaves home to start college, I know that Antonio was leaving the safe confines of the hospital to return to the mean streets of adolescence. No longer could a physician, nurse, or therapist be there to protect him or help him make decisions. While I wish I could always be there to guide him, as an occupational therapist I know that Antonio must be responsible for the decisions he makes in life. Antonio must now rely on himself and his family to be strong and to resist the pull of his previous life.

As he was leaving the hospital for the last time, we gave Antonio a t-shirt with the hospital name emblazoned on the front to remind him of the physical and mental challenges he had faced and conquered. With our prayers and support and his newly acquired physical and mental skills hopefully Antonio will make the most of his new start in life.

Chapter Eighty-Three

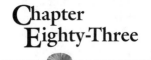

Rambo

Lt. Col. Len Cancio, MPH, OTR/L

By 1986, the civil war in El Salvador had gone on for 7 years. The FMLN (Frente Faravundo Marti de Liberacion Nacional), a Marxist insurgency group, continued to harass the population and government troops with guerrilla tactics. They attacked small outposts with regularity and indiscriminately planted homemade antipersonnel mines called quita pata, slang for "foot cutter." Although the mines had the potential to kill, they were designed to maim, removing a portion of the foot of any unfortunate soldier, civilian, or cow that stepped on them.

The land mines were effective weapons in a war of attrition and had a demoralizing effect on the Salvadoran soldiers. By 1986, there were thousands of Salvadorans, primarily soldiers, with foot amputations, most without any hope of ever receiving a modern artificial limb. At best, the soldiers were fitted with a prosthesis made of plaster and steel poles, with carved wooden feet in order to maintain a sense of wholeness. In the Salvadoran army, soldiers with amputations remained on active duty until their enlistment was up, doing whatever they could in units to the rear. While the efforts to keep these young men working was exemplary, because they remained in the midst of other troops where they could be seen every day, the soldiers with amputations also became symbols to their fellow soldiers of their own possible fate.

Chapter Eighty-Three

I met "Rambo" at the Hospital Militar, in San Salvador, El Salvador, in 1986. He was one of hundreds standing in line waiting for an evaluation by the American Advisors for an artificial leg. He had lost his foot while setting an ambush on a special operation. Ironically, it was his own unit that was subsequently ambushed. While running for cover, Rambo stepped on a mine, shrapnel tearing into his foot. Salvadoran surgeons removed the mangled foot.

Rambo became one more of the unfortunate soldiers who lost his foot to a quita pata. His real name was Luis Martinez DeCampo. He was given the nickname Rambo, from the popular movies of the time, by his fellow soldiers for his tenacity in battle. Rambo was a member of the Atlacatl Battalion, an elite fighting force in the Salvadoran Army, trained by United States military advisors and modeled after American's Special Forces. He was all of 19 and already a seasoned veteran. He was poorly educated, a child of the campesinos. He now represented the thousands of maimed veterans of the war without a limb and without hope.

As a U.S. Army occupational therapist, I was a member of a multidisciplinary mobile medical training team, or MTT. The MTT was composed of an occupational therapist and a physical therapist, a dietitian, a nurse, civilian prosthetist/orthotists, and several orthopedic technicians. In an effort to keep a low profile, all of the team members were Hispanic and spoke fluent Spanish. I was the exception, being of Filipino ancestry. Having a Spanish last name was apparently close enough, so I was selected for the team. We were sent on a humanitarian mission to train host nation health care workers in the management of the thousands of combat casualties.

My mission, as an advisor, was to train the host nation occupational therapists in upper extremity rehabilitation. The hospital employed two excellent occupational therapists, trained in Argentina. What these therapists lacked in supplies and equipment, they made up for with enthusiasm and creativity. They had an old typewriter that the patients used constantly. I realized that in their situation, activities of daily living had to begin with such basic skills as learning to read and write. The therapists even made homemade exercise devices from pieces of wood and rubber bands. They were certainly not lacking in patients. The 70-bed military hospital held 500 wounded soldiers. Several were on the floor for lack of bed space. "Terapia occupacional (OT)" was located next to the emergency room. Helicopters ferried in freshly wounded soldiers daily. The scenes were reminiscent of "M.A.S.H." television shows, only the screams and blood were real.

Military trucks delivered Rambo and many others like him to the military hospital daily. They attended physical and occupational therapy, socializing with others who shared similar injuries. They also came to see what the "Norte Americanos" could do for them, thinking we would work some miracle for them. We could not. Their futures looked grim; they had no skills, no education, and they were missing a limb. Depression was a common reaction of these young men with amputations. We desperately needed something to boost morale and give these men hope.

One day, Col. Fred Thill, our officer-in-charge, came to me with an article from the *San Francisco Examiner* that told of an amputee soccer league. The idea was exactly what we had been searching for. The opportunity to play soccer, or "futbol," the national sport of El Salvador, was sure to motivate these men to strengthen their upper bodies and develop dexterity, while hopefully regaining confidence by doing something meaningful and fun. I wrote to the league president, and he forwarded the rules of play. With the help of the hospital recreational director, we selected 14 soldiers with lower extremity amputations and, following league rules, one soldier with an upper extremity amputation to be the goalie. Funds were solicited from an officers' wives' club for uniforms and soccer balls.

Naturally, at first the wounded soldiers were reluctant, but they soon regained a smile, then a laugh, as they passed the ball and practiced dribbling. Soon the MTT challenged the American Special Forces assigned to La Primera Brigada (First Brigade). They selected 15 of their soldiers with amputations for a soccer match.

Rambo was our star forward. He had always been athletic, a virtue that had made him a good soldier. The soccer match became a media frenzy. Salvadoran television stations covered the event. The American Ambassador and the commander of all Salvadoran troops came to present medals to the victors. More importantly, hundreds of troops from the Primera Brigada were in the stadium, cheering the team members. The pride was evident in the faces of the soccer players. The play was intense. The hospital team had the advantage of forearm crutches, giving them greater mobility, the result of a last minute arrival of supplies. The team members of the First Brigade fought hard, with an intensity that could only remind me of the combat they had seen. A forward from the First Brigade threw down his crutches, hopping on one leg, forcing the ball toward the goal. Bodies collided, and crutches flew. In the end, the hospital team won, on a goal scored by Rambo. Both teams celebrated with jubilation, for everyone on the field won that day.

Years later, I had the opportunity to meet with Rambo again in an international amputee soccer tournament held in Seattle, Washington. El Salvador sent an all-star team with their best athletes. For many of the Salvadoran team members, it was their first time in the United States. You could see in their eyes a mixture of wonderment and envy, as they witnessed things they had only seen in movies in a country without fear of civil war. Rambo was their starting forward. I brought my family this time, giving them an opportunity to meet the team. They played against teams from Seattle, Calgary, Vancouver, Portland, and Los Angeles. El Salvador won it all, winning all their matches easily.

Chapter Eighty-Three

The team's victory was particularly satisfying to those of us who had worked with the men and had organized the amputee league as an occupational therapy activity years before. But even more important, after their win, the team returned to El Salvador as national heroes, not only because they served as an inspiration and hope for the fellow countrymen with disabilities, but because the people of El Salvador take football very seriously, and a winning team of any kind—with or without disabilities—brought glory to the entire country. Not a bad achievement for a group of men whose futures looked bleak before the Army-issued soccer balls and uniforms gave them a chance to play a game and become real winners.

Chapter Eighty-Four

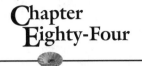

Getting
Back to Life

Wendy Elliman

Atalia Elbaz is a statistic: one of the hundred people injured when a suicide bomber blew up a Jerusalem bus and one of the 23 most seriously hurt. So seriously, in fact, that she was initially taken for dead and put on that far grimmer list along with the four people actually killed in the attack.

But statistics have their limits. Three years later, the slender young woman is sitting cross-legged on her bed in the student dormitory on Mt. Scopus, a student in the occupational therapy program at the Hebrew University. Barefoot on a blustery February morning, she's between exams and clearly at peace with the world.

Even though she is still in the middle of her occupational therapy education, she has already learned things that have helped her immensely in her recovery, physically, mentally, and emotionally. She credits some of her occupational therapy courses for keeping her focused and for enabling her to practice on herself, doing what she would do if she were treating a patient.

"What happened to me has changed my sense of proportion," she says in a voice that's hoarser than before she was injured. "I don't take everyday things so seriously. Many of my friends get hysterical about their exams, for example. I don't. Yes, it sets me apart a little. But in the end we're all alone, aren't we?"

Atalia was alone on the crowded No. 26 bus on her way to the Hebrew University. It was August 21, 1995; she was 20 years old and had just finished her Israel Defense Forces service, the mandatory tour of duty for most Israeli high school graduates before they start college.

"I'd been assistant to the commander of an air force base," she says. "Now I had 2 months before starting at the university. There were a couple of compulsory courses in English I had to take as part of my BA in occupational therapy, and I decided to get them out of the way that summer. So I went to stay with my grandmother, who lives closer to Jerusalem."

Atalia's grandmother saw her safely to the bus that morning, as she did every day, and waved goodbye. The crowded No. 26 chugged slowly through the city's morning traffic.

"I wasn't paying any particular attention to the other passengers," she recalls, "although I did notice the bomber. He came and sat next to me. I remember thinking he was kind of weird, strung out, the way he kept looking all around. Then he got up and pushed his way to the back of the bus. I didn't consciously think he was a terrorist. But the moment the bus went up, I knew with certainty that it was him."

Atalia remembers the explosion clearly, but after that everything is hazy. The sights, the sounds, the smells are hardly there. She remembers getting up and staggering out of the twisted burnt skeleton of the bus, scarcely aware she'd been hurt.

And then her mind is blank for the next 4 days. Nails from the bomb and hot flying metal from the bus had lacerated her body in several places. One piece had severed a major artery on the right side of her neck. She got as far as the sidewalk, the blood pumping out, when her right lung collapsed. She lay there, the right side of her brain slowly being starved of its vital oxygen.

A passerby pulled off his shirt and wrapped it around her leaking neck. An ambulance hurried her to the nearby Hadassah-University Hospital on Mt. Scopus, where ER staff clamped the artery and did a massive emergency blood transfusion. Stabilized sufficiently for the race across town, Atalia was rushed into the operating rooms of the Hadassah-Hebrew University Medical Center at Ein Karem. Urgently, vascular surgeons tried to graft in a vessel from her leg to replace the ruined artery in her throat. When their first attempt failed, they tried again with synthetic material and it held.

After long hours in surgery, Atalia was wheeled into the critical-care unit. With a ventilator doing the breathing for her, she spent the next 4 days fighting for her life. "I remember waking up and seeing a lot of faces around my bed," she recalls. "I had no idea what was going on. Then I recognized my mother and I gestured to her, 'what's happened?' She said there was an explosion. It all came back to me then. Later, when the security people brought photographs of terror suspects to the hospital, I had no trouble identifying the man who'd sat next to me."

Atalia quickly began healing in body and in mind. "Only 6 days after I awoke, I was released from the hospital. I went back every day for a long time, of course. My body was all covered with cuts. The long rip down my neck needed plastic surgery. There was nerve damage to my throat and I had no voice. That was really worrying me, because no one could guarantee it would ever come back.

"But after 3 or 4 months of therapy, it was there again, just huskier than before. As well as voice therapy, I needed physical and occupational therapy for my right hand and leg, damaged when my brain lost its oxygen supply. That, too, has come back." Atalia's hand injuries were the focus of her self-prescribed occupational therapy treatments for the next year as well. She practiced doing various activities for strengthening the muscles and in particular concentrated on redeveloping her fine finger dexterity and coordination through appropriate games and crafts. She was able to get advice about what she needed to do from faculty, clinical supervisors, and from the textbooks she was using in class. All in all, the therapy and the "figuring out what to do" part were quite helpful; she learned in addition about how the patient receiving the occupational therapy feels, so it was a worthwhile experience, she recalls.

For over a year, Atalia remained closely connected to the hospital. As she grew stronger, she'd travel there by bus. Although as time passed, her fear of bus rides grew, and she began saving up for a car.

"It was a difficult year, because it was the start of my degree course in OT and I missed classes because of hospital appointments," she says. "But I have no complaints. The doctors, the nurses, everyone at Hadassah, they couldn't have been kinder, more understanding, or more supportive. I don't know if everyone gets the treatment I did, but they cared for me wonderfully, from my smallest complaint to my largest request. I don't have enough good words for them in my vocabulary."

In fact, she would later refer to her care through that year as having been "born at Hadassah once again." She subsequently changed her name from "Atalia" to "Gabi" as a symbolic gesture to mark what she considers her "rebirth."

Twenty years earlier, when her mother had gone into labor, she had insisted on making the hour's journey to Jerusalem to give birth to Atalia in Hadassah, rather than in her local hospital in Kiryat Gat. Atalia was her second, the middle child in a family of three daughters.

"My parents came to Israel as young children, my father from Morocco and my mother from Egypt," Atalia explains. "They did well here. Dad was a school principal and my mom did clerical work in the local health clinic.

"We've always been a close family, but when I was recovering from the explosion, they'd call me 20 times a day. They'd ask: 'Have you slept? Have you eaten? Where are you going? How are you getting there? When will you be back? How will you get back? What will you do then?' I understood why of course, but it began to get a bit much after a while! Again my occupational therapy training helped me realize what trauma the families of people who are injured go through, so I was able to be a bit more understanding of their pain and concern for me and my welfare."

For Atalia's mother, Sara, Hadassah Hospital is a worker of wonders. "There's only one word for what happened to Atalia at Hadassah, and that word is 'miracle.' There is no other way to put it. Hadassah saved our daughter and gave her back to us as a gift from heaven. They worked a miracle."

It took about 2 months for the phone calls and the anxiety to subside to a manageable level. As for Atalia, the psychological distress receded quite quickly.

"I think it's partly because I remember so little of the bomb's aftermath that I don't dwell on it," she says. "I had some social problems afterward. At first, my friends surrounded me, but as time passed and I couldn't relate to their daily concerns seriously, a communication gap opened between us. But then we got back to normal again. I was also very involved in my studies." In fact, the studies also helped her deal with some of those psychological issues because she learned how normal it is to have stress reactions following such a trauma and some helpful ways to deal with those reactions.

After 6 years as a volunteer with Magen David Adom in Kiryat Gat (Israel's Red Cross), Atalia had selected the profession of occupational therapy and secured a much-sought-after place at the Hadassah-Hebrew University School of Occupational Therapy. "I love it," she says, "especially working with children. But it's a heavy studyload and I work very hard. Now I'm doubly glad I am studying it."

To what degree is she just another student?

"Look, I take my studies very seriously," she explains. "I live in the student dorms here on Mt. Scopus. I have friends, go out with them and go home regularly to Kiryat Gat to see my family. What happened to me is in the past. But I don't try to pretend it never happened. I was badly hurt and I nearly died. I was afraid and in pain for a long time. I suffered and so did my family and my friends.

"That has left me with greater insight, a greater understanding. When I heard of terror attacks before, I'd always wanted to help. Now when something happens, I know there are things I can do and that I can help. Every time something happens now, I go to the hospitals and talk to the survivors. I try to bolster them for the fight to recovery ahead of them. It's not hard for me to do. I've been there myself. I know the language of pain and fear, and the new victims can see from what happened to me that it's possible to build a life beyond it."

Chapter Eighty-Five

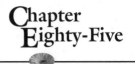

After the Explosion

Michal Magnes Raveh, MA, OTR

I divide my life into before the bomb exploded and after the bomb exploded. I was in my early 50s when it happened, and the event marked a turning point in my professional life and in my view of myself. It was the classic case of being in the wrong place at the wrong time. I am an Israeli, but I rarely ride the public buses as do so many of my fellow Jerusalemites. That day my car was at the repair shop, so I hopped onto the No. 26 bus for the short ride to my office at the Hebrew University's Mt. Scopus campus where I teach in the Occupational Therapy School. As we neared Mt. Scopus, there was a big bang. There was no doubt in my mind what had happened. I remember saying to myself, "Once in a lifetime you take a bus and this has to happen!"

August 21, 1995, was a beautiful summer morning in Jerusalem. Since it was still the summer holiday at the University, I was in no great hurry and was even looking forward to the leisurely adventure of taking a public bus, which in Israel can be a very social experience. The driver's radio is invariably turned on loudly to the news broadcasts, so you are never out of touch with the world around you, and the ethnic variety of the other passengers provides wonderful people-watching opportunities. When I relive that day in my mind, I often think about the number of circumstances that had to occur precisely in turn in order for me to have been on that particular bus at that particular time. I took my time taking money out of the automatic bank machine. I spent several minutes helping a blind man get onto the right bus. I strolled around a bit taking in some sights that I don't normally see from my car. When the No. 26 bus pulled up, I was surprised to see that it was a double bus and that it was so full. I found a seat behind the rear door on the aisle. At first, it was a routine ride. People were getting on and off. There were many summer school students on it speaking many different foreign languages, and I was enjoying listening to their conversations in the languages that I understand. As we neared Mt. Scopus, there was that very big bang.

When I came to, I felt as though a huge wave had swept over me, and now I was coming up again. When the flying glass stopped and the smoke dispersed and things settled down, I evaluated the situation. I was in the aisle, low, but crouched on my own two feet. In front of me, I could see that the rear door of the bus was blown out. I had lost my left shoe, but saw my handbag a few feet to the left. I knew that I had to get myself out of there as quickly as possible but that if I could reach my handbag it would make things much easier later. I somehow got it and got out of the bus; I saw a wall at the edge of the sidewalk nearby, so I sat leaning against it. Then for the first time I saw the bus and what was going on around it. It was totally burnt. The rear end was only a skeleton of a bus and there were some scorched bodies hanging over it. At my side, there was a lot of commotion; people were taking off their shirts in order to use them to stop someone else's bleeding, and a young girl stripped to her underwear was lying face down on the ground with two holes in her body.

I vaguely heard what was going on but realized that I wasn't hearing well. In the movies, however, when there is a big bang, you lose your hearing temporarily, so I didn't take much notice of it. My professional occupational therapy knowledge made me realize that the people around me were injured much more severely than I was and needed immediate care; yet after a while, I felt very lonely and didn't really know what I was waiting for, but somehow I couldn't muster the energy to move.

Out of the blue, a rescuer suddenly materialized. It was Eran, the son of good friends of mine, who lived nearby; a medic in the Army, he had rushed to the scene to help. Like an angel from heaven, he sized up the situation, borrowed a cell phone from a policemen, and called his mother to tell her I had been in the blast but was okay and would soon be evacuated. Somehow it felt better that someone I knew now knew where I was and what was happening to me, and I felt less alone. He then began helping me up, but we immediately realized that something was very wrong with my left foot. He carried me like a baby to a stretcher and I was taken to the hospital.

I relate these scenes that are imprinted indelibly on my mind, even several years later, because the psychological impact on me would prove to be a critical part of my transformative experience. In order to understand that, it is important to understand what I saw and what I went through.

My recollections of the first few days following the bombing are, mercifully, fading. What happened to me was the greatest approximation to death I have ever encountered. I have reacted to that near-death experience in ways that I have since learned are quite common to others who have had similar occurrences. Perhaps it is for the best that although the actual traumatic experiences may remain vividly imprinted, the all-encompassing emotional connections can eventually fade from conscious memory, enabling us to get on with our normal lives. I am, nonetheless, amazed at the ways in which the bomb, and the near-death experience it caused me to undergo, have altered my life and refocused it in dramatic ways.

My physical injuries, while serious, were relatively minor compared to the four people who died and the more than 100 others who were horribly burned or who suffered permanent disabilities. I had several bone breaks, some minor burns, and some serious cuts from flying glass that acted as shrapnel, all of which have healed, and a major hearing loss in one ear, the residual of which remains with me to this day. The psychological trauma, unrecognized at first as posttraumatic stress, took some time to be relieved, but has been under control for a long time now. I believe that this is largely due to my occupational therapy professional training in recognizing and dealing with psychological trauma, treating physical disabilities, and navigating the medical system effectively in order to get the appropriate kinds, quantity, and quality of restorative services. It is also due to my firm belief in the value of purposeful activities and meaningful occupations in restoring normal functioning.

I had previously taught courses that dealt with the ideal treatments for various disabilities and with how to handle the medical establishment to recognize and obtain the correct services. It was time to go into action to secure those very things for myself! I became very assertive in always expecting the appropriate services and obtaining things to which I knew I was entitled but which I was not yet receiving. Never in my career was I more eager to help a client obtain medical and psychological services than I was to get these for myself; never did a client have a more determined advocate than I had with myself as my own therapist. It was not always easy and I sometimes had to spend a lot of time arranging to get what I needed. Furthermore, as extensive and cutting-edge as the medical care is in Israel, I still sometimes had to go elsewhere, such as to the United States, to receive certain specialized services.

I was a whirlwind as my own occupational therapist in my home, adapting everything in sight that gave me any trouble, so that I could manage all my daily activities. I decided it would be best for me to resume my regular routine as quickly as possible, so I returned to work at the university only 3 weeks after the bus attack, even though I could have stayed at home and received

Chapter Eighty-Five

compensation from Israel's national insurance system for a much longer period of time. I believe that my finding it necessary to do this was a sign of my need to define myself as a healthy and productive person rather than as a person who was recovering from injuries. My prior lifetime as an assertive person helped me persevere with the tasks necessary to obtain the rehabilitation services I needed; on the other hand, one of the surprises to me was that having been a basically healthy person before the attack made it unbelievably difficult in many ways to be "on the other side" as a patient; I did not know what to expect and there were times when I "didn't know the language" of even what questions to ask. There were also times when logic, and my therapists, told me that I should move toward a new goal, but I simply could not move forward, because I just did not feel ready.

So, for example, it took many weeks, far longer that anyone had predicted, before I could resume driving again. Although I was physically capable, I wasn't confident in my ability to do it; yet, one day, I "knew" it was time, and off I went. On the other hand, I took on one of the largest responsibilities possible when I was offered the position of Chair of the Department of Occupational Therapy at Hebrew University 2 years after I experienced the bomb explosion. No one, me included, could figure out why I was willing to undertake that enormous job after being injured in the attack when previously, I had refused the job. Yet, as with driving, my mind and my body "knew" it was the right time, so I had the confidence in myself to take the position.

My near-death experience heightened my awareness of what was really important. It helped me separate the tasks I most value from those that reflect other people's agendas. Most important, it made me aware of the value of listening to myself and of having faith in my own feelings of confidence in my abilities. My own rehabilitation process shaped my insight. I found during the course of my rehabilitation that I was ready to undertake a new task, such as driving, only when I felt confident to do so rather than when the logic of a rehabilitation professional suggested that it was "time" to move forward. This showed me, as an occupational therapist, the critical importance of taking cues from the patient rather than setting goals for the patient. It made me realize that the feeling of confidence to do something is very complex, probably impossible to analyze, and of course different for every client.

And what about becoming Chair of the Occupational Therapy Department, a job I had never had the confidence to accept before the bomb exploded on the bus? What made me feel confident enough to do so after the attack? Perhaps it is because after surviving a terrorist attack, other kinds of tasks don't seem quite so tough. Or maybe it is because a near-death experience puts all aspects of life into perspective. Or it just could be that surviving the near-death experience gives you the confidence to take on other life-affirming challenges.

316

Chapter Eighty-Six

Fire Fall
and Therapy Ball

Christine Gaspar, OTR

Thursday, April 4, 1991, began as an ordinary, bright, sunny day at Merion Elementary School and ended in tragedy. At noon that day, children who had finished eating lunch hurried outside onto the playground behind the school for recess. In the warmth of the sun, they tossed their jackets to the ground. Among the children was a red-haired second-grade boy whose mother had sent him to school in a new pair of shoes that morning and a first-grade girl who was wearing her favorite pink sweatshirt.

In the clear skies above southeastern Pennsylvania, U.S. Senator John Heinz of Pennsylvania was traveling to a speaking engagement in a small private plane. At 12:04 p.m., the pilot of the Senator's plane radioed to Philadelphia International Airport that he could not tell if his landing gear was down. Nearby, two pilots in a helicopter overheard the radio call and offered to assist by flying around the plane to inspect the landing gear. What happened next made national news headlines.

A few moments later, the two aircraft—the Senator's airplane and the helicopter trying to help—collided in mid-air above the school. Three people in the plane, including U.S. Senator Heinz, were killed in the crash. So were the two pilots in the helicopter. Fiery debris from the impact came crashing down all around the school building.

Chapter Eighty-Six

As the school's occupational therapist, at 12:15 p.m. I was chatting with the school's physical therapist near a large window at the front of the school. Suddenly, we felt a tremendous explosion and in horror saw a flaming piece of airplane crash yards in front of the building. The physical therapist ran toward the auditorium in the front of the building where children were rehearsing a play, and I ran immediately to the back door to reach the children outdoors in the playground behind the building. We did not know then that the helicopter had crashed directly onto that playground.

As the doors from the playground into the building were thrown open, I saw screaming children running inside for safety, an inferno behind them. The girl in her pink sweatshirt ran into the building, her hair and arm on fire. My occupational therapy training in emergency measures made me respond automatically with stop, drop, and roll; I grabbed her and put out her flames by rolling her on the floor. At that moment, the second-grade boy entered the building totally engulfed in fire from his red hair to his new shoes. As I assisted in moving the girl to safety away from the area, I saw the school custodian and a teacher leaning over him, frantically beating out his flames with the custodian's jeans jacket.

Outside, teachers tried to organize the children by class groups as sirens wailed and frantic parents rushed to the scene searching for their children. Emergency vehicles arrived along with the press and hundreds of onlookers from the community. A helicopter flew in to take the second-grade boy to Chester-Crozier Hospital Burn Center, while the first-grade girl was transported to a local hospital in an ambulance. When the school principal announced that we should go back inside the building, we all reentered, dazed. Children and teachers began to try to talk about what they had seen.

Later, on the evening news, we learned that all the men aboard the plane and the helicopter died in the accident. On the ground, two first-grade girls on the playground were killed, hit by debris from the crash. The second-grade boy with new shoes was severely burned over 70% of his body. The pink-shirted first-grade girl was only mildly burned, thanks to the immediate dousing of her flames. Many other children suffered varying minor external physical injuries that were expected to heal.

The internal healing of emotional injuries would take longer for all of us. As an occupational therapist, I had often seen the power of talking about traumatic experiences to help make sense of them. Psychologists would be available to help us talk. For those not able to talk yet, I realized I could provide ways for children to express their feelings. For those children who are too young to find words for their emotions or who are not yet ready to talk about their fears, occupational therapists use various play activities and games that allow them to express their feelings. These could be included in the daily classroom routines.

Over the weekend following the accident, transportation investigators worked quickly to clear the wreckage from the crash site. A tremendous outpouring of community volunteers donated materials and labor to restore the areas around the school. By Monday morning, new shrubbery had been planted and the school reopened. Counselors and psychologists were called in to meet with parents, children, and staff who were experiencing the predictable posttraumatic stress reactions.

During this time, I found myself unable to sleep and cried uncontrollably, preoccupied with the things I had seen. What made me saddest was that the children had experienced this dreadful event at a place where they should feel safe. I found it helpful to allow myself to cry, to talk about it to my family, and to write down my thoughts and feelings. A psychologist I knew acknowledged the horror I felt, but also helped me realize that the impact of this event might be used in my life for a good purpose. I knew that I could not heal on my own and that part of the healing process would have to occur with those who had shared this experience. I went to the support sessions for teachers and found that being together with them helped me.

I knew that I would need to be strong. As their occupational therapist, in addition to working with those who needed outward physical healing, I would be encouraging the children who were not able to talk about what they had seen to express themselves through play and to begin their inner emotional healing.

I arranged to meet the girl whose flames I had put out, and for a few days we spent recess time together indoors. While we played games together, we talked about what had happened and how we were both feeling. When it was suggested that she return to recess outside, she was extremely reluctant to do so. I was aware that many of the other children were also afraid to go outside. One little boy even hid under a stairwell to avoid going out onto the playground. Many of the children who did go outdoors lingered close to the school building. Only a few ventured out onto the field where the crash had taken place.

There was occupational therapy work to be done on that playground. I began to go outside during recess. At first my goal was to help the girl feel more comfortable outside by playing games with her that would focus her attention on having fun. She sat and tried to balance herself on my four-foot-in-diameter blue rubber therapy ball while we played catch with another ball. She loved the challenge and began to develop skill at it. As I had hoped, some of the other children were attracted to the balls and wanted to join us. Each day the number of participants in the ball games increased. Two weeks after the crash, when I brought the blue therapy ball outside, I deliberately began kicking it onto the area of the playground that the children had been avoiding. As I anticipated, several of the children began to chase the ball and eventually they ran all over the playground, replacing the trauma they had recently associated with the space with safe and successful experiences there. Having fun while chasing the ball around the yard helped them regain their confidence in the outdoors as a safe place to play and to be.

I spoke with the teachers about the games and my goals to help the children feel comfortable again on their playground, and I loaned them several of the large balls at recess time. These additional balls provided needed distraction and a sense of accomplishment for many children and helped them feel safe in their environment again. The teachers and I loved seeing the children reclaiming their playground.

To our great relief, most of the children seemed resilient and returned to their usual activities. However, in time I realized that despite their outward happy behavior, many children constantly thought of the accident for months afterwards. The teachers and I continued our work to encourage these children in their emotional healing. The children were given opportunities to draw pictures, write stories, and to play with toys such as airplanes and fire trucks to replay the accident over and over. We knew that for many it would take time.

The second-grade boy who was severely burned returned to school the following year. He received extensive occupational therapy treatment in school for both his physical injuries and his emotional trauma. In some of his occupational therapy sessions, he played with paper airplanes and helicopters. During these activities he was finally able to talk about what had happened. It has been many years, and he is now a college student and doing well.

Over the past several years, the children have talked about and written about their memories. To this day, though we each remember the event differently, none of us will ever forget the day the airplane fell from the sky— the day that changed us forever.

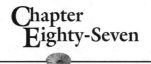

My
12-Story Plunge

Brett T. Duffey, OTR/L

On a breezy spring evening in 1989 in Myrtle Beach, South Carolina, I was a 20-year-old Marine air traffic controller on leave, enjoying a vacation with my dad in a posh high-rise hotel overlooking the beach. When I stepped out onto the balcony of our 12th-floor room to view the sunset, I noticed some attractive young ladies on the balcony two floors above me and leaned out to exchange friendly greetings. As I was talking, my foot slipped, and this 6'3" Marine lost his balance and plummeted through space, 12 stories down to the ground below.

I knew in that split second as I plunged from the balcony that my life was probably over. So casually, so quickly, so incredibly impossibly. I had only intended to watch the sunset and flirt with some cute girls, and now I was going to die. And yet, miraculously, I did not die. I landed... with 16 broken bones and a closed head injury that left me in a coma for 6 weeks... but alive.

Before that fall, I had it all—youth, confidence, a promising career, a loving family, and supportive friends. In that one instant, however, everything changed forever. That day, I literally hit bottom. I survived the 12-story fall, but what began that day was an uphill battle, first to heal my broken body and then ultimately to return to a "normal" life. 12 years later, I am glad to be alive and able to tell my remarkable story.

Chapter Eighty-Seven

When I awoke from the coma 6 weeks later, my world had been turned upside down. I broke 16 bones in the fall, three ribs and 13 bones in my legs because of the way I hit the ground. Luckily, my spine was not broken and, while I suffered a closed head wound, I did not suffer from any permanent brain damage. But all that I had learned in my life and all of my future plans were affected somehow. I would spend the next 13 months recovering in four different hospitals. My parents were informed by my doctors that I had less than a 5% chance of surviving, and that even if I did survive, my chances of recovery were slim.

After I came out of the coma, I was partially paralyzed for 9 months. I couldn't walk, and I couldn't move my right arm or leg. This was especially difficult for me because I was right-handed, and I had to learn to write with my left hand. Additionally, I was unable to speak for 3 months because my vocal cords had been nicked during a tracheotomy. So my immediate rehabilitation needs were to relearn how to walk, talk, write, and use my right leg, hand, and arm again. The fact that I couldn't speak made it hard for the doctors to determine whether I had any brain damage; even after I regained my speech, they were uncertain about whether my ability to think and reason would return to normal. These were the biggest physical obstacles I had to overcome during my recovery, although there were many other smaller challenges as well. The psychological issues of facing my future—life with possible disabilities—also needed attention.

The support of my family and friends really helped me through my ordeal. My many months of recovery took place far from home and my military base. My family and friends were too far away to visit frequently, though my parents were at my side nearly every week. Because of the distance they had to travel, any and all visits from friends and other family members were especially meaningful to me. I credit my friends with breaking me out of the shell of my new disabilities. They helped me by not treating me any differently than before, even though I now had some disabilities. Whenever they visited, they would take me out of the hospital for a bite to eat, shopping, and the movies. They never complained about the inconvenience of hauling around my wheelchair. I am forever indebted to my friends for showing me the love and companionship that was vital for my "social" recovery.

At the Oteen Veterans Administration Hospital in Asheville, North Carolina—the last of the four hospitals in which I stayed—I was lucky to meet James White, OTR/L, who was like a second father to me. He laughed and joked with me and constantly provided friendship accompanied by just the right level of challenge in everything that I did. He kept me motivated during my occupational therapy, and through his leadership I learned to become a fighter again and to pursue my dreams. I visit him whenever I am in the area, but I don't think he realizes how much I value having had his mentorship throughout my recovery, nor does he know what a lasting influence he had on my choice of a career.

Jim was a dedicated, no-nonsense therapist, but he always was sensitive to my moods. If I wasn't having a good day, he would change the therapy to match my feelings. Although I was having physical therapy and speech therapy as well as occupational therapy, whenever I got bored in the hospital, I would go back to the occupational therapy area, often six times a day, and I liked it the most. Jim and the other occupational therapists spent hours ranging my stiff right arm, moving it from the close-to-my-chest position in which it seemed locked, through all the normal movement patterns, in order to prevent the muscles from becoming too stiff to ever allow return of normal movement again. Jim then encouraged me to try to move my arm, even though it was extremely painful for me to do so. Jim became an expert at distracting me with conversation and jokes during those sessions, so that I wasn't focusing solely on the pain, and this was very helpful. It took several weeks to get the full range of passive motion back, and it took another 6 months for me to be able to move my arm actively through all of the normal muscle patterns, but with Jim's encouragement for my mind and his skilled fingers moving my body's joints, I was able to do it! Next, I needed to regain strength in the arm, and again Jim found the right activities to help develop overall strength and also to improve my fine finger dexterity. I believe that my previous excellent physical shape and my Marine training helped me stay focused on getting well, but Jim's own "Marine can-do" attitude kept me going.

Following my release from Oteen, I was living at home and trying to figure out what to do with my life. Before my unexpected fall, I had planned to work for the Federal Aviation Administration as an air traffic controller, but, understandably, no one who has had a closed head injury is eligible for this demanding and fast-paced work for the federal government. So that was no longer an option for me. I had been honorably discharged from the Marines, and I was now attempting college again at Forsyth Technical Community College in Winston-Salem, North Carolina. While I was there, my grades gradually improved from B's and C's to straight A's over five quarters. With grades like those, I was pleased to let my doctors know that I didn't seem to have any lingering cognitive problems. During this period of my physical recovery, I "graduated" from a wheelchair to walking wearing only a supportive brace on my right leg. And on the social front, while at Forsyth, I also met my future wife.

My career goals came into focus one night while at dinner with my mother. We were discussing my occupational therapy experiences at Oteen and what I could do with my life now that my original career plans needed to be altered. Hearing me extol Jim's virtues and the great job he had done with my rehabilitation, she suggested that I consider becoming a therapist. "Just think about it," she told me, "other people will listen to you because you've been there."

Chapter Eighty-Seven

My mother was right. It was there in front of me all this time, but I had never thought about it before. Back at school the next day, I put in motion plans to transfer to the occupational therapy department at Lenoir-Rhyne College in Hickory, North Carolina. I then began concentrating on completing the 2 years of prerequisite courses. I entered the occupational therapy program at Lenoir-Rhyne in 1995 and graduated in May 1998.

Meanwhile, during this time, I married and fathered a son, now 2 years old and the joy of my life. Although that marriage ended after 5 years, I am now seriously involved in a new relationship that has promise of being an important long-term one.

I now work as an occupational therapist with people who have the same kinds of physical rehabilitation needs that I had, and I find this incredibly rewarding. With hindsight, I realize that one of the reasons I became an occupational therapist was to help other individuals the way James White helped me. I hope that I will be able to help others achieve as much success in their struggles with impairments and disabilities as I have achieved. It has been a long journey back following that 12-story plunge, and I am very grateful to all of the people who have supported me throughout the years since my very long fall.

I also realize that my mother was right. I have been able to make a major impact on patients when they find out my story—the extent of my original injuries and how I have been through the rehabilitation process myself—and when they can see for themselves my full recovery. They say I give them hope.

Chapter Eighty-Eight

September 11, 2001: Ambiguous Loss

Judy Grossman,
DrPH, OTR, FAOTA

Susan was at the Head Start program on the Lower East Side of Manhattan dropping off her two young children at 8:47 a.m. on September 11 when the first plane hit the World Trade Center North Tower. As she and the rest of the parents and staff watched the flames and smoke in shocked horror, at 9:03 a.m. her own world burst into flames. When the second hijacked airplane rammed the South World Trade Center Tower, and its entire middle section exploded, Susan knew immediately that her husband, Juan, a food service worker on the 82nd floor of that building, was in grave danger.

Before their horrified eyes, in the scene replayed endlessly on the TV sets of the entire world, it was clear that those working on the floors where the planes hit and on the floors above the fires in both buildings had virtually no chance to escape. Trapped first by the heat, smoke, and flames, and then buried in the rubble by the unexpected catastrophic collapse of the South Tower, Building Two, shortly after 10 a.m., and the North Tower, Building One, a short time later, nearly 3000 people lost their lives. When 3000 people die, it is an almost unimaginable statistic. When one individual person dies, it is an unimaginable tragedy for the family and friends left behind. And so it was for

Chapter Eighty-Eight

Susan and her family. Juan, her beloved husband and the father of their two preschoolers, did not return from work that fateful day.

I sat in front of the television both drawn to and repelled by the images of the World Trade Center disaster. The Twin Towers were collapsing, and people were expecting the casualties to overwhelm the local hospitals. My sense of grief and disbelief grew as the rescue efforts continued and the death toll rose. Still, the impact was secondhand because at first I did not suffer any direct loss. One week later, the phone rang.

It was Christine, an occupational therapist who had been my research assistant last year working with Head Start families as part of a University-Head Start Partnership grant between New York University and four Head Start centers on the Lower East Side of New York City. She and I together had provided occupational therapy services to the children, teachers, and parents at two of the centers.

Christine had been contacted that morning by the Head Start director at one of the centers because of her relationship with Susan, the Head Start mother whose husband had worked at the World Trade Center. He had not returned home from work the day of the attack and was still considered among the missing in the World Trade Center tragedy. Christine's connection with Susan was strong, and Susan now needed comfort and support as she tried to sort out and deal with her family's fate. Unfortunately, Christine was moving to the West Coast that very day. Relieved to know that I would contact Susan and provide some of the comfort and support Susan needed, she reached Susan by phone and told her that I would call her. Christine promised Susan that she would continue to stay in touch with her from her new location.

For the past 2 years, Susan had participated in the "Mother's Club" at the Center while her children attended Head Start. At first she had appeared shy and depressed. She was hesitant to come to the group and would spend most of the day at home alone after she dropped off her children. Over time, as she attended the group, she developed confidence and friendships with some of the other mothers. We helped her set some personal goals, she completed her high school equivalency diploma, and she applied for a position as an assistant teacher. We saw tremendous growth in her capabilities and had shared her and her husband's delight in her new accomplishments.

I immediately contacted the Head Start program to offer my services to Susan as well as to provide support for the staff who had been close enough to view the flames and smoke directly. I knew it would be difficult work. Fortunately, my occupational therapy education and practice have been supplemented by training and certification as a family therapist, and I have had many years of experience providing family services as part of my occupational therapy and family therapy practice. I also have done research on the promotion of family resilience and the prevention of social, emotional, and developmental problems in high risk children and families, and I teach courses on these topics at local university occupational therapy educational programs. But nothing in my past experience could possibly have prepared me for the magnitude of this disaster and the horrifying aftermath effects on the grieving families. I anticipated that it would take all of my combined skills to help Susan and her family in this crisis situation. I was right.

Susan was anxious to meet with me but was still in a state of shock and denial. She had spent her days at home, crying, since the attacks. Frustrated in my attempts to meet with Susan at the family assistance center that wass set up for the families of those missing by the city of New York or my office, I decided to rely on the Head Start staff to tell the family I would be coming to see her at the program. Our work together began the very next day.

Susan explained tearfully that her husband Juan had worked in food services on the 82nd floor of Tower Two. On September 11th, he had left early for work and they did not have time for their usual morning goodbye. Susan was at the Head Start program when she saw the attacks, heard the news, and feared the worst. With no actual body or any physical remains, however, the finality of his death was difficult for her to accept.

Our first session included Susan, her children, her mother-in-law, and several other family members. My primary objective was to create a safe place to talk about the husband, father, and son who was missing. There was a sense of urgency since some family members were returning to Puerto Rico, and they were anxious to have a memorial service. Previous family traumas surfaced as Susan's mother-in-law related other unanticipated deaths in her family. Sorrow and compassion were evident as tender words were shared between Susan and her husband's mother. Naturally, the children needed special attention to help them understand what had happened to their father.

My ongoing work with Susan has been difficult and frustrating because there are so many competing demands. Most pressing is the need for her to express grief and the need for the children to express their fears and feelings through play. Just as important is the pressure on Susan to deal with the business of dying and the maze of paperwork required by the Red Cross and other federal, state, and city agencies. She has had to learn new skills to become self-sufficient and to secure resources for her children's future after having been dependent on her husband since their courtship began.

The work with Susan took many forms. She shared her recurring thoughts about her husband's unimaginable final moments as the plane exploded in the tower. She had had no chance for closure and a final goodbye. She now had new kinds of fears and insecurities, and many unanswerable questions. "Will my children grow up in a safe world?" "How could the terrorists act so cruelly?" "Will I be able to manage?" I encouraged Susan to share her sorrow and anger and to capture special memories of her husband and their time together.

Susan's children, ages 4 and 6 years, came to my office every week to play and spend time with their mother, engaged in normal childhood activities. Their reactions to the trauma were different: one child was tearful and reluctant to talk, the other was a frenzy of activity and somewhat aggressive. Play and art activities were used to understand the children's concerns. We created photo albums and the children drew pictures for Daddy's memorial service. Family rituals were encouraged. Six weeks after the tragedy, we celebrated Susan's birthday with her children and her mother and brother who had just arrived from overseas. Intergenerational connections were strengthened and the children began to experience the normal activities of everyday life. It was important for them to know that even though Mommy cried a lot, she could still provide comfort and share the joys of the moment.

Another therapeutic goal was to encourage Susan to recognize her personal strengths and help her move toward self-sufficiency. She was asked to identify and begin to utilize sources of emotional and practical support. I referred her to a group for family members who lost a partner or child in the World Trade Center attack, and this experience was very meaningful. Susan also needed to prioritize tasks, pace herself, and make deliberate decisions about her future. She had to cope with increased responsibilities and with being a single parent. She missed Juan; her loneliness was coupled with a perceived lack of control and a sense of helplessness. Susan needed to learn some new skills, such as how to budget and keep a bank account, and how to seek out help when she was despondent. Our time together was always precious and filled with hints of change and personal growth.

The work demanded compassion and empathy. I joined Susan and her family in their sorrow and pain and listened to their stories with humility. I worked closely with the Head Start staff to allay their fears and anxiety and to help them meet Susan's immediate needs. Some of them experienced personal loss; all of them felt vulnerable after the terrorist attacks. My work with Susan, her family, and the Head Start staff has been challenging and rewarding. It has contributed to my own healing process in the wake of the tragedy and to my belief that people are resilient and capable of good deeds.

The story is not over. I continue to work with Susan and her children to help the grieving process and bring some normalcy back to their lives. As Susan and all the other people who lost loved ones on that awful day try to deal with their very real but still ambiguous loss, the entire country shares their pain and grief. It was a day no one will ever forget, and the healing process is just beginning.

Chapter Eighty-Nine

September 11, 2001: Getting Through Trying Times

Elisabeth Refn, MA, OTR

I n the aftermath of the horrific World Trade Center attacks on September 11, 2001, all New Yorkers seemed to crave extra touches of healing and kindness. An understanding police officer gave both to Mrs. Adams in her moment of greatest anxiety following the terrifying attacks. This is the story of one of New York's finest, a police officer who became a very special kind of hero by helping a frightened New York woman calm down using handout materials from an occupational therapy treatment session in a very unusual venue—the local police station—after she had just been taken into custody.

On the Upper West Side of New York City, there is a psychiatric day treatment center for chronic mentally ill adults who live in the surrounding Manhattan community. I work as an occupational therapist with Wendy Sobelman, a dance therapist, in a program there that is focused on helping a particular group of patients: those who become so uncontrollably panicked that frequently they must go to hospital emergency rooms, searching for help.

The "Coping with Anxiety" skills group that we run tries to help these patients help themselves by teaching them specific

329

coping strategies and skills to use to avoid an anxiety attack and to reduce their anxiety if they are in the midst of a one. The group provides the opportunity for patients to practice those skills twice a week in the group treatment sessions. Patients learn how to observe and monitor their own breathing, to practice deep-breathing skills, to do slow-walking to their breathing (called walking meditation), and to focus on counting their breaths.

To make it easier for our members to remember and to practice the necessary skills, we give them handout sheets with step-by-step instructions, which they carry around with them at all times. The idea is for them to have with them always a means to control their own anxious behavior. Our first task at each treatment session is hearing reports from patients who practiced their new skills at home or had to use them in real-life situations.

Never had I been more concerned about my patients than at our session on Thursday, September 13, 2001. Two days earlier, as the world watched in horror on TV, and New Yorkers watched in shocked disbelief from their street corners or windows, terrorists had attacked our city, destroying the World Trade Centers, and leaving everyone frightened, sad, and angry. How would my patients, New Yorkers all, with their additional special problems and anxieties, cope with these terrifying events?

Despite the unusual circumstances, we began our session by following the normal routine of our group, which calls for first checking with the participants to acknowledge and encourage those who did their "homework" and/or had to apply the skills to real-life situations. When I asked my group how they were handling the events, Mrs. Adams immediately raised her hand. I expected to hear the worst from her. Mrs. Adams is extremely committed to our group, but she is always very anxious. She takes events very personally, hears voices, and has attempted suicide numerous times. She has had to be rehospitalized frequently.

Although used to all kinds of unusual adventures related by Mrs. Adams, the group was nonetheless astonished to hear her story. It seemed that on September 12, the day after the attack, Mrs. Adams was extremely anxious about what had happened and what might follow, but she decided to go anyway to her planned appointment at the psychiatric day treatment center. On her way home on the bus, she suddenly heard very insistent voices telling her that there was a bomb on the bus.

"I was so frightened, I had to scream," she explained to us. Terrified, she shrieked, "There's a bomb on the bus, there's a bomb on the bus!"

Her screams were met with immediate action. The bus driver called for assistance, and police arrived swiftly. The bus was searched, and Mrs. Adams was taken to the police station, where her belongings were searched.

At the police station, Mrs. Adams stopped her continuous screaming, but she remained very frightened. She asked questions at a furious rate, not listening to answers or words of reassurance. She paced continually, breathing quickly and nervously. She didn't seem to know what to do next or how to calm herself down.

The police officers at the station were obviously extremely busy. They were emotionally distraught at the extent of the tragedy and at the number of their comrades in the fire department and the police department who had been killed or were missing in the rubble of the collapsed buildings. The last thing their frayed nerves needed that afternoon was a screaming, out-of-control person in their midst.

Suddenly, a police officer came to her rescue in a most unexpected way. The officer searching her purse discovered the handouts that she always carries with her from the "Coping with Anxiety" skills group. Hoping that he'd found a cure for Mrs. Avila's screaming outbursts, he brought them to her. Slowly and deliberately, he began to read aloud to her the instructions for deep breathing and walking meditation. Calmly, carefully, he recited to her, "Breathe in, one; breathe out, one. Breathe in, two; breathe out, two." He followed along, doing the breathing exercises himself, as he read the step-by-step instructions to her; he seemed to find this routine helpful, and he gently encouraged Mrs. Adams to join in.

As he read to her, Mrs. Adams was surprised and relieved to find that the familiar words were calming to her. She became stable enough to remain at the police station and quietly wait for her family to pick her up. This time, despite the extreme circumstances and her high anxiety level, she didn't have to be rehospitalized.

"So now I know that I may need other people to tell me what to do when I get out of control," she concluded her report. "And I know that the instructions really work for me."

Being taken into custody by the New York Police proved to be the best thing that could have happened to Mrs. Adams that frightening day after the World Trade Center disaster. She will always remember the extraordinary kindness shown by the police officer who, in the midst of his own pain, reached out to help her by reading and practicing the advice from our occupational therapy group. The enormous public heroic actions of New York's police and firefighters during and after the terrorist attacks were already apparent to the entire nation; the smaller private heroic actions, like reaching out to people in need and being kind and helpful, would become apparent as the days passed. These would begin the healing process.

Mrs. Adams' experience was reassuring to all of us. Even in the days immediately after September 11, when so many people throughout New York were coping with anxiety and fear, we were comforted knowing that our special patients were gaining solid skills to help get them through the trying times. That made all of us breathe a little bit easier.

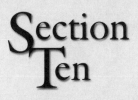

Section Ten

Reflections of the Journey

Review of Lives Well Lived

Review of
Lives Well Lived

Reminisce with seven people whose initial outlooks seemed bleak due to diseases like polio that were "incurable" years ago when they were first diagnosed or to cancer and other progressive diseases. Instead of succumbing to despair and giving in to the certainty of a life of limitations, these brave and resourceful individuals and their therapists succeeded in creating full lives of productivity and happiness for many years or full lives of productivity and serenity for the time remaining. Their lives and accomplishments will inspire everyone.

Chapter Ninety

Therapy Begins at Home

Anitta Boyko Fox, BS, MA, OTR

"It's a boy! It's a boy—another beautiful baby!" When we arrived home with our newest bundle of joy, our 1-year-old daughter greeted us, her arms outstretched to welcome us. We showed her the baby and guided her small hand to David's cheek. She was delighted, bewildered, and surprised all at the same time. Her puzzled look gave way to a broad smile as she groped for the little bit of hairy fuzz on top of David's head. She exclaimed, "Titzi!" which was the way she lovingly pronounced our cat's name. For us, it meant her official acceptance of the new arrival into her world and into our family. Things seemed perfect.

But in fact, they weren't. Within 2 months, I was certain that David's spine curved to the left. During diapering, I noticed that he moved only his left leg, while the right one rested on the table. When I tickled his belly, the tiny stump of umbilical cord moved to the left, showing an imbalance in his abdominal muscles. It became clear to me that there was something very wrong with David, and my husband, a physician, agreed. The following month, x-rays revealed an extra half vertebra wedged between the first and second vertebrae in his middle back, forcing his spine into a C-curve. He also had a congenital "leaking" bladder, which is usually caused by a neurological problem. My heart began to sink.

However, because of my training as an occupational therapist, I

immediately considered therapies to help our son. As an occupational therapist, I was able to recognize, evaluate, think, and act constructively. I began
that day, and for the next few years, I worked hard with David right in our own
home to prevent serious deformity, forestall disability, and halt psychological
trauma and maladjustment.

I started with his diapering, carefully rolling his leg in and holding his hips
tightly in place to prevent any malformation of the hip joint. I used a splint
to hold his feet in a more natural position. I also used another diaper or strap
to hold his knees together to prevent outward rotation at the hip and inward
rotation at the knees. I made long play and swimming sessions in the bathtub a part of David's daily therapy routine. I believed that swimming would
become an important part of David's treatment and his lifelong maintenance
program.

By the time David was 2 years old, we had made numerous visits to
Boston's Children's Hospital, Babies Hospital at Columbia-Presbyterian
Medical Center, NYU Medical Center, and others. The general consensus
among the doctors was to operate, but because David was so young, my husband and I decided to wait before attempting any radical procedures. I wanted the chance to help David learn to walk. We concluded that if all of my
efforts failed to help him, there still would be plenty of time to consider surgery.

Our daughter became part of David's occupational therapy routine. She
took great pride and pleasure in entertaining her baby brother. They played
together in the yard, chasing each other, rolling on the grass, and playing
peek-a-boo with the cat. In the winter, they played together on the ice on a
nearby pond. They slipped and fell frequently, and fell again while trying to
get up, but had fun nonetheless. Chasing, crawling, falling, and pulling himself upright were important exercises for David; the naturalness and purpose-
fulness of these activities as he roughhoused with his sister made them fun as
well and motivated him to keep them up in the house each day. Continuing
the home-based occupational therapy activities when we had our next child,
she and David were thrilled to be able to help with the same kind of healthy
exercise and bathtub program as they had experienced. To me it was more
exercise for David, for all of us, though, we were also having fun!

By age 3, David was crawling on his hands and knees. He then learned to
walk fairly well with the help of an elastic twister, a stretchy elastic band that
acted like a rubber band to rotate his right leg inward, to help his hamstring
muscles in his thigh bend his knee, and to pull up his foot. He enjoyed riding his tricycle and playing outdoors with other neighborhood children. As
he got older, he outgrew the need for the elastic twister and walked well on
his own. David had developed into a bright, happy, and active child who was
physically quite independent.

I was concerned about the rapid growth period David would undergo as an adolescent. During such periods of physical development, spinal curvatures usually tend to worsen, so I urged David to use crutches to help strengthen his muscles. He cooperated willingly, to him it was fun to zip along on crutches when he really didn't need them to walk. By the end of the summer, David's expertise with crutches had brought about all the results for which I had hoped. His spinal curve had lessened by 4 degrees. His upper body muscle tone improved overall. David's stronger arms and shoulders compensated for a weak kick when swimming. He became a strong swimmer of the crawl, breaststroke, and butterfly, and he was invited to return to his summer camp as the new swim counselor. Additionally, his more developed back muscles leveled his shoulders and pulled his shoulder blades back and together to help him stand more fully erect. Finally, exercise to strengthen his abdominal muscles, back muscles, and diaphragm also dramatically improved his kinesthetic sense of where his body was in space. Meanwhile, his extra vertebra fused solidly on its own.

Not surprisingly, after learning of these improvements, his doctors re-evaluated the need to operate. While we no longer considered orthopedic surgery, we still had to deal with the accompanying difficulty of his congenital leaking bladder. As an infant, his bladder capacity had needed to be increased and maintained. At first it used to have to be emptied every 1 or 2 hours, but we worked to lengthen the time between toilet visits at night until he was able to hold it until morning. Even so, he still needed to use absorbent padding at all times. We treated this absolutely matter-of-factly and considered it part of his ordinary underwear routine. As a result, he never became self-conscious or gave it a second thought. Over the years, with patience and persistence, we explored new treatments, and as a young adult, after two benign nonsurgical procedures, David finally gained control of his bladder.

As David grew into a teenager and then an adult, he continued his athletic approach to the world in which he lived. As a family, we all contributed to David's therapy as we hiked, skated, skied, rode bicycles, and played tennis, leading healthy physical and mental lives in general. David took on leadership positions in school, and colleges began recruiting him for their swim teams. He was an excellent student, earning several academic awards to prove it.

Today, David is a gracious, multitalented, compassionate, and modest man who lives a completely normal life. At home in Florida, he still swims everyday. He works as an attorney, and in his spare time writes beautiful prose and poetry. He is married to a lovely young woman who is as gracious as he is. We suspect that their children, our grandchildren, will benefit greatly from the nurturing we provided to David.

David moved out of our house many years ago, and when he vacated the premises, the impromptu occupational therapy home-based program that I set up especially for him closed its doors. However, vigilant occupational therapist that I remain, I am ever ready to open those doors to a niece, nephew, or grandchild who might need occupational therapy services. You see, when it comes to occupational therapy, you can always go home again.

Chris
Leaves a Legacy

Mary LeChene Bennett,
OTR/L Retired

Sometimes it takes death to reveal fully the success of a life well lived, no matter how short and full of overwhelming personal suffering. Fifteen-year-old Christopher DiBiasi lived that profoundly successful life. Contributing to this story about Chris gave his mother, Rosalind, a chance to share the meaning of Chris' life with others, while at the same time it provided her the opportunity to reconnect with me, the occupational therapist who had helped Chris live his life as fully as possible. Recalling Chris's courage, as she helped me write, helped Rosalind to find comfort in reliving her memories of his life.

On the morning of November 4, 1994, I arrived as usual at the home of my 15-year-old patient, Chris, for his daily occupational therapy appointment. I entered the living room and found his hospital bed empty. His completely distraught grandmother greeted me with the news: "I think Chris is dead, but I'm not sure."

My eyes darted quickly from room to room, half-expecting and half-fearing that I'd find his body lying somewhere. But the house was empty; Christopher's grandmother filled me in on the details. An hour earlier Christopher had trouble breathing during his morning bath routine, and a substitute home health aide suddenly had to resuscitate him. A desperate race to the hospital to save his life followed. Grandmother had barely had time to bid Chris a quick goodbye before the ambulance had rushed him and Rosiland off, only 30 minutes before my arrival. I immediately drove his grandmother to the hospital where we met Chris' mother, Rosalind, who confirmed our worst fears: Christopher, indeed, had died at the hospital.

It has now been many years since I heard those chilling words and focused on the empty hospital bed he usually occupied, but to this day I still remember Chris with fondness and awe.

Because of his terrible illness, we all knew this inevitable day would come. Even so, each of us felt shock that the day indeed had come now, so soon. We could not believe that Chris was gone. We could not imagine that Chris was free from his painful struggles. His rare, genetic neurological illness called Hallervorden-Spatz disease (or "stiff-man syndrome") had taken its final toll. But not before Chris had already had the chance to demonstrate his rare gifts of courage and understanding to his family, friends, and the professionals who worked with him.

Stiff-man syndrome damages the brain of those unfortunate enough to have it, resulting in severe twisting muscle spasms that are extraordinarily painful. The person suffers uncontrollable spasms that cause strange postures at first, eventually leading to loss of muscle control for balance and purposeful movements. It is progressive—it gets steadily worse—and degenerative—the body keeps breaking down more and more over time—and it most often results in death during the teenage years.

I had worked with Chris as his occupational therapist for more than 5 years. Chris started out as a charming, intelligent, lively, and capable 10-year-old boy who was full of mischief. At first he only needed help with adaptations to make dressing himself easier and needed suggestions for positioning himself at a table to make schoolwork possible and to make his handwriting more legible. We even brainstormed a few ideas to keep him independent in making a light lunch for himself in the kitchen. Each week he came to see me at my occupational therapy clinic for therapy. Each week Rosalind supplied fresh observations on the challenges that Chris faced and his ever changing needs. When spasms in his arms grew more severe, we tried various splints to protect the joints of his fingers, wrists, and elbows. We were well aware that as the disease progressed, he would need more and more help to cope with his newly developing limitations. Through it all he remained charming and intelligent, if not quite so lively and capable, even though he felt fearful about the changes.

When his whole trunk became involved with spasms that pulled him backward, he began suffering frequent falls. No longer were a hard protective helmet and a full-time personal attendant sufficient to ensure his safety. So a team was mustered. This group of rehabilitation professionals worked together to solve Chris' unique needs for getting around by himself. I, as the occupational therapist, provided measurements for a computerized electric power wheelchair and designed the special cushions Chris needed in the chair to support his skeleton yet protect his thin body. We found the best placement for the joystick control unit he would use to propel the chair. Lastly, attached to the power unit, we hooked up a computer with synthesized speech, because by then Chris' facial and jaw muscles had become affected, preventing normal speech, eating, and facial expression.

Though Chris was treated with strong medications to relax the spasms, the spasms never really went away. On especially bad days when his pain and fatigue made it impossible for him to function in school, Rosalind was called from her teaching job in another district to take him home. Yet remarkably Chris still maintained his marvelous sense of humor. Even on those tough days, she remembers that Chris would lock himself in the car to play a little joke on her. It was a favorite little trick to make her laugh. We were constantly amazed that during those days of despair Chris so often found a way to escape through his sense of humor and to make those around him laugh too.

Rosalind remembers that occupational therapy provided hope when too many little losses compounded and threatened Chris with hopelessness. She told me that occupational therapy provided an opportunity for Chris to exercise some control over the illness. Occupational therapy made him aware that like all children, he had important responsibilities in life and that he was still a vital part of life. I agreed that occupational therapy was a profound acknowledgment of our respect and love for Chris. But throughout it all, Chris supplied all the courage. Furthermore, it was the kind of courage that exceeded all of our expectations. He was always willing to try new treatments, no matter how painful, no matter how hard, and his positive attitude touched all who came in contact with him.

Shortly after his 15th birthday, Chris was admitted to a hospital 65 miles from home to undergo a procedure that would wean him off oral medications and test a new procedure of administering medicine directly into his body through a pump. If the test procedure was successful, a small pump would be inserted under the skin of his stomach to administer medicine in measured doses to better control the debilitating spasms. But there were no guarantees.

In order to prepare his body to receive the constant measured dose using the pump, and to test whether this new system would work, his body had to be clear of all other medicines. As pills and other oral medications were withdrawn, Chris endured the torture of unmitigated pain and relentless tightening and twisting of his muscles. But he never complained. Then we all suffered a crashing disappointment. The pump couldn't work for Chris. High enough medicine levels could not be achieved and sustained in his body; ultimately the pump test procedure had to be ended and the pump removed. As a result of the test procedure, yet another setback was in store for Chris—he developed meningitis. Very tense hours and days passed. Rosalind, a single mother whose life revolved around Chris, kept her vigil with her son, essentially having "moved in" to the hospital. Finally, Chris responded to antibiotic treatment and he survived the meningitis.

Then the neurosurgeon offered a different solution to control the muscle spasms, called selective thalamotomy. In this procedure, a part of the brain, the thalamus, is surgically cauterized or given tiny electric shocks that seal off the nerve endings. This selectively reduces the nerve signals sent to skeletal muscles and is often helpful in relieving intractable pain. Chris underwent that difficult brain surgery and important gains were achieved. Following surgery, nourishing him became a priority, so a tube was surgically inserted into his small intestine through which liquid nourishment was pumped. After 2 months in the hospital, Chris really wanted to go home. But only if a way could be found to care for him at home, could he leave the hospital. It was, and so he did. Again Rosalind came to the rescue!

Rosalind was taught to manage the feeding tube. A hospital bed was set up in the living room. A virtual pharmacy of medications had to be given to Chris in just the right doses and order. Rosalind took a leave from her job, and so Chris was discharged the first week of October. In spite of his need for round-the-clock care, Chris was motivated to learn to sit in a chair again and put weight on his legs. He even hoped to go back to school. Just 5 days before his death, Rosalind and Chris repeated their annual fall tradition of going to a farm market to buy gourds and a pumpkin for Halloween. Chris truly enjoyed the trip. Smiling in the crisp fall air, he let his mother know that he was still looking forward to getting back to school to see his classmates' Halloween costumes. His optimism cheered Rosalind and she smiled back.

As we stood in the emergency room together trying to find words to say goodbye to Chris, I was struck with a profound awareness of what a privilege it had been to be so closely involved in his life and in the life of his family and to be one of the beneficiaries of his legacy. "We'll take good care of your mom," I spoke on that day and made that promise to his still-warm body. His legacy that lives on is this: Christopher brought out the best in every life he touched. And he touched ever so many lives.

Now, nearly 3 years later, I was able to fulfill that promise. Writing Chris' story gave me the opportunity to reconnect with Rosalind on a new level that extended the relationship we had when Chris was alive. When I called her to discuss the idea of memorializing Chris by telling his story, I found her still in the throes of grief even though almost 3 years had passed. Working with me to write Chris' story helped Rosalind deal with her loss and channel her grief; it helped her to continue to heal as she reviewed Chris' life and shared its special meaning. Working together on this story allowed Rosalind to bring her grieving to another level of resolution. For we both saw Chris' ultimate legacy: a life counts, a life matters, no matter how short or limited it may have been. Even after death, Chris' life remained an inspiration.

What an achievement and what a legacy for a 15 year old.

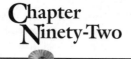

The Music Lady

Anitta Boyko Fox, BS, MA, OTR

Today, for most of us, the word "polio" brings to mind one of the great medical success stories of the 20th century. It is the devastating disease that was conquered by Dr. Jonas Salk and his seemingly miraculous vaccine. But for Esther Breslau, who is now in her 60s, it was a disease that could have defined the rest of her life, if she had let it. What makes Esther's story so special is that with early occupational therapy intervention, she did not let that happen.

Esther was born in 1937, at a time when childhood polio was every parent's nightmare. Within a few years of her birth, Esther was stricken with polio. As a child, she became partially paralyzed in her upper body and almost totally paralyzed in her lower body. She spent a year in a rehabilitation hospital and another year at home undergoing daily occupational and physical therapy. Esther pushed herself extremely hard and struggled fiercely to conquer all tasks during her rehabilitation. But she never wasted time feeling sorry for herself and always strived toward loftier goals. I was quite privileged to work with Esther from the very beginning to provide occupational therapy that was focused on achieving independence and leading a normal and productive life. As you read her story, you will see that Esther accomplished these goals better than anyone ever could have anticipated.

The Music Lady

As Esther got older, she became very self-sufficient, using leg braces and crutches to get around on her own, even commuting to high school on public transportation. As a teenager, a spinal fusion allowed her to regain sufficient balance so that she could move about indoors without crutches, and she secretly began walking through the house without her left leg brace. Her parents gave Esther much more freedom than most girls her age got in those days because they wanted her to become as independent as possible and Esther made the most of her freedom during high school and her early college years. She made frequent trips to Manhattan on buses and subways. Some weekends, she would visit a museum in the morning, return home to change, go out to parties in the evening, and possibly return to Manhattan in the wee hours of the following morning.

Esther met her future husband during her last semester of high school. During their courtship, they went on long hikes, climbed the Statue of Liberty, and wandered Book Row on the Lower East Side of Manhattan, among other things. Esther never believed that any of these activities were beyond her reach or that she shouldn't have been doing these things with her "condition." Esther and her husband were married in 1957. Esther spent the next several years as a stay-at-home mom for their three children. Of course, this meant doing housework, cooking, and taking care of the babies—responsibilities she took in stride. Virtually everything she did required some degree of creativity. They lived in married student housing at Rensselaer Polytechnic Institute, which was located in very hilly terrain. Even "normal" activities like getting the kids in or out of the apartment was quite a tricky endeavor. The house was on the upper end of a slope, which required Esther to get the carriage down the stairs one step at a time to the porch, and then required some very innovative maneuvers to get down the slope. But Esther was always up for the task.

The family later moved to New Jersey, where Esther had a much bigger house to take care of. She joined the peace movement in 1963 and even went on 5-mile marches without much difficulty. Esther later returned to college to study psychology, and she also began to work part-time. Between her family, the peace movement, school, and work, Esther led quite a busy life!

In 1971, Esther began working in the music business as a billing clerk for a classical music publisher/library supplier/store. Within 2 years, she gave up her psychology major and dropped out of college for the second time, this time to devote herself to the music business. She had found her calling in the music field and never looked back. In 1976, after another move and several months of unsuccessful job hunting, she started her own music business, which now employs seven people. Her company—The Yesterday Service—is known for its worldwide distribution of classical sheet music to schools, orchestras, choruses, and individuals, as well as for its resources and efficiency. Today, Esther continues to encourage many people with her confidence and positive attitude. Although she can't get around as well as she once did, she still enjoys running the business and expects to continue for quite some time.

Esther really has made the most of her abilities without dwelling on her physical limitations. Her "can-do" attitude made up for many of the constraints of her disability. Her untiring efforts and support from her family made many of her successes possible. I believe that Esther applied the basic tenets of occupational therapy to her life in general, focusing her efforts on specific goals to attain.

Working with Esther, watching her conquests and achievements for so many years, has been an inspiration to me personally. Throughout the years, we learned a lot from each other. Most importantly, Esther taught me to become a better therapist and a better person overall. Thank you, Esther, and more power to you. You proved that you don't have to let polio keep you from making beautiful music your whole life through.

Chapter
Ninety-Three

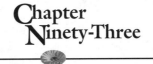

Hello, Can I
Help You?

Jacqueline Goldberg

"Hello, doctor's office. Can I help you?" For 25 years, 7 days a week, I repeated those words, or others like them. And each time I did, I said a silent thank you to Florence Stattel, the Chief of Occupational Therapy at the Kessler Institute for Rehabilitation in West Orange, New Jersey. Even though I am paralyzed from the chest down, being able to answer the phone with those familiar phrases allowed me to support myself all those years and now to enjoy my retirement in Florida. But it never would have happened without Florence.

In September 1948, at the age of 20, while preparing to return from summer vacation for my junior year at the University of Pennsylvania, I was stricken with Bulbar polio. In those days, it was still called "infantile paralysis." Polio did mostly strike children as the name suggests, but in 1948 many teens and young adults like me were affected. Many young people died that summer in Atlantic City where I was stricken; I fortunately survived.

However, I was totally paralyzed and unable to breathe without the help of an "iron lung," a large, ugly cylinder in which I lay on my back, with only my head protruding. I spent 2 years in hospitals getting hot packs, passive exercise, and other therapy. Eventually, I was weaned from the iron lung, but I was still paralyzed from the chest down, except for a slight return of function in my arms and hands.

In October 1950, I was very fortunate to be accepted as a patient at the Kessler Institute. The Institute had been founded a few years earlier by Dr. Henry Kessler, a pioneer in the field of rehabilitation, and was considered one of the best rehabilitation facilities in the country. Florence Stattel was the very intelligent, hard working, and devoted Chief of Occupational Therapy.

Florence and I discussed my future, what I could do with my very limited mobility to earn a living and experience some measure of self-sufficiency and fulfillment. Returning to college was not an option. Those were the days before the Americans with Disabilities Act, curb cuts for wheelchairs, ramps, and vans with lifts. Florence and I had to face the fact that it would be almost impossible for me to secure employment outside my own home. That's when Florence and I came up with the idea that it would be possible for me, with specially designed equipment, to operate an answering service from the apartment that I shared with my extraordinary parents.

Florence contacted New Jersey Bell Telephone. The Bell representative was extremely encouraging and cooperative. He, Florence, and I visited several answering services in the West Orange area so that I could see what was involved. Above and beyond his job requirements, the strong, young phone executive lifted me gently in and out of the car. Florence convinced New Jersey Bell to adapt telephone equipment that I could operate with my limited muscle function. A unique switchboard was installed in our apartment, and I learned to use it.

Over the next 25 years, I serviced about 75 clients, mostly doctors and businesses. It was a 24 hours a day, 7 days a week operation. I employed a night operator, and my wonderful parents also pitched in when necessary. Over all those years, I only missed one day of work, and that was due to an occupational hazard—laryngitis. I must have been doing a good job, because I always had a long waiting list for service.

Thanks to Florence and New Jersey Bell, not only was I financially self-sufficient, but I was able to carefully invest the money I earned. In 1976, I sold the business to one of my competitors and used the proceeds to purchase a condo in Florida for me and my parents. They are now deceased, but I continue to live in the condo with a live-in aide. Thank goodness I can afford it. I shudder to think how different my life would have been without the determination, guidance, and inspiration afforded me by Florence. She was a tremendous influence in my life, and I will be eternally grateful to her.

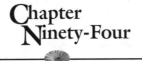

Chapter
Ninety-Four

The First Two
Clowns in Iceland

Diane J. Jones, RN

Children in the hospital in Iceland laugh more often due to a mysterious visitor named Disa and to a very special but very funny-looking medical specialist named Dr. Oliver. The two are award-winning clowns who have been visiting sick children at both of the hospitals in Reykjavík, Iceland's largest city, since 1990. Both Disa and Dr. Oliver are actually the same person—a creative occupational therapist who has discovered that clowning around with seriously ill children is a great way to boost their morale, distract them from their pain, and speed their recovery. She has also discovered that clowning around is a great way to help herself at the same time.

When Peggy Helgason gets herself ready for work, her efforts are a real labor of love. It takes 1½ hours to transform pretty, petite Peggy into her alter ego, Disa, a delightful and charming clown. Peggy considers her job as a professional clown very serious business, even though she receives no pay for her work. Disa's creation is a story that goes back more than 20 years.

Peggy is a 49-year-old American who now lives in Iceland. She is a native of North Carolina who attended the University of North Carolina at Chapel Hill. It was there, while studying for a master's degree in early childhood education in 1972, that she met Sigurdur ("Siggi") Helgason, an Icelander who was also at the University where he was studying for a master's degree in business administration.

In 1973, Peggy and Siggi were married in a tiny, historic church in Iceland, and Peggy began her life there. Adjusting to life in Iceland was not easy, but having a supportive husband, whom Peggy claims is also her best friend, helped Peggy face the many challenges, including learning a new language and adapting to a new culture. Peggy teases that Siggi wanted an American souvenir and a cook who could make good fried chicken that he learned to appreciate while in the South!

In 1983, the Helgasons moved to Manhattan, New York where Peggy earned her master's degree in occupational therapy at New York University, while Siggi worked for Icelandair's office at JFK Airport in New York. In 1985, they returned to Iceland, where Peggy became one of only 40 occupational therapists in all of Iceland.

1988 was a turning point in Peggy's life. It was then that she became very ill, and subsequently, suffered a stroke in 1989. The stroke left her without speech and paralyzed on one side. At the same time, she was diagnosed with another incurable progressive disease that she was told would continue to get worse, with possible periods of quiet remission between active acute episodes. After spending 3 months in a rehabilitation center, Peggy recovered her speech and regained use of the affected side. She decided that wondering "Why me?" was pointless, and she channeled her energies into fighting the effects of her disease. She accepted what could not be changed and also accepted the responsibility of developing her potential so that her life would be meaningful. Peggy says, "I feel as though my illness is a gift from a Higher Being. It has allowed me the freedom to do all of the things I've wanted to do and to live each day to its fullest without looking at yesterday or at what tomorrow may bring."

Because of her background in early childhood education and in occupational therapy, which she had practiced with hospitalized children, and because of her skills in dealing with psychological problems, Peggy decided on a new vocation—clowning in a medical setting. Specifically, Peggy wanted to develop a character who could talk on a one-to-one basis with seriously ill and terminally ill children. It was not easy getting started, since information on clowning was almost nonexistent in Iceland. In fact, she was the first professional clown in the whole country. Peggy received her first professional training for clowning at Richard Snowberg's Clown Camp, where she met veteran clowns who helped her with make-up and costumes. Later that summer she met Jim Roberts, a.k.a. "Strutter," who was most instrumental in Peggy's developing "Airplane Disa," so named for her early work aboard aircraft. She once entertained 120 passengers on an Icelandair Boeing 757 while at an altitude of 30,000 feet. Talk about having a captive audience!

Strutter became Peggy's mentor and a very important friend. The year after attending the Clown Camp, she attended Laugh Makers and learned a great deal from Bob Gibbons.

Peggy decided that because of her own frequent hospitalizations, her work would be on a volunteer basis. Interestingly, volunteerism as such does not exist in Iceland, and Peggy found the medical staff very cautious about allowing her to begin her clowning program. She wrote a proposal outlining what she wanted to do that was accepted by both of the hospitals in Reykjavík, and she is now considered to be an integral part of the medical teams at both places. Because initially Peggy wanted to keep her identity a secret, and because she speaks Icelandic with a decidedly American Southern accent, she decided that Disa must be mute. In 1992, Peggy developed a second character, Dr. Oliver, who works mainly with children with cancer and teenage patients. He also is silent except, like Disa, when he is in the room of a patient and the door is closed. This is the magic the child possesses—making the clowns talk.

Both of Peggy's clown characters are very "soft" both in their make-up and in their actions. It is important to Peggy that no child be frightened by the clowns' antics. Because Peggy is petite, her characters are not overwhelming. Disa is a typical lady white-face clown, with an unruly mop of blond hair and a soft red hat. She is dressed in an oversized blue blouse with white sleeves and a full blue skirt with a red bow at her neck, red cummerbund at her waist, and red gloves. Completing her outfit are red tights, neat white lace-trimmed socks, and black patent leather Mary Jane shoes. Dr. Oliver is more European-styled, with a polka-dot shirt, large red spotted bowtie, baggy plaid pants held up by red suspenders, and oversized "medical instruments" including a humorous giant searchlight on "his" headband.

Disa entertains large groups in the hospital once or twice a week. Her program is 20 minutes in length and her routines contain some delightful magic. Parents enjoy the shows as much as the children do. Before her performance, she goes into the children's rooms to spark their interest. After the show, she interacts with each child individually. She then visits the children in the intensive care unit and those in isolation. Disa is a real charmer and is known to be a little flirtatious. Peggy says that Disa has Siggi wrapped around her little finger. When Peggy decides that Disa needs a new outfit, she always has Disa herself do the asking! Oliver is a little more mischievous and loves to make people laugh. He has a large medical bag complete with all the equipment needed to do a thorough "medical examination" which he performs on members of the medical staff, the patient's parents, and the patient, if the child gives permission. Teenagers especially like the medical examination. Peggy often entertains patients in her home when their condition permits such visits. She has also been known to give wonderful birthday parties, complete with generous gifts, to individual patients. Both of the Helgasons enjoy shopping for the perfect gift for the children, and they are amazingly good at this endeavor.

Peggy routinely updates her acts and keeps her characters in top form for performing. She has studied with some of the best clowns in the business. All of this hard work is evident in her class acts. Siggi is very supportive of Peggy's continuing training. In the early stages of her planning to become a clown, he insisted that, if she embarked on this profession, she should become the best clown possible. Over the years, Peggy has learned that Icelanders tend to be quite reserved. Keeping this in mind, her characters do not make loud noises or throw water or pies, and she does not make fun of anyone except herself. Dr. Oliver has learned to ride a unicycle and he now juggles and spins plates. A dog who is exceptionally good with terminally ill children has joined the "therapeutic team," and they are very busy doing hospital and home visits. Siggi remains very helpful, but, according to Peggy, he has drawn the line at the unicycle and the slack rope.

An Icelandic friend, Lilja Sigurdardottir, often accompanies Peggy on her hospital visits. She reads the signs that introduce Peggy's acts and participates in many of Peggy's routines. Lilja is in remission from leukemia, and she and Peggy both know what it is like to be sick and how it feels to be a patient in an unfamiliar environment. They can both empathize with the children. During the performances, for a short time, the children can forget about medical procedures, pain, and fear. The children easily relate to Peggy's fantasy characters. They feel sorry for Disa because she cannot speak; they are delighted after the show when, in the privacy of their own rooms, she will talk with them and help them express their fears and hopes.

Peggy's clown characters keep a very low profile. Iceland has only 250,000 inhabitants and it seems as if everyone knows everyone else. Peggy shuns publicity for the clowns because she feels strongly that the clowns belong to the hospitalized children and not to the public. For a very long while Peggy was successful in keeping her identity a secret, but she is now comfortable with having her identity known, especially since she has received recognition and numerous awards over the past 8 years for her work. Siggi is now President of Icelandair, which has sponsored trips abroad for dying children and their families and has granted over 40 "Make-a-Wish" wishes for them as well.

Each year Peggy performs at the Christmas party given for seriously ill children by the President of Iceland. This party takes place at the Bessastadir, the Icelandic White House. For 3 years, Peggy has volunteered in the United States at camps for children who have cancer and chronic illnesses. She performs for the children and teaches them some clowning and magic tricks. She has been known to become actively involved in the physical care of the children and also has prepared Icelandic specialty treats for the campers. In

1993, Peggy received the Partnership Award, given for her work with children, from a former American Ambassador to Iceland. In 1996, the National Hospital in Iceland recognized her for her work as Dr. Oliver, and the same year she was also cited by the Children's Cancer Society of Iceland. She has lectured for the Scandinavian Oncology Nurses about the therapeutic value of humor with children with cancer.

Peggy becomes very close to the children and their parents. Many times children talk with Peggy/Disa/Dr. Oliver about things they cannot discuss with their parents or the staff. Peggy thinks that this happens because her characters are not "real" and therefore are safer for the children to confide in. Her professional education as an occupational therapist with a background in psychology is an important factor in her ability to encourage the children to talk and to respond to them therapeutically, as is her empathy and understanding because of her own frequent bouts with illness. Peggy readily admits that the most difficult thing for her to deal with is the death of a child. She realizes, however, that losses in life are inevitable and she finds comfort knowing that she made a difference in that child's life.

Clowning has helped Peggy deal with her own illness, which periodically relapses, requiring regular hospital stays. She believes that the children give more to her than she could ever give to them. "In them I see courage and the determination to go on. Children are so sensitive to the life around them, and they are so trusting in God. From my clowning with children, I have learned to accept today for what it is and to be happy for each moment that I have." Peggy's deep faith in God helps her deal with death. She believes that loss can sometimes help people grow and become stronger. "By having this faith, I can enjoy life to its fullest, especially by clowning with the hospitalized children and making them laugh in the midst of their pain. I pray that God will allow me to continue this work." Peggy's work is indeed a labor of love that touches deeply those who need it most—the young recipients, their families, and the dedicated healer herself.

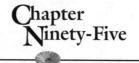

The Power of Joy

Judith E. Bowen, MPA, OTR

The old man rolled over. It was time to start the day, his early rising driven by habits of years gone by. His legs moved slowly, rigidly toward the edge of the bed and then over. He did not want to disturb his still sleeping wife. Pushing himself up to a sit, arms moving stiffly, he found his balance, then moved bent toes into familiar slippers. He sat for a moment, getting ready for the effort. Slowly he began to rock, first a little, then a bit harder, and finally up. The momentum helped him begin to move, shuffling, then a bit steadier. First to the bathroom and then into the kitchen.

His morning ritual of making the coffee began. While the coffee perked, he counted out his pills, being careful to make sure the right number were there. In the effort and concentration of fixing and bending and counting, he felt the drooling begin, arms moving too slow to bother to wipe it away.

When the coffee was done he carefully poured it into his mug, added some sugar and milk, and stirred. It took a long time, moving in slow motion. He made his way to the table with his cup, bent over, in the rhythm that allowed forward movement with no spills. Carefully moving around the corner of the table, he set his cup down and lowered himself into the chair. It was time to rest now and sip his coffee. He tried to ignore the familiar pain that seemed everywhere.

The first few sips went down easily. But then the liquid was suddenly stopped and went back up through his nose, dribbling out and down his chin. He reached for a napkin and dabbed. The stubble of beard did not hide the expression of disgust and misery.

His wife appeared from the bedroom, trying to wake up. She was slow at that in the morning. She went into the kitchen, poured herself a cup of coffee, black, and joined him at the table.

"I feel dead," he said.

She knew this mood and tried to struggle out of her fog to meet it.

"What would you like for breakfast?"

"Nothing. I can't eat."

"How about some prunes?"

"No, I can't eat."

She got up and went into the kitchen and busied herself getting the dark purée out of the refrigerator. She always had some made up, knowing he liked the sweetness. For later, she thought. Then, she stepped outside the apartment door and picked up the morning paper.

"Do you want the sports page?" she asked.

"I feel like my body is dead. I can't do anything."

"Did you take your pills?" she asked.

"Yeah."

"They should help in a little bit. Here's the paper."

He slowly opened the paper and spread it out on the table. The tap, tap, tap of his hand on the table began as a tremor moved through his arm. It did not seem to interfere. It went on for a while and then stopped.

Looking up from the paper he said, "The Phillies play this afternoon. A double header. They won yesterday."

"They do? What channel?"

"Three," he said. "They have a chance at the playoffs."

She saw the energy. "How about trying some prunes now?"

"Okay," he said, and she brought the dish to him.

He ate. It took him a long time, perhaps half an hour, but the purée did not come back through his nose. The concentration it took to coordinate breathing and chewing and swallowing, body bent forward so as to shorten the distance the rigid muscles had to travel to move the spoon from dish to mouth, left him exhausted.

"How about watching Perry Mason? It'll be on soon."

"Okay."

In slow motion, using the table edge to pull up on, he began to get up and out of the chair. Finding his balance, he started the bent over shuffle to the chair and the slow descent into it. He picked up the remote and turned on the TV and she knew he would soon be asleep and would not wake until noon. Soon after that, the game would start, and then it would be a better day, especially if the Phillies won.

This man was my father. The woman is my mother. He had Parkinson's disease. It is hard to remember where lines of myself as daughter or occupational therapist were drawn. Most of the time the roles seemed to blend as our family moved through time together. Perhaps I was therapist when I suggested that rocking might help him rise from the bed or chair. Perhaps I was therapist when I suggested that an electric razor might be easier to manage than a safety razor. Or when I designed a special holder for his spoon and for his mug handle so that his tapping, tremulous hands could hold them firmly. Often I was reminded that I was a daughter and my suggestions were ignored, but sometimes the therapist was heard.

The father of my childhood was a tall, vigorous, athletic man. Like many others during the Depression, he was forced to leave school early to find work. Most of his adult life was spent working for the Bethlehem Steel Company in southeastern Pennsylvania. His work was hard, outdoors, and physical. He worked swing shift, rotating from days to middle shift to nights, in a predictable pattern. He seemed to find no joy in his work and rarely talked about what he did when at home. It was simply what he had to do to support his family. He worked there from his teens until he was 58, when he announced he was retiring because he was afraid that his slowed reflexes might cause an accident that would harm someone else.

I was proud of my handsome, gregarious dad. He had a creative mind and took great pleasure in his skill with tools. He rebuilt the kitchen in our small house and built much of the furniture for our home. His basement workshop was immaculate with each tool in its proper place. A favorite pastime was sketching his baseball heroes.

The last time I saw my father, Christmas of 1994, he was very frail and so very tired. In his prime, he weighed 200 pounds. At the time of that visit, he weighed 132 pounds. When I hugged him he felt bony and fragile. We who had lived our lives with him understood his speech, but others often did not. It took him at least an hour to eat even small amounts of food because of his difficulty with chewing and swallowing. Severe degenerative joint disease, causing deterioration of the spine, left him bent forward at a 45-degree angle, and he could no longer look people in the face when standing.

During that Christmas visit, I sat with him for many hours. We talked sometimes and sometimes just watched TV. He asked me if he had been a good father, and I told him that he had indeed been a very good one. I also told him my sister and I would take care of my mother. I felt like the therapist again when I encouraged his process of life review to help him understand and organize his life experiences in preparation for the impending end of his life. But in the end, it was the daughter that gained the understanding.

We watched sports. The NFL playoffs were in progress. We talked about the teams and about the Major League Baseball strike that had prevented a World Series that fall. He remembered amazing details about the teams and stayed very current, even when he had trouble remembering what he had for breakfast that morning.

During one such conversation, he looked directly at me and suddenly said, with passion and energy and sudden fire in his dark eyes, "I live for sports! I mean it."

I was startled by that sudden and powerful rush of life force from this frail man who seemed so very tired. The intensity of the statement came from somewhere deep inside of him and was meant for me. The power of his energy stayed with me. It drew me. I needed to know what his meaning might have been in the context of my search, as an occupational therapist, for meaning-making in the lives of those whom I treat. I did not fully understand then, but in searching I have found his gift to me.

I had known about the Depression and its toll on both my parents' lives. Both had come from large families. My father was the oldest of 11, the son of Austrian immigrants. He had told me that as a child his lunches were often nothing more than lard sandwiches. I later learned that sometimes when he came home from school he was so hungry that he went into the pigeon coop kept by his father, took the pigeon eggs, cracked them, and ate them raw.

His father, my grandfather, had been a hardworking, undemonstrative, and unaffectionate man who was unable to give any emotional support to his oldest son. He was most likely overwhelmed himself at having to take care of such a large family in such hard times.

I also was aware of my father's natural athletic ability. As a young man he played city league basketball and soccer. He was a strong swimmer and competed successfully in local meets. He played baseball well enough to be signed by the old Washington Senators to play on their Class A farm team in the Maryland shore league.

Sometime during the year after my father's death my mother told me something I had not known. She said that as a young teen he had become involved in the local YMCA. He had once told her that the "Y" became his home and the people who ran it became his family. It was there that he found nourishment for his spirit and affirmation of his life. It was through this organization that he became involved in sports and because of his natural ability became successful on a local level.

And then I understood. It was in these activities that he had found his identity, his value, and his joy. It was his continuing connection with this thread of sports that saw him through the many bad times in his life. It was the part of his life that gave him pleasure and joy and accomplishment.

Chapter Ninety-Five

When he could no longer participate, it was the imagery allowed by radio and then television that allowed him to still "live" in that world of sports.

Suddenly I was flooded with memories of the shape and form of our relatedness. It never involved his "work." It always involved his joy. The time he took to teach me how to swim. His patience in trying to teach me how to swing a bat. His playing first base at church picnics. There were other shared joys. Standing by his elbow in the basement as he replaced our shoe heels on his shoemaker's last or as he began building a new piece of furniture. Watching him sketch his favorite baseball heroes.

His work was what he had to do to support his family. But his life fire came from his joy in his own creativity, in the playing of sports, and in the creative process of working with his hands.

I reflect on this understanding, this gift, within the context of the world in which I work as an occupational therapist. There is no longer a Depression, but we still have starving children and young people living in poverty. We have an abundance of self-help books but we still have young people who live without hope and without a nurturing family. We still have people who find little meaning beyond the wages in low-paying, uninteresting, and unsatisfying work, jobs they must hold to support their families. In looking at the life-saving impact a community program had for my father, based on organized sports, I see opportunity and possibility for my profession of occupational therapy. In looking at the life-saving impact that caring adults had, most unknowingly, on a young boy impoverished in spirit and soul, I reflect on where our involvement as health "care" professionals might lead us. In looking at the power of imagery to sustain a life identity in a deteriorating body, I understand the power, richness, and resource inherent in the miracle of mind/body/spirit. I now understand more about the need for people to have creativity, beauty, and pleasure in their lives and the role that art, music, literature, and sports play in making us human. My father's gift to me is the awareness that his life meaning was not within his work, but within his joy.

Chapter Ninety-Six

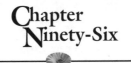

Back to Life, Work, and Happiness

Anitta Boyko Fox, BS, MA, OTR

My dining room is home to a beautiful painting of a young woman in a royal blue velvet gown with heavy cream-colored lace at the shoulders. She is fanning herself with a light blue ostrich fan that she holds in her right hand. The background canvas is delicately textured in pastel colors. But the pleats and folds in the long skirt are outlined with only a few rough brush strokes in sharp contrast to the smooth and carefully detailed technique of the rest of the painting.

The canvas reminds me of a still life into which my father carefully placed me. I can still hear his voice of so long ago "This is the way I see the world—young and promising. For I am yesterday, but you are my tomorrow."

My father was a very successful professional portrait artist in his native Europe and later in his adopted country, America. Our family had managed to survive Hitler's Nazi regime for several years. Then we were fortunate enough to get out of Vienna, Austria, to start a new life in America in March 1939. Unfortunately, despite his 1939 escape from the outside peril of the Nazis, a few short years later my father could not escape a slower but insidiously more destructive inside force—a vicious cancer that ultimately attacked every part of his body.

Chapter Ninety-Six

By 1951, at the age of 57, he was clearly dying from the disease. In September 1951, several weeks after he had put the finishing touches on his last customer's portrait, it was obvious that he could no longer travel every day to his studio in Carnegie Hall, even with my mother's help. Nor could he accept any more portrait order commissions. He was too weak and in too much pain. Even worse, he was bored, discouraged, almost defeated, and resigned to waiting for the inevitable, his death.

As his daughter, I found his noticeable, almost daily, decline nearly impossible to watch and even harder to accept. I cried for the artist he had been and for his anguish at losing his beloved vocation. I remembered him at his young and energetic best, when he and I spent hours together, he painting the walls of my room with colorful birds, butterflies, grasshoppers, dragonflies, and ladybugs, while I contributed little brush strokes along the bottom with my childish hands to indicate the grass. How could I help him now? My adult love alone clearly was not enough.

Suddenly I had the perfect idea. I remembered how many times my father had told me how eager he was to paint my portrait, but both of us had always been too busy to devote the time that such a major project required. My education as an occupational therapist gave me the wisdom to ask him, "Do you still want to paint me?" His eyes lit up. "Do I want to paint you? Of course I do! You know it's the one thing in life I have always wanted to do, but we never before could take the time for it." Then he became thoughtful. "So everything in life is good for something," he mused, "perhaps even having cancer."

Full of anticipation, we planned our project. We both knew that the time left to him was limited. We had to get started right away, while he was still able to paint. I hoped that it was not already too late. "Not a portrait," I said, knowing how exacting and demanding painting a portrait was for him even under the best of circumstances. "Paint only a still life, something that you will really enjoy painting, with me in it just incidentally," I suggested, trying to ease the task for him. Thankfully, he agreed.

At once I took a leave of absence from my occupational therapy private practice. I explained to my regular patients about my need to spend this time with my father and arranged for a substitute therapist. I was about to begin an even more private practice, providing occupational therapy for my most beloved patient as my last gift to him and to myself. My other patients and their families understood my father's need and my task. They all promised to continue with their respective occupational therapy activity programs and planned to surprise me with their progress. They all wanted to help me accomplish my labor of love.

So we began. Every day my mother helped as my father struggled to get dressed and get himself out of the house. Every day, I drove my father to his

Carnegie Hall studio and helped him struggle to get inside. Every day, the journey from the car, through the revolving doors, in and out of the elevator, and down the hall to his studio was so difficult for him that he immediately collapsed into his chair, completely exhausted. But we both knew there was purpose in the struggle. We had a goal to reach that went far beyond his painful present reality.

In the beginning, he was still able to squeeze the right amount of color from each tube of oil paint onto the artist's palette in the precise order characteristic of a professional artist. He could still stand erect, holding the palette in his left hand and the brushes in his right hand as usual. He could work for an hour or more. Then he rested. Then he worked and he rested again. Over and over, the pattern was repeated.

We talked about many things during the rest periods, which became longer and longer as the work periods became more difficult for him and therefore shorter and shorter. We happily reminisced about his childhood and mine and his years with my mother before I was born. We talked about life in Vienna, the Nazi horrors, our life in the United States, and my plans for the future. We talked about his hopes and dreams for his family's life after his own death.

So the days and weeks passed. After a while, when he could no longer hold it, I adapted a music stand to serve as support for his palette. When his fingers became too weak for their task, I began to squeeze the colors onto the palette under his direction. Then I made elastic bands to tie to his belt and loop around his right thumb, which helped to control his ever-increasing hand tremor. He marveled at my ingenuity and my occupational therapy "know-how" that helped him happily and successfully to continue with his determined quest. Eventually I made him a long, thin, wand-like stick to support the weight of his right arm holding the brush. I fashioned a special headband to absorb the pearls of perspiration which would otherwise have clouded his eyes. That is the way it went. He painted; I adapted his world to make his painting possible.

Three months went by, months that were intensely arduous, yet months that passed too swiftly. They had been the most difficult but most meaningful 3 months of our lives together. He knew he wouldn't be able to complete the entire painting with the same fine detail of the early weeks. Ever the professional painter, he knew exactly what he had to do to finish his work. He asked me to help him prepare his brushes for their final task. I did as he directed.

One day he wanted to talk about my choice of profession, occupational therapy.

"I am so happy that you studied it. It's a perfect profession for you. It combines all your interests, and it suits your personality. I can see that you love working with people and with other medical professionals. Only, why is it called 'occupational therapy'? It should be called 'back to life, work, and happiness therapy,' because that's what you do." We laughed together. Yet at that very moment we both realized that it was he who had guided me toward my profession, toward life, work, and happiness. Then we tried to embrace. His tremor made it almost impossible.

He insisted on getting up and continuing to work. "You must never give up," he struggled to whisper. Then I helped him out of the chair, steadied his hand on the wand with the elastic band looped around his thumb, and adjusted his headband. I positioned myself in my pose on the podium for the last time for the last few strokes of his brush which we had trimmed and shaped so carefully for this purpose. Laboriously and with obvious love, he applied a few of the finishing brush strokes to the pleats and folds in the long skirt of his "masterpiece." A minute later, he fell back onto his chair for the last time and all I could do was kiss his hands that could no longer hold the brush to finish painting the blue velvet skirt. Trying to hold back my tears, I held him and whispered, "Thank you for the painting. It is so beautiful and through it you will always be with me. No one will ever know it is not quite finished. It's our secret—yours and mine."

Looking at the painting now, I can still hear his voice which by then had dwindled to a mere whisper, "I'm glad you will have this painting to help you remember that this is the way I see the world—young and promising. For I am yesterday and you are my tomorrow."

Epilogue

J ust as there is no one way or right way to read this book, there is no one way or right way to finish it. Some readers may want to know more about occupational therapy or how to contact an occupational therapist. The best source of information is the American Occupational Therapy Association, Inc. Contact the association at 4720 Montgomery Lane, Bethesda, MD, 20814-3425, 301-652-AOTA, or visit online at www.aota.org.

If any reader thinks that he or she may want to consider a career as an occupational therapist, he or she can locate colleges and universities that have occupational therapy educational programs and learn how to contact them through the American Occupational Therapy Association, Inc., as listed above.

For myself, compiling this book has been an exhilarating and rewarding experience. In person, by telephone, by mail, and via e-mail, I met so many wonderful colleagues and a group of very special people who generously shared their ordinary miracles with me. Their messages of hope and their stories about the large and small miracles of their lives reinforced my faith in the ability of people to deal constructively with adversity.

To express my appreciation, and hopefully to help bring about many more ordinary miracles, a portion of the royalties from the book will be donated to the following funds.

Epilogue

The Frieda Behlen Scholarship Fund of the Department of Occupational Therapy at New York University. Perpetuating the memory and lifelong activities of a remarkable educator and founding Department Chair, the Fund provides scholarships for occupational therapy students to complete their education at New York University. For information about the fund or to make a contribution, contact occupationaltherapy@nyu.edu or visit online at www.nyu.edu/education/ot/alumni.htm

The AMBUCS Investing in the Future Campaign. A national organization with local chapters all over America, AMBUCS "is dedicated to creating independence and opportunities for people with disabilities." It distributes rehabilitation equipment to individuals on a person-to-person basis through its membership chapters, provides scholarships for future therapists, and maintains a Resource Center in High Point, North Carolina. It can be reached at P.O. Box 5127, High Point, NC 27262, 336-869-2166, or online at www.ambucs.com.

Collecting these stories and compiling this book has had a profoundly positive effect on me; I sincerely hope that some or all of these stories will touch you in the same way, and that you, too, will come away with renewed optimism about the ability of ordinary people to overcome obstacles and survive catastrophes.

ACKNOWLEDGMENTS

Producing a book of this kind requires the help of countless people whose valuable input I gratefully acknowledge. Foremost are the contributing authors and the individuals whose stories have been told. They have generously shared their life experiences with me and with you, the reader. I thank these authors for making this book possible. Through them, I also thank the people whose stories these are. Without you all, obviously there could have been no such book. I also thank the hundreds of others who submitted stories that, for reasons of space, could not be included here. Every story was about a person whose life was touched by the important experience of coping with adversity, and all those stories were gratifying to read. I hope that those who could not be included here will still have the satisfaction of knowing that they dealt with tough situations in their own lives and that they were a part of the meaningful work that occupational therapists do on a daily basis.

I also owe a huge debt to those who worked behind the scenes to help with the various production tasks associated with putting together such an ambitious project. The dedicated group of early reviewers—colleagues, family, friends, and volunteers—who read and rated the hundreds of stories initially submitted deserve credit for their generous contribution of time and energy and their perseverance as batch after batch of stories flooded their mailboxes. Thank you to Susan Bachner, Leah Gittel Labovitz, Kathryn Labovitz, Joan Lyons, Harry Wolovitz, and Pearl Haber for their always insightful comments and their faithful adherence to deadlines. I thank Ellen Greer and Christine Peters in addition for their help with cataloging, reproducing, and distributing the stories as well as reading and critically reviewing them, and Phyllis Ginsberg for her insightful reviews of stories and for her ongoing administrative work distributing and tracking materials and helping to keep me and the entire project organized.

For their invaluable help in the later stages of production, I gratefully thank Gregg Geller and Bethany Walls, whose editorial assistance greatly enhanced my ability to complete the editing of several of the stories. I also thank my student assistant, Jessica Cline, for her always-cheerful keyboarding of my edits of the stories as well as her help with many other aspects of the project.

My colleagues in the occupational therapy profession have been incredibly enthusiastic about this book and have generously supported my work on it. My initial "Calls for Stories" were published as a professional courtesy in *Advance for Occupational Therapists*, for which I thank Merion Publications, Inc., and in the various publications of the American Occupational Therapy Association, Inc., to which I owe special thanks for its unwavering support of

Acknowledgments

this endeavor. Because this book has been years in the making, I am grateful to several presidents of the association: Mary Evert, in whose term this began with her endorsement of my initial idea, and Mary Foto, Karen Jacobs, and the current President Barbara Kornblau, for their continuing encouragement over this time. I thank association executive directors Jeanette Bair, who helped me initiate the book, and Joe Isaacs, current executive director, who has made resources available to help me with some administrative aspects. I also thank and acknowledge the pivotal encouragement and help provided at the outset by Maureen Muncaster, formerly acquisitions editor for the AOTA. Her belief in the necessity for this book and the eventual market niche for it were critical in shaping the book as it is now. Her referral of my work to Peter Porosky, editorial consultant, was also instrumental in the development and organization of my ideas into a product attractive to publishers, and I thank him for the time he devoted to critiquing my work and referring me to appropriate contacts.

SLACK Incorporated, my publisher, and the individuals I have worked with during the publication process have made this one of the most pleasurable professional experiences I have ever had. I will be forever appreciative of the confidence in me and in this book that their publishing it has shown. I am particularly grateful to John Bond, vice president of book publishing, for his initial enthusiasm about my proposal and his willingness to persuade SLACK Incorporated to undertake a book that is somewhat different from the usual books it publishes. I have very much enjoyed working with him; with Amy Drummond McShane, editorial director; Debra Toulson, managing editor; Jennifer Stewart, managing editor; Lauren Plummer, design editor; and April Johnson, project editor. Their constant availability and helpful suggestions have helped me clarify my ideas and refine this material in ways that have been extremely valuable, and I thank you all. In addition, the many behind-the-scenes people at SLACK Incorporated, such as Michelle Gatt, marketing manager, and others whose names I do not know, have helped in countless ways, large and small, and I thank you all as well.

I thank my colleagues in the Department of Occupational Therapy at New York University, the administration, faculty, and students, who have been supportive of my work on this book and who have taught me a great deal about the power of occupational therapy to work miracles in people's lives. I also thank my colleagues in the occupational therapy professional community, the members and officers of the statewide New York State Occupational Therapy Association, and its local affiliate, the Metropolitan New York District of NYSOTA, for the many opportunities they have given me to solicit stories and to publicize this book and for the response of the members in submitting stories.

Acknowledgments

Finally, I acknowledge and thank my family for the unwavering love, encouragement, and support that has made my life so rich and has enabled me to accomplish so many professional achievements like this book. My parents, the late Samuel Rubin and Clara Rubin Levy, were always proud of me and gave me confidence in myself, as well as being wonderful role models. My mother-in-law, Leah Gittel Labovitz, has encouraged me for the past 40 years to achieve professionally as well as to establish a home and regularly feed her son and her grandchildren; after participating in this project at the age of 90 by reviewing stories, she is now, at age 95, waiting excitedly to actually hold the printed book in her hands. I have always appreciated this vote of confidence from a woman whose continuing active long life has reinforced my belief in the values of occupational therapy. To my children, Gail, Bruce, and Daniel, and to the in-law spouses whom they have brought into our family, William Seligman, Katie Labovitz, and Natasha Labovitz, I acknowledge and value your love and your support of my professional activities over the years. Katie and Daniel, thank you for your review and editorial activities, and I appreciate your tolerance for the endless discussions we have had about the progress of this book and the helpful advice you all have given me. To my grandchildren, Hannah and Joel Seligman; Jennifer, Jacob, and Sarah Labovitz; and Samuel Labovitz, thank you for keeping me aware of what is truly important in my life, and, to those of you able to read and to appreciate the importance of books, for being impressed that your grandmother is writing one. Finally, to my husband, Judah Labovitz, my partner in life and in all other activities, who after all these years with me can define occupational therapy as easily as I can, thank you for tolerating my late night work on this project and bringing me coffee when I toiled well beyond midnight, for using your proofreading and editorial talents on these stories, and for loving and supporting me in everything I do. None of this would have been possible without you.

Deborah R. Labovitz, PhD, OTR/L, FAOTA
New York, New York
March 2002

About the Editor

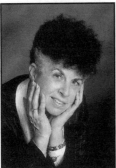

Deborah R. Labovitz, PhD, OTR/L, FAOTA, an occupational therapist for 40 years and chair of the department of occupational therapy in the Steinhart School of Education at New York University, New York, New York from 1980 to 2000, is currently a professor at NYU and an avid collector of stories about people who have had the kind of miraculous experiences found in this book. She earned her undergraduate degree in occupational therapy and her master's degree and doctorate in sociology from the University of Pennsylvania and is a fellow of the American Occupational Therapy Association.

As a daughter, wife, daughter-in-law, mother of three, mother-in-law of three, and grandmother of six, she has seen ordinary miracles of coping and courage in both her professional and personal life. She continues to be amazed, energized, and awed by the achievements of the ordinary people in this book who have accomplished so much and by the occupational therapists who have helped them to do so. At this time in our society, when hope and optimism are so necessary, she hopes that this book of triumphs over adversity will provide you with both.

ABOUT THE CONTRIBUTORS

Bobbie Andrews is a resident of an assisted living facility in Massachusetts. She enjoyed writing her story, and she and her husband are pleased that it has been included in this book.

Elizabeth A. Haluska Ankney, OTR/L, PC, is a rehabilitation director and occupational therapist with a concentration in dysphagia and feeding disorders. She is now challenged daily with worsening multiple sclerosis, from complications of which her sister died and with which her eldest son has recently been diagnosed. Liz tackles her busy life with the help of her very supportive husband, Mark. Between them they have four children and three grandchildren. Liz enjoys archery and writing informational articles and true life stories.

Susan Bachner, MA, OTR/L, FAOTA, CEAC, is an occupational therapist with over 38 years of clinical and consultation experiences. She received her master's degree in sociology/anthropology in 1970 and this area of study has been a major influence on her practice perspective. The American Occupational Therapy Association recognized Susan for "clinical excellence" and honored her with membership on the Roster of Fellows. In 1999, she completed all requirements for certification in environmental access consulting.

Mary LeChene Bennett, OTR/L, Retired, is a 1984 graduate of the State University of New York (SUNY) at Buffalo's occupational therapy program. She is certified in sensory integration therapy and had a private pediatric practice for 9 years in western Pennsylvania before retiring from occupational therapy practice to have a family. Currently, she helps her self-employed husband, is very involved in homeschooling their three sons, and is active in the life of her church. She is very grateful to God for the lessons she learned from Christopher and remains in touch from time to time with his mother.

Toby Black, MA, OTR/L, graduated from Washington University, St. Louis, Mo, in 1971. She moved with her husband to Bowling Green, KY, in 1976 and established her pediatric occupational therapy practice while raising their two children. She initiated several support groups. She is a cofounder of a transdisciplinary team offering evaluations and consultation services. She is a 10-year miracle survivor of breast cancer. She enjoys writing and traveling.

About the Contributors

Michelle Anne Blackburn, OTR/L, has worked as an occupational therapist for 18 years since graduating from Utica College of Syracuse University, Utica, NY, in 1985. Her primary area of practice and interest is the geriatric and neurologically challenged patient. Michelle resides in Granby, CT, with her 9-year-old son. She works for Genesis Eldercare Rehabilitation Services and stays diversified through contracts with Sub-Acute and intensive rehabilitation programs in Hartford County.

Judith E. Bowen, MPA, OTR, has been nourished and taught by all of those she treated throughout her 25 years of clinical practice and by all of the students in her 10 years in academia. She has given numerous workshops, has been published, and practices healing touch. She and her husband enjoy their children and grandchildren and make their home in deep south Texas.

Ann Burkhardt, MA, OTR/L, BCN, FAOTA, is an occupational therapist who "wears many hats"—board certified in neurorehabilitation, an administrator at a large university-based medical center in New York City, a faculty member at two metropolitan area colleges and universities, a researcher, and a director of the AOTA. Ann also sings, kayaks, paints, dances, travels, writes, and is a doctoral student.

Lt. Col. Len Cancio, MPH, OTR/L, has been both an active and a reserve Army occupational therapist for 23 years. Len is chief of occupational therapy at a large Army medical center in Hawaii. He is married and enjoys being a soccer dad.

Paula D. Carey, MS, OTR/L, is the occupational therapy program director at Utica College, Utica, NY, and has been in occupational therapy in a variety of roles for more than 20 years. She continues to be affirmed by the resiliency and power of the human spirit in her work with occupational therapy clients and students. Paula values being a wife, mother, grandmother, and daughter and receives strength and support from these relationships.

Ron Carson, MHS, OTR/L, graduated from the Medical University of South Carolina, Charleston, SC, in 1997. Since graduating, he has worked in acute care rehabilitation, community-based mental health, and private practice. Currently, he is an assistant professor at the University of St. Augustine, St. Augustine, FL. He is also the founder of the internet web site and list serve, OTnow, which can be found at www.OTnow.com.

Julie Chelte, OTR/L, completed her BS degree in occupational therapy at the University of Minnesota, Minneapolis, MN. She practices in the area of

physical disabilities with special interest in spinal cord injury and stroke rehabilitation. She has worked as an occupational therapist in Las Vegas, NV, and
San Antonio, TX. She is currently the occupational therapy department
supervisor at HealthSouth Rehabilitation Hospital in Henderson, NV. Julie
enjoys hiking, reading, music, creative writing, and traveling.

Ronda Christopher, OTR/L, MEd, LNHA, while she loves working with
children and still volunteers with local children's groups, has found a career
in long-term care as a regional manager. She continues to advocate for the
use of woodworking, pottery, ceramics, and other occupations for her current
clients as a way to promote higher quality of life for the elderly. She resides
in West Chester, OH, with her husband and daughter and often reflects on
the profound influence that summer fieldwork experience had on her.

Laura Faye Clubok, OTR/L, has a private occupational therapy practice, "On
the Other Hand Therapy," located in Columbus, OH. She works with a variety
of children's issues, including Down syndrome, autism, sensory processing, handwriting, and hand anomalies. She also gives workshops and is a certified weight
trainer. Laura thanks her amazingly supportive husband and her network of dedicated family and friends for helping her to fulfill her life's calling.

Josephine Cohen, MA, OTR/L, has had an extensive career as a clinician
and educator teaching at Columbia University, New York, NY; University of
Pennsylvania, Philadelphia, PA; and Elizabethtown College, Elizabethtown,
PA, where she was chair of the department of occupational therapy. Her area
of expertise is hand therapy and her master's degree in human relations
enabled her to have a second career in development and alumni affairs. She
enjoys traveling, Jewish archival work, and contributing to this book.

Vera Cohen, BS, OTR/L, has been an occupational therapist treating the
geriatric population for 19 years. A recipient of the Novacare Corporation
Chairman's Award, she is presently pursuing a master's of science degree in
occupational therapy (with a specialization in gerontology) and is employed at
Willow Ridge Subacute Center, Genesis Elder Care Corporation in Hatboro,
PA.

Donna Conley, OTR/L, graduated from the University of Florida,
Gainesville, in 1973. She retired in September of 2001 after a 27-year career
working for the Veterans Administration, primarily in mental health. Donna
is currently enjoying her long-neglected passions of quilting, gardening, and
traveling, as well as her own "ordinary miracle," having recently married for
the first time at age 52.

About the Contributors

Beth Cooper, OTR, graduated from the University of Alabama at Birmingham's occupational therapy program in 1988. She has worked primarily in acute care and rehabilitation with neurologically involved clients and is NDT certified. Beth resides in Virginia with her husband and two sons, ages 6 and 8. Currently, she is enjoying using all of her therapy skills and God-given gifts in her most challenging position yet, homeschooling mom.

Lisa E. Cyzner, PhD, OTR/L, received her doctoral degree in occupational therapy from New York University, New York, NY. She is the owner of Carolina Pediatric Therapeutic Resources, a private practice dedicated to providing services for infants, toddlers, children, adolescents, and their families. Lisa resides in Charlotte, NC, with her husband, Ronnie, and their son, Benjamin.

Peggy Dawson, OTR/L, is an occupational therapist who works in the area of adult mental health. She has four great children and an extraordinary husband. Peggy loves being an occupational therapist, and in her spare time makes handmade paper and does creative design work for local schools.

Mary V. Donohue, PhD, OT, FAOTA, is currently a clinical associate professor at New York University in the department of occupational therapy. She is Coeditor of the journal Occupational Therapy in Mental Health and cochair of the Metropolitan New York District/NYSOTA OT Research Committee. She developed the Group Level of Function Profile, a research instrument that is used to study group interaction in hospitals, preschools, and senior centers.

Brett T. Duffey, OTR/L, is a true Tarheel, born and bred, who loves the outdoors, sports, fitness, and the Marine Corps. He has been able to use his personal experience to work in a variety of settings and is currently doing home healthcare occupational therapy in the Winston-Salem/Forsyth County, NC, area as well as in all adjacent counties. He has a 3-year-old son and is currently involved in a very loving relationship. He is grateful for the path his misfortune has led him and enjoys using this experience to influence others in their recovery.

Kimberly Eberhardt, MS, OTR/L, is an occupational therapist at the Rehabilitation Institute of Chicago. She is a member of the adjunct faculty at the University of Illinois-Chicago, IL, where her emphasis is on technology and the environment and spinal cord injury. In addition to her teaching and research interests related to home modifications and assistive technology, she is an active board member of the Illinois chapter of the National Spinal Cord Injury Association.

About the Contributors

Joshua M. Eisenstein, MA, BS, was born in 1975 in Livingston, NJ. He completed his master's degree in 1998 at New York University and is pursuing a PhD in educational psychology at Temple University, Philadelphia, Pa, researching cross-national attitudes toward corporal punishment of children. As well as being a researcher, he is a poet and songwriter. He currently resides in the suburbs of Philadelphia.

Wendy Elliman is a free lance science writer. Born in Britain, she has lived in Israel since 1974 and has contributed a monthly medical article to Hadassah Magazine since 1979. Her greater claim to fame, however, is as mother to identical 11-year-old triplet daughters.

Rhona Feldt-Stein, BSc OT, OT Reg (Ont), is an occupational therapist, owner, and CEO of York Pediatric Therapy Services Inc, Richmond Hill, Ontario, Canada. She has worked with children for over 25 years and holds a faculty status position at the University of Toronto. She has lectured extensively both in Canada and abroad. Rhona is married with two children and has three cats and a dog whom she has incorporated into her therapy practice.

Patricia H. Findlay, OT, is an occupational therapy graduate of the University of Manitoba, Winniped, Manitoba, Canada, with more than 35 years of experience, primarily spent enjoying the many aspects of geriatric rehabilitation and administration. Now semiretired, Pat has returned to her first love, mental health, where she can explore her recently developed interest in the use of multisensory environments as a treatment modality.

Anitta Boyko Fox, BS, MA, OTR, is a Holocaust survivor. She received her professional occupational therapy education at New York University where she met, studied under, and worked with Dr. Howard A. Rusk and others who became her mentors and friends. She worked at the Veteran's Administration Regional Office in Manhattan and at the Rusk Institute of Physical Medicine and Rehabilitation, New York, NY. She visited homebound patients privately. She is married to a radiologist (now retired), has three grown children, and is president of her local Hadassah chapter.

Anne Gaier, OTR/L, CHT, has been working to create a legacy of hope and functional independence by treating patients in physical disabilities and hand rehabilitation her whole career. She is a graduate of the University of Puget Sound, Tacoma, WA.

About the Contributors

Christine Gaspar, OTR, has been a pediatric occupational therapist for 27 years. She has worked in rehabilitation and school settings. Christine dedicates this story to Merion Elementary School, her family, and friends.

Deborah Goldberg, MA, OTR/L, is a pediatric occupational therapist in private practice. After completing her BA at Barnard College, New York, NY, and MA in occupational therapy at New York University, Deborah worked in a variety of acute, subacute, rehabilitation, and chronic care settings. She is trained in both neurodevelopmental and sensory integration treatment and is certified in SIPT administration. Deborah currently resides in Teaneck, NJ, with her husband and two children.

Jacqueline Goldberg has been enjoying her retirement in South Florida after operating her answering service for 25 years. She keeps busy with surfing the web, doing crossword puzzles, playing scrabble and canasta, and spending time with family and friends.

Judy Grossman, DrPH, OTR, FAOTA, is a health, education, and research consultant. She also has a private practice in couples and family therapy in New York City and Westport, CT. During her career, she has held many academic appointments in occupational therapy, and she continues to be an enthusiastic advocate for the profession.

Peggy Lee Gurock, OTR, was a member of the last graduating class of the certified occupational therapy program at New York Medical College, Valhalla, NY, and the first graduating class at Quinnipiac College, Hamden, CT. Peggy has enjoyed working with children for more than 30 years. Peggy presently works as a school-based occupational therapist with Trinitas Children's Therapy Services in Elizabeth, NJ. She enjoys being a parent and a partner to her husband, Noah, and together they have been writing articles on occupational therapy for a local community newsletter.

Elizabeth (Betsy) J. Healey received her OTR at age 45 from the Medical College of Virginia, Richmond, and launched a career with the Powhatan School System, which she has pursued for the past 15 years. Although engaged in a variety of roles and interests, such as batteau captain, therapeutic riding instructor, carriage driving groom, mountain hiking, rock hounding, investment club, and playing the guitar, most significant in her life are four amazing children, Mary Beth, Jerry, Tim, and Meg.

Judi Hoggatt, MA, OTR, is an occupational therapist in a neonatal intensive care unit at Woman's Hospital in Houston, TX. After receiving her mas-

378

ter's degree in occupational therapy, Judi knew she had found her calling working with preemies, infants, and young children. Judi also enjoys teaching continuing education classes about NICU and therapy with infants. She is happily married with four grown children, one wonderful granddaughter, and a very supportive mother. She enjoys babies, crafts, fishing, and traveling.

Donna Holt, BS, has worked in the field of dietetics. She is currently attending graduate school. Donna lives in Ohio with her husband and two dogs. She enjoys traveling, painting, and writing.

Barbara E. Joe was a staff writer for the American Occupational Therapy Association and a frequent contributor to OT Week, formerly a weekly professional AOTA news magazine now published biweekly by the AOTA as OT Practice. She lived in the Washington, DC area.

Diane J. Jones, RN, received her BSN from the University of Minnesota and her MSN from Boston University, Boston, Mass. She served in the United States Army Nurse Corps, taught nursing at a university, and served as a consultant on a state board of nursing. Diane met Peggy Helgason through her son, Matthew, who attended a camp for children with chronic illness. The clown with a heart of gold made a sterling impression on the Jones family.

Jan Johnson, OTR, and her husband now enjoy a wondrous retirement in the rural mountains of Southern Arizona—writing, weaving, weeding, and watching grandchildren grow. Jan's former life in Ohio was filled with nearly 40 years of practice in academic teaching and as a school-based occupational therapist.

Jean M. Kassnel attended the University of Tampa, Tampa, FL, and Goddard College, Plainfield, VT, and was a human resource manager prior to staying home to raise her two children. She currently does volunteer work at their school while pursuing a writing career. Jean has published numerous essays and is working on a novel, in addition to a collection of short stories.

Jan Keith, COTA/L, AP, is a graduate of the occupational therapy assistant program at Fox Valley Technical College in Appleton, WI. She earned her Advanced Practice credential in geriatrics and currently works with children in an early intervention program. She and her husband live and play in Wyoming.

About the Contributors

Margret I. Kingrey, MA, OTR, graduated from the University of Puget Sound in 1975 and received her master's degree in early childhood special education from New Mexico State University, Las Cruces, NM, 20 years later. Having worked in six states, her career has spanned the continent and most areas of occupational therapy practice. She has one grown son and lives with her husband in Maryland. She is a doctoral student in occupational science at Towson University, Towson, MD, and writes short stories.

Ellen L. Kolodner, MSS, OTR/L, FAOTA, has been an occupational therapy practitioner, educator, and administrator for more than 30 years. At present, she is professor and founding director of the occupational therapy program at Philadelphia University, Pennsylvania, PA. Ellen is passionate about her profession, her family, cooking, travel, and flower arranging. In 1997, Ellen received the American Occupational Therapy Association Award of Merit.

Lesley Larsen Kountz, COTA, has achieved advanced practice credentials in pediatrics and worked in early intervention for 9 years. Lesley currently works as a program manager supervising the service coordinators for the Waukesha county birth to three program in Waukesha, WI. She enjoys gardening, reading, and traveling with her family.

Donna Langmead, COTA, lives in Westminster, MD, with her husband, daughter, and stepson. She also has an older stepson who lives on his own. She works for the Carroll County Public School System where she has been a therapist for the past 9 years. She works with infants, toddler, and students of all ages.

Beth Larson, PhD, OTR, is currently a faculty member in the occupational therapy program in the department of kinesiology at the University of Wisconsin in Madison, teaching future occupational therapists and doing research on families' management of daily life activities when parenting children with disabilities. Although she has left the community in which Elizabeth and her family reside, the artwork described at the beginning of her story still hangs in her home and reminds her daily of her life before graduate school.

Linda Lorentzen, OTR/L, has worked as an occupational therapist for 24 years, mostly at Fairview University Medical Center, Minneapolis, MN, specializing in seating and wheeled mobility, assistive technology, and home accessibility for neurological and neuromuscular outpatients. Linda resides in Robbinsdale, MN, with her husband and two active teenagers. Her primary interest area is writing, and she receives daily inspiration from the people with physical challenges with whom she works.

Karen Crane Macdonald, PhD, OTR/L, is a lecturer at Housatonic Community College, Bridgeport, Conn. She also has several volunteer roles that involve purposeful occupations to continually increase her functional skills. Karen plans to continue involvement in the occupational therapy profession through writing and teaching. She is married and enjoys outdoor, spiritual, and handcraft activities.

Deborah Mandel, MA, OTR, was a researcher and occupational therapy clinical supervisor in The Well Elderly Study, a randomized clinical trial undertaken by the department of occupational science and occupational therapy at the University of Southern California, Los Angeles, CA. The study was supported by a grant from the National Institute on Aging and several other agencies, foundations, and private corporations, and the study results were published in the Journal of the American Medical Association in October 1997. Roland was a participant in the study.

Allison Brown Mann, OTR/L, received a BS in occupational therapy in 1993 from the University of Alabama at Birmingham. She has worked in outpatient rehabilitation and rehabilitation oriented nursing homes. Allison was also instrumental in developing and implementing occupational therapy programs in home health and in hospital in- and out patient rehabilitation. She currently lives in Cartersville, GA, as a stay-at-home-mom with her husband and two small children.

Cindy Martin, COTA/L, works for Appalachian Therapy Pediatric Services in Maryville, TN. Cindy is a skilled seamstress and gardener, and she enjoys folk crafts and antiques. She often incorporates her love of crafts into therapeutic patient treatment activities.

Constance Martinez-de la Vega, OTR/L, received her MA in occupational therapy from New York University in 1993. Currently a pediatric therapist (outpatient) at Norwalk Hospital in Connecticut, Mrs. de la Vega also works with the elderly at HoneyHill Care Center in Norwalk, CT. Mrs. de la Vega has been an occupational therapist for 91/2 years. She loves her job as a pediatric therapist and also enjoys the rewards of working with the geriatric population. She was born and raised in New York and now resides in Westchester County, NY, with her husband and two children.

Denise McCormick is a third-grade teacher and has taught for 13 years. She is currently working on her master's of arts degree in education. Denise has been married for 26 years and her husband farms. They have a daughter in medical school at the University of Sydney in Sydney, Australia, and another daughter working on her master's degree in education at the University of Iowa, Iowa City, IA. Denise enjoys playing the piano, singing, composing music, traveling, reading, swimming, and her family.

Zoe McGrath, COTA, acquired her occupational therapy assistant certification in 1992. In 1999, Zoe took a break from conventional occupational therapy to take over full-time care for her significant other, Cruz, who is quadriplegic following a traumatic brain injury, and to manage "Their Bullet, My Life," a presentation program to educate youth about the effects of gun violence. In 2000, Zoe and Cruz adopted their son, Aidan, 2 days after he was born.

Valnere McLean, OTR, is an occupational therapist who started her training in Melbourne, Australia before continuing her education and work in the United States. She is married and had one daughter who died of cancer in 1995. This sadness brought out depths of feeling and knowing. She has learned that coping with loss can be overwhelming, but profound and deeply enriching as well.

Stephanie M. Milazzo, MA, OTR, CHT, is an occupational therapist who earned both her BS and advanced master's degrees at New York University. She became a certified hand therapist in 1997 and has been specializing in hand and upper extremity rehabilitation for the past 12 years. She has also taught courses at Touro College, New York, NY, on the master's degree level. Her favorite leisure time activity is scuba diving.

Deborah Morawski, OTR/L, has worked as an occupational therapist for 24 years, is a generalist, but has specialized in NDT with hemiplegia, dysphagia and vestibular rehabilitation. She recently moved from a metropolitan area and now lives in a rural community in California, working part-time for several different companies. She enjoys scuba diving, traveling, mycology, back packing, running, and beekeeping with her spouse.

Linda Carver Morse, OTR, is a 1978 graduate of Utica College. She is certified in neurodevelopmental treatment and complete decongestive therapy. She has two children and is a volunteer for the American Cancer Society and a comfort ministry.

Laurie E. Nelson, MA, OTR, is the director of the occupational therapy program at Mariposa Women's and Family Counseling Center in Orange, CA, in partnership with Santa Ana College occupational therapy assistant program. She loves to sing, create dance choreography, and watch God perform miracles in her own life.

Janet Christhilf O'Flynn, OTR/L, BCP, has been a pediatric occupational therapist for close to 20 years. She is a graduate of St. John's College, Annapolis, MD, and earned a post-baccalaureate certificate from the University of Pennsylvania in occupational therapy. She has worked in Washington, DC, Virginia, Connecticut, and is currently employed by the Martha's Vineyard Public Schools. She is married to Donnel O'Flynn, an Episcopal priest, and has two great young adult offspring.

Jane C. Chamberlain Olsasky, OTR/L, received her BS in occupational therapy in 1986 from the University of Kansas, Lawrence, KS. She has worked in a variety of settings in Des Moines, IA, with pediatric and adult populations. For 6 years she evaluated and treated infants and children perinataly exposed to drugs/alcohol. Jane is married and has a daughter and son who are twins. She enjoys writing poetry, gardening and playing guitar.

Nina Paris, OT/L, formerly associate director of occupational therapy at the Kessler Institute for Rehabilitation in West Orange, NJ, is now director of occupational therapy at the Miller Health Care Institute for Performing Artists in New York City, NY. She is also the founder and president of the International Foundation for Performing Arts Medicine.

Bhavisha H. Patel is an attorney in New York City. She still continues her daily commute to New York City from Philadelphia. She has been made partner at the firm in which she worked at the time of her injury. She spends most of her spare time painting the landscape of Philadelphia, a hobby that she developed during her recovery.

Patricia Petersen, MA, OTR, returned to school following the birth of her youngest child (Fayda) and received her degree in occupational therapy in 1998. She has worked as an occupational therapist with children, adults with chronic pain, and persons with mental illness. She enjoys writing essays and inspirational pieces.

Irene Phillips, MPA, MA, OTR/L, is assistant professor in the department of occupational therapy at Winston-Salem State University, Winston-Salem, NC. She has worked as an administrator in the public arena before changing careers to occupational therapy. She has been an occupational therapist for over 10 years and teaches subjects in gerontology, mental health, and spirituality. She is a doctoral candidate in pastoral community counseling at Argosy University, Sarasota, FL.

About the Contributors

Michelle Ponsolle-Mays, MS, OTR/L, has worked in a variety of settings. Michelle is presently a self-employed practitioner and busy mother of two young toddlers. Her professional interests have grown to encompass the evaluation and treatment of preschool- and school-aged children, in addition to her natural inclination for aiding individuals with hand injuries. Her hopes are to one day teach on a college or university level.

Wayne S. Pusatero entered the automotive field after completing his tour of duty with the United States Air Force. He retired after 25 years, 15 of which were spent as a Chevron dealer. He currently enjoys doing "stuff" on the computer, entertaining grandchildren, and watching sports.

Michal Magnes Raveh, MA, OTR, is currently the program director of the Hebrew University and Hadassah School of Occupational Therapy in Jerusalem, Israel, where she has been working since 1976 as a lecturer, program coordinator, and student advisor. She completed her undergraduate studies at that same school and an advanced master's degree in occupational therapy at New York University. She lives in Jerusalem and is a mother of two.

Elisabeth Refn, MA, OTR, a Danish New Yorker, has worked with chronic mentally ill New Yorkers in various outpatient settings for over 25 years. In addition to a degree in cultural sociology, she has a Danish degree in occupational therapy and an advanced master's degree in occupational therapy from New York University, where she is currently an adjunct instructor. She likes gardening, painting, and cartooning.

Rhona Gorsky Reiss, PhD, OTR/L, FAOTA, left Philadelphia's Widener Memorial School in 1972 to teach occupational therapy in Tokyo, Japan. For the next 30 years her career adventures included clinical and academic positions in Chicago, Sydney, Dallas, and Washington, DC. She served for 5 years as the education director of the American Occupational Therapy Association and completed a PhD in higher education in the year 2000. Dr. Reiss now resides in North Potomac, MD, and and is the director of clinical services at the Spectrum Center, a Tomatis Auditory Training Center in Bethesda, MD.

Laura Rutherford Renner, OTR/L, is a school occupational therapist in southern New Jersey. She has worked in adult rehabilitation centers throughout the region. Also, Laura is an artist whose paintings and drawings have appeared in galleries in the Philadelphia area. She enjoys writing children's stories and spending time with her husband and daughter, Sara.

Margaret D. Rerek, MS, OTR/L (Retired), completed her education as an occupational therapist at New York University in 1954. Although most of her 42 year career was spent as a treatment team administrator in the New York State mental hospital system, she has also worked as an occupational therapist in the clinical areas of physical disabilities, cerebral palsy, adult and child psychiatry, and learning disabled children. Among "Peg's" retirement activities is acting as cochair of the alumni board of New York University's programs in occupational therapy.

Rebecca L. Rogers, MEd, OTR/L, is currently working at Good Samaritan Hospital, Cincinnati, Ohio, as a senior occupational therapist. Rebecca attended Xavier University, Cincinnati, OH, receiving both a master's of education and an occupational therapy degree. She also received her bachelor of business administration degree from Eastern Kentucky University, Richmond, KY, with a double major in management and marketing. Rebecca enjoys reading, being outdoors, and coordinating an annual week-long camp for traumatic brain injured adults through Good Samaritan Hospital.

Leslie Rubman, MPH, OTR, has been working with young children for over 20 years and currently is involved in early intervention in Hudson County, NJ. In 1976, she received her BS in occupational therapy from Boston University and an MPH in maternal and child health in 1981 from the University of Minnesota.

Richard J. Russ, MA, OTR/L, earned a master's degree from New York University in 1981. He currently provides occupational therapy to children in public schools and to adults in their homes. He also manages www.HealthCareJobsUSA.com, a web site listing jobs and continuing education workshops for occupational therapists, physical therapists, and speech therapists.

Joyce Sabari, PhD, OTR, BCN, FAOTA, is an associate professor and chair of the occupational therapy program at SUNY Downstate Medical Center. Joyce lives in Brooklyn, NY, with her husband and three children. Her experience working with Julia Tavalaro has profoundly influenced her clinical practice, teaching, and academic work.

Fred Sammons, PhD, OTR, entered the profession of occupational therapy in 1955 at the Rehabilitation Institute of Chicago. In 1960 he became a research associate in prosthetics at Northwestern University, Evanston, IL. In 1965, he formed a mail order business to supply aids of daily living to the profession. The business was successful and was later merged with another such business to form

About the Contributors

SammonsPreston Inc. He continues to do public relations and to help with new product development. Fred is a director of the American Occupational Therapy Foundation and is professionally active nationally and internationally.

Julia Waggoner Santini, OTR/L, received her degree in occupational therapy from Thomas Jefferson University, Philadelphia, PA. Since then, she has worked in several inpatient rehabilitation hospitals along the east coast. She enjoys spending time with her husband, Joe, and her dog, Maggie, as well as hiking, reading, and traveling.

Barbara Schroeder had a very enjoyable and successful albeit short career as a COTA in the state of Wisconsin. However, life threw her another curve and she once again returned to school for yet another career change and currently does clerical work for the state of Wisconsin. Her training and experience in occupational therapy continue to serve her well in life as she also cares for her elderly parents.

Kathy Swoboda is a COTA/L currently practicing in geriatrics. She and her husband, Barry, live in Poland, OH, with their two children. This story is now in memory of their Joey. Dance with the angels little boy!

Jacqueline Davis Templin, OTR/L, has been an occupational therapist in private practice for the past 20 years, with a special interest in hand rehabilitation. She owns Handstand, which can be found at www.justhands.com, a company selling hand-shaped jewelry and other items to therapists and surgeons all over the world. She lives just outside of Philadelphia with her husband and four children, who range in age from first grader to college freshman.

Jill E. (Anderson) Van Dyke, OTR, graduated from occupational therapy school in 1988. She then became a staff occupational therapist at Good Samaritan Hospital in Cincinnati, OH, where she specialized in arthritis, spinal cord injury, cerebrovascular accidents, and dysphagia. In 1992, Jill began a career with the rehabilitation division of Smith & Nephew, Inc (located in Germantown, WI), where she had multiple roles—technical service representative, clinical research manager, and global product manager. She transferred to the wound management division of Smith & Nephew, Inc in 2001, where she became an account manager in the acute care market segment covering the state of Wisconsin. Jill resides in Menomonee Falls, WI, with her husband and daughter.

Bethany S. Walls, MA, is a professional writer and editor who has worked in the health care industry for over a decade. She has earned national recognition for her work in magazines, newspapers, and on web sites. A native of Maryland, Bethany has also lived in Connecticut and Massachusetts, where she earned a master's degree in journalism. When she is not writing, she enjoys traveling and spending time with friends and her German shepherd, Jammer.

Mary-Kay Webster has a BS in Accounting from Virginia Commonwealth University in Richmond, VA. Along with her varied positions in finance, she has served on the Board of Independent Living Centers, State Commissions for Persons with Disabilities, and helped develop the Virginia personal assistance program. Currently, she is an independent financial consultant who also enjoys writing.

Gwen Weinstock, MA, OTR/L, treats individuals with hand injuries at New York Presbyterian Hospital, New York, NY. She has completed her advanced master's degree in occupational therapy with a focus on ergonomics and biomechanics at NYU and is currently working on her doctorate there as well. Gwen lives in Riverdale, NY, with her husband, Ira, and her daughters, Davi and Kayla.

Amy B. Westerman, OTR/L, is an occupational therapist working for the Ashland Public Schools, Ashland, MA, and is the therapy coordinator for ACCEPT Collaborative in Framingham, MA. She and her husband, Michael, have three children, Ben, Taryn, and Becca.

Valerie B. Whiting, OTR/L, LMT, teaches in an occupational therapy assistant program in Oak Ridge, TN. She maintains a private practice in therapeutic bodywork. Her favorite healing modalities are structural integration, thai massage, and yoga.

Denise E. Williams, OTR/L, CHTP, is a pediatric occupational therapist, certified healing touch practitioner, and classical vocalist. She is a graduate of the University of Illinois at the Medical Center and has been an occupational therapist for 26 years. Ms. Williams has recorded a compact disc that includes text on the benefits of music on the parasympathetic nervous system with classical and spiritual selections. She employs her musical acumen as a therapeutic technique in her pediatric occupational therapy and healing touch practice.

About the Contributors

Peggy Prince Wittman, EdD, OTR/L, FAOTA, has practiced, taught, and researched occupational therapy for 30 years; long enough to frequently experience its healing powers on both herself and many others. Music, scrapbooking, reading, camping, writing, traveling, and beach-sitting are occupations she engages in for fun and well being. The presence of family, friends, and God are also critical to her life satisfaction.

Margaret Mary (Mimi) Wolak, MA,OTR, has been a practicing occupational therapist for the past 32 years. She presently works in public schools with students who are blind or visually impaired and has recently adopted a retired guide dog. Now that her only son is raised, she is active in various church ministries and has completed her master's degree in pastoral leadership. Mimi has been published in an ecumenical worship resource magazine.

Cindy Wright, MA, OTR, was formerly assistant professor of occupational therapy at Louisiana State University Medical Center in New Orleans. She currently lives in Baton Rouge with her husband, Terrell Martin, and is an at-home mother to Sam, now 10, and Jack, 13. Sam is a fifth grader in the gifted magnet program at Brookstown Elementary and is a talented artist. He hopes to be a paleontologist when he grows up. He continues to receive occupational therapy services through his school.

Submit Your Story

Do you have your own experience with occupational therapy that you would like to share and submit for a possible future book? If so, please e-mail your story to **miracles@slackinc.com** or via our website at **www.ordinarymiracles.net**

Be sure to include your name, address, telephone number, fax number, and e-mail address. If you prefer to send your story by mail, please submit it (including a diskette version if possible) to:

Ordinary Miracles
SLACK Incorporated
6900 Grove Road
Thorofare, NJ 08086